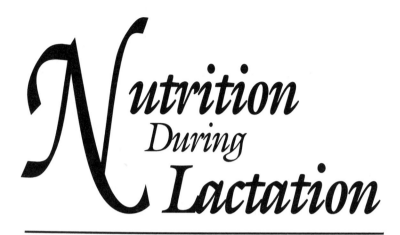

Nutrition During Lactation

Subcommittee on Nutrition During Lactation
Committee on Nutritional Status During Pregnancy and Lactation
Food and Nutrition Board
Institute of Medicine
National Academy of Sciences

NATIONAL ACADEMY PRESS
Washington, D.C.   1991

National Academy Press ● 2101 Constitution Avenue, NW ● Washington, DC 20418

NOTICE: The project that is the subject of this report was approved by the Governing Board of the National Research Council, whose members are drawn from the councils of the National Academy of Sciences, the National Academy of Engineering, and the Institute of Medicine. The members of the committee responsible for the report were chosen for their special competences and with regard for appropriate balance.

This report has been reviewed by a group other than the authors according to procedures approved by a Report Review Committee consisting of members of the National Academy of Sciences, the National Academy of Engineering, and the Institute of Medicine.

The Institute of Medicine was chartered in 1970 by the National Academy of Sciences to enlist distinguished members of the appropriate professions in the examination of policy matters pertaining to the health of the public. In this, the Institute acts under both the Academy's 1863 congressional charter responsibility to be an adviser to the federal government and its own initiative in identifying issues of medical care, research, and education. Dr. Samuel O. Thier is president of the Institute of Medicine.

This study was supported by project no. MCJ 116011 from the Maternal and Child Health Program (Title V, Social Security Act), Health Resources and Services Administration, U.S. Department of Health and Human Services.

SUBCOMMITTEE ON NUTRITION DURING LACTATION

MARGIT HAMOSH (*Chair*), Division of Developmental Biology and
Nutrition, Georgetown University Medical Center, Washington, D.C.

KATHRYN G. DEWEY, Department of Nutrition, University of California,
Davis, California

CUTBERTO GARZA, Division of Nutritional Sciences, Cornell University,
Ithaca, New York

ARMOND S. GOLDMAN, Department of Pediatrics, Division of
Immunology/Allergy, The University of Texas Medical Branch,
Galveston, Texas

RUTH A. LAWRENCE, Department of Pediatrics, School of Medicine and
Dentistry, University of Rochester, Rochester, New York

MARY FRANCES PICCIANO, Department of Nutrition, The Pennsylvania
State University, University Park, Pennsylvania

SARA A. QUANDT, Department of Anthropology, University of Kentucky,
Lexington, Kentucky

KATHLEEN M. RASMUSSEN, Division of Nutritional Sciences, Cornell
University, Ithaca, New York

DAVID RUSH, Epidemiology Program, USDA Human Nutrition Research
Center at Tufts University, Boston, Massachusetts

Staff:

CAROL WEST SUITOR, Study Director
YVONNE L. BRONNER, Research Associate
MARIAN M. F. MILLSTONE, Research Assistant (until July 1990)
GERALDINE KENNEDO, Senior Secretary
WILHELMENA TAMALE, Senior Secretary (until August 1990)

Preface

The biological importance of milk to all mammals, including humans, is evident from historical and physiologic perspectives. The survival of human infants depended on breastfeeding until early in the twentieth century when substitutes for human milk were developed, leading to a marked decrease in breastfeeding. Subsequent reports of lower morbidity and mortality among breastfed infants compared with formula-fed infants stimulated a reexamination of infant feeding practices. Questions have also been raised concerning the role of breastfeeding in promoting optimal infant growth, nutritional well-being of the infant, and bonding between mother and infant. Relatively little attention has been given to the mother and her needs.

Growing concerns among health professionals led to the first Surgeon General's Report, *Healthy People: The Surgeon General's Report on Health Promotion and Disease Prevention* (Department of Health, Education, and Welfare, 1979), and subsequently to publication of *Promoting Health/Preventing Disease: Objectives for the Nation* (Department of Health and Human Services [DHHS], 1980). The latter report set breastfeeding of 75% of all infants at hospital discharge and 35% at 6 months of age as an objective to be attained by 1990. Shortly thereafter, the Surgeon General's Workshop on Breastfeeding and Human Lactation further emphasized that objective and provided a framework for its implementation. The breastfeeding objective has not yet been achieved; in fact, the rate of breastfeeding at hospital discharge has decreased since the time of the Surgeon General's Workshop. Factors such as lack of specific policies for paid maternity leave, lack of child care facilities at the mother's place of employment, or lack of adequate facilities for pumping and storing human milk might have contributed to the failure to reach the breastfeeding objective. The objective is reaffirmed and expanded in the *Year 2000 Objectives for the Nation* (DHHS, 1990).

Since 1980 there has been a marked increase in research on human milk, with special emphasis on its composition and role in promoting or sustaining the well-being and development of the infant. Six workshops on human milk and lactation were sponsored by the National Institute of Child Health and Human Development between 1982 and 1990. The third workshop was dedicated to maternal and environmental factors that affect human lactation, but the influence of maternal nutrition on lactation was reviewed only briefly.

Many studies of maternal and child nutrition have been conducted by committees of the Food and Nutrition Board under the sponsorship of the Office of Maternal and Child Health of the DHHS. However, the study reported in this volume is the first one directed specifically toward maternal nutrition during lactation.

Although great progress has been made in understanding the process of lactation and in characterizing and quantitating the composition of human milk, less progress has been made in linking the nutritional status of lactating women with various outcomes of breastfeeding. The subcommittee carefully examined evidence pertaining to the demographics of breastfeeding; lactation performance, including milk volume, duration of lactation, and milk composition; infant outcomes such as nutritional status, growth, development, morbidity, and mortality; and maternal long-term health outcomes. Special effort was made to search for studies to investigate the impact of maternal nutrition on these outcomes and studies of the effects of breastfeeding on maternal nutrition.

This volume provides information that will help researchers, students, and health care providers understand how nutrition of healthy women relates to various outcomes of lactation in the context of many other contributing factors. It is also intended to aid in formulating guidelines for clinical application in the United States. Finally, the report highlights gaps in knowledge and recommends directions for further research.

ORGANIZATION OF THIS REPORT

This volume begins with a summary of the report and its principal recommendations. Chapter 3 addresses the question, "Who is breastfeeding?," identifying breastfeeding rates in the United States by different demographic characteristics (such as age, ethnic background, region of the country, and employment status). It also provides a historical perspective of the incidence and duration of breastfeeding in the past century.

Chapter 4 examines anthropometric, biochemical, and dietary methods for assessing the nutritional status of lactating women and points out their uses and limitations. Since most interventions designed to improve nutritional status act to increase intake of nutrients in short supply in the diet, the subcommittee tabulated and interpreted nutrient intake data from studies of lactating women. Chapters 5 and 6 contain discussions of the volume and composition of human milk and explain factors that must be considered when evaluating the impact of maternal nutrition on these two lactation outcomes. These chapters also provide the basis for estimating the range of the mother's nutrient losses resulting from breastfeeding.

Although infant growth, development, and health are key outcomes of breastfeeding, the effects of maternal nutrition during lactation on these outcomes have been largely ignored in the literature. To the extent possible, Chapter 7 reports links between the nutrition of the mother and the nutrition and growth of the nursing infant. Since a slower than expected rate of infant weight gain may be given as a reason to discontinue breastfeeding, the subcommittee paid special attention to the assessment of the growth of breastfed infants. The possibility that maternal nutrition may influence infant health through altered immunologic function and the links between maternal food intake while lactating and infant health are also considered in Chapter 7 as they relate to allergic diseases and environmental toxins. To provide a balanced overview of infant health, the risk of transmission of infectious agents via human milk and the presence of drugs in human milk are also covered. In addition, there is brief mention of the development of obesity and atherosclerosis in later life in relation to the method of infant feeding.

Chapter 8 explores ways that maternal health can be influenced by lactation, with special emphasis on obesity, osteoporosis, and breast cancer, as well as the impact of lactation on ovulation and fertility. In Chapter 9, information from preceding chapters is synthesized in a discussion of ways to meet the nutrient needs of lactating women. Chapter 10 includes a brief review of recent research recommendations concerning lactation and breastfeeding and then presents the subcommittee's recommendations for research concerning nutrition during lactation. The conclusions and recommendations of the subcommittee are presented in the Summary, Chapter 1.

ACKNOWLEDGMENTS

The subcommittee acknowledges the outstanding contribution of Carol Suitor, Study Director for this report. Her dedication, skill, and attention to all aspects of this report have been invaluable at all stages of its preparation.

The committee and subcommittee also appreciate the support provided by many other members of the Food and Nutrition Board staff, especially Dr. Alvin Lazen, Dr. Catherine Woteki, Mrs. Frances Peter, Dr. Yvonne Bronner, Ms. Marian Millstone, Ms. Wilhelmena Tamale, and Ms. Geraldine Kennedo. Mr. Michael Hayes ably served as copy editor.

The subcommittee benefitted from advice and suggestions provided by the Committee on Nutritional Status During Pregnancy and Lactation, from the sharing of information with the Subcommittee on Nutritional Status and Weight Gain During Pregnancy and the Subcommittee on Dietary Intake and Nutrient Supplements During Pregnancy, and from the assistance provided by the Food and Nutrition Board and its Subcommittee on the Tenth Edition of the Recommended Dietary Allowances.

Many people made important contributions to this combined report by giving presentations, providing the subcommittees with data or special written reports or analyses, sharing their views during workshops, commenting on drafts, or otherwise serving as resource persons. In particular, the committee and subcommittees wish to thank Dr. Thomas A. Arcury, University of Kentucky; Dr. Kenneth Brown, University of California, Davis; Ms. Becky Catey, Ross Laboratories; Dr. Catherine Cowell, Bureau of Nutrition, City of New York; Dr. Jan Dodds, Bureau of Nutrition, New York State; Dr. J. David Erickson, Centers for Disease Control; Ms. Linda Friedman, University of Rochester School of Medicine and Dentistry; Dr. Jean-Pierre Habicht, Cornell University; Dr. Suzanne Harris, Food and Consumer Services, U.S. Department of Agriculture (USDA); Mr. Jay Hirshman, Food and Nutrition Service, USDA; Ms. Patricia Jensen, Santa Clara County Department of Health, California; Ms. Lynn Kuba, Childbirth Educator, Fairfax County, Va.; Ms. Alice Lenihan, National Association of WIC (Supplemental Food Program for Women, Infants, and Children) Directors; Ms. Brenda Lisi, Food and Nutrition Service, USDA; Ms. Ruth Lubic, Maternity Center Association, New York City; Ms. Shelly Marks, Harbor University of California at Los Angeles Medical Center; Dr. Gilbert Martinez, Ross Laboratories; Dr. Margaret Neville, University of Colorado; Dr. Alan S. Ryan, Ross Laboratories; Dr. Rebecca Stoltzfus, Cornell University; Dr. Rita Thomas, Bristol-Myers; and Ms. Colette Zyrkowski, Centers for Disease Control.

ROY M. PITKIN
Chair
Committee on Nutritional
Status During Pregnancy
and Lactation

MARGIT HAMOSH
Chair
Subcommittee on
Nutrition During
Lactation

Contents

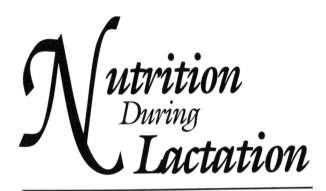

1
Summary, Conclusions, and Recommendations

During the past decade, the benefits of breastfeeding have been emphasized by many authorities and organizations in the United States. Federal agencies have set specific objectives to increase the incidence and duration of breast-feeding (DHHS, 1980, 1990), and the Surgeon General has held workshops on breastfeeding and human lactation (DHHS, 1984, 1985). At the federal and state levels, the Special Supplemental Food Program for Women, Infants, and Children (WIC) has produced materials designed to promote breastfeeding (e.g., Malone, 1980; USDA, 1988). Furthermore, the Office of Maternal and Child Health has sponsored breastfeeding projects (e.g., The Steering Committee to Promote Breastfeeding in New York City, 1986), as have state health departments and others. However, less attention has been given to two general topics: (1) the effects of breastfeeding on the nutritional status and long-term health of the mother and (2) the effects of the mother's nutritional status on the volume and composition of her milk and on the potential subsequent effects of those changes on infant health. The present report was designed to address these topics.

This summary briefly describes the origin of this effort and the process; provides key definitions; reviews what was learned about who is breastfeeding in the United States and if those women are well nourished; discusses nutritional influences on milk volume or composition; and describes how breastfeeding may affect infant growth, nutrition, and health, as well as maternal health. It then presents major conclusions, clinical recommendations, and the research recommendations most directly related to the nutrition of lactating women in the United States.

ORIGIN OF THIS STUDY

This study was undertaken at the request of the Maternal and Child Health Program (Title V, Social Security Act) of the Health Resources and Services Administration, U.S. Department of Health and Human Services. In response to that request, the Food and Nutrition Board's Committee on Nutritional Status During Pregnancy and Lactation and its Subcommittee on Nutrition During Lactation were asked to evaluate current scientific evidence and formulate recommendations pertaining to the nutritional needs of lactating women, giving special attention to the needs of lactating adolescents; women over age 35; and women of black, Hispanic, or Southeast Asian origin. Part of this task included consideration of the effects of maternal dietary intake and nutritional status on the volume and composition of human milk, the appropriateness of various anthropometric methods for assessing nutritional status during lactation, and the effects of lactation both on maternal and infant health and on the nutritional status of both the mother and the infant.

APPROACH TO THE STUDY

The study was limited to consideration of healthy U.S. women and their healthy, full-term infants. The Subcommittee on Nutrition During Lactation conducted an extensive literature review, consulted with a variety of experts, and met as a group seven times to discuss the data and draw conclusions from them. The Committee on Nutritional Status During Pregnancy and Lactation (the advisory committee) reviewed and commented on the work of the subcommittee and helped establish appropriate linkages between this report and the reports on weight gain and nutrient supplements during pregnancy contained in *Nutrition During Pregnancy*—a report prepared by two other subcommittees of this advisory committee (IOM, 1990). Compared with earlier reports from the National Research Council, *Nutrition During Pregnancy* recommended a higher range of weight gain (11.5 to 16 kg, or 25 to 35 lb, for women of normal prepregnancy weight for height). In addition, it advised routine low-dose iron supplementation during pregnancy, but supplements of other vitamins or minerals were recommended only under special circumstances.

In examining the nutritional needs of lactating women, priority was given to energy and to those nutrients believed to be consumed in amounts lower than Recommended Dietary Allowances (RDAs) by many women in the United States. These nutrients include calcium, magnesium, iron, zinc, folate, and vitamin B_6. Careful attention was given to the effects of lactation on various *indicators of nutritional status*, such as measurements of levels of biochemical compounds; functions related to specific nutrients; nutrient levels in specific body compartments; and height, weight, or other indicators of body size or adiposity. The subcommittee took into consideration that weight gain recommendations for pregnant women have been raised (see *Nutrition During Pregnancy* [IOM, 1990]) and that average weight gains of U.S. women during pregnancy have risen over the past two decades.

When possible, a distinction was made between *exclusive breastfeeding*, defined as the consumption of human milk as the sole source of energy, and *partial breastfeeding*, defined as the consumption of human milk in combination with formula or other foods, or both.

The nutritional demands imposed by lactation were estimated from data on volume and composition of milk produced by healthy, successfully lactating women, as done in *Recommended Dietary Allowances* (NRC, 1989). When it was feasible, evidence relating to possible depletion of maternal stores or to a decrease in the specific nutrient content of milk resulting from low maternal intake of the nutrient was also addressed. Because of the complex relationships between the nutrition of the mother and infant, the subcommittee examined the nutrition and growth of the breastfed infant.

The terms *maternal health* and *infant health* were interpreted in a broad sense. Consideration was given to both beneficial and adverse consequences for the health of the mother and her offspring, both during lactation and long after breastfeeding has been discontinued. For the mother, there was a search for evidence of differences in outcome related to whether or not she had breastfed. For the infant, evidence was sought for differences in outcome related to the method of feeding (breast compared with bottle). The possible influences of breastfeeding on prevention or promotion of chronic disease were addressed.

To the extent possible, this report includes detailed coverage of published evidence linking maternal nutrition, breastfeeding, and maternal and infant health. Because breastfeeding is encouraged primarily as a method for promoting the health of infants, considerable attention is also directed toward infant health even when there is no established relationship to maternal nutritional status. Recognizing the serious gaps in knowledge of nutrition during lactation, the subcommittee gave much thought to establishing directions for research.

The members of the subcommittee realized that nutrition is not the sole determinant of successful breastfeeding. A network of overlapping social factors including access to maternal leave, instructions concerning breastfeeding, availability of prenatal care, the length of hospital stay following delivery, infant care in the workplace, and the public attitudes toward breastfeeding are important. Given the goals of this report, the subcommittee did not specifically address those factors, but it recognizes that they should be considered in depth by public health groups that are attempting to improve rates of breastfeeding in this and other countries.

WHAT WAS LEARNED

Who Is Breastfeeding?

The incidence and duration of breastfeeding changed markedly during the twentieth century—first declining, then rising, and, from the early 1980s, declining once again. Currently, women who choose to breastfeed tend to be well educated, older, and white. Data on the incidence and duration of breastfeeding in the United States are especially limited for mothers who are economically disadvantaged and for those who are members of ethnic minority groups. The best data for any minority groups are for black women. Their rates of breastfeeding are substantially lower than those for white women, but factors that distinguish breastfeeding from nonbreastfeeding women tend to be similar among black and white women. Social, cultural, economic, and psychological factors that influence infant feeding choices by adolescent mothers are not well understood. In the United States, where few employers provide paid maternity leave, return to work outside the home is associated with a shorter duration of breastfeeding, but little else is known about when mothers discontinue either exclusive or partial breastfeeding. Such data are needed to estimate the *total* nutrient demands of lactation.

How Can It Be Determined Whether Lactating Women Are Well Nourished?

The few lactating women who have been studied in the United States have been characterized as well nourished, but this observation cannot be generalized since these subjects were principally white women with some college education. Women from less advantaged, less well studied populations may be at higher risk of nutritional problems but tend not to breastfeed.

To determine whether women are adequately nourished, investigators use biochemical or anthropometric methods, or both. For lactating women, however, there are serious gaps and limitations in the data collected with these methods. Consequently, there is no scientific basis for determining whether poor nutritional status is a problem among certain groups of these women. To identify the nutrients likely to be consumed in inadequate amounts by lactating women, the subcommittee used an approach involving nutrient densities (nutrient intakes per 1,000 kcal) calculated from typical diets of nonlactating U.S. women. That is, they made the assumption that the average nutrient densities of the diets of lactating women would be the same as those of nonlactating women but that lactating women would have higher total energy intake (and therefore higher nutrient intake). Using this approach, the nutrients most likely to be consumed in amounts lower than the RDAs for lactating women are calcium, zinc, magnesium, vitamin B_6, and folate.

Data for U.S. women indicate that successful lactation occurs regardless of whether a woman is thin, of normal weight, or obese. Anthropometric measurements (such as weight, weight for height, and skinfold thickness) have not been useful for predicting the success of lactation among the few U.S. women who have been studied. The predictive ability is not known for anthropometric measurements that fall outside the ranges observed in these limited samples.

Lactating women eating self-selected diets typically lose weight at the rate of 0.5 to 1.0 kg (~1 to 2 lb) per month in the first 4 to 6 months of lactation. Such weight loss is probably physiologic. During the same period, values for subscapular and suprailiac skinfold thickness also decrease; triceps skinfold thickness does not. Not all women lose weight during lactation; studies suggest that approximately 20% may maintain or gain weight.

Biochemical data for lactating women have been obtained only from small, select samples. Such data are of limited use in the clinical situation because there are no norms for lactating women, and the norms for nonpregnant, nonlactating women may not be applicable to breastfeeding women. For example, there appear to be changes in plasma volume post partum, and there are changes in blood nutrient values over the course of lactation that are unrelated to changes in plasma volume.

Does Maternal Nutritional Status or Dietary Intake Influence Milk Volume?

The mean volume of milk secreted by healthy U.S. women whose infants are exclusively breastfed during the first 4 to 6 months is approximately 750 to 800 ml/day, but there is considerable variability from woman to woman and in the same woman at different times. The standard deviation of daily milk intake by infants is about 165 ml; thus, 5% of women secrete less than 550 ml or more than 1,200 ml on a given day. The major determinant of milk production is the infant's demand for milk, which in turn may be influenced by the size, age, health, and other characteristics of the infant as well as by his or her intake of supplemental foods. The potential for milk production may be considerably higher than that actually produced, as evidenced by findings that the milk volumes produced by women nursing twins or triplets are much higher than those produced by women nursing a single infant.

Studies of healthy women in industrialized countries demonstrate that milk volume is not related to maternal weight or height or indices of fatness. In developing countries, there is conflicting evidence about whether thin women produce less milk than do women with higher weight for height.

Increased maternal energy intake has not been linked with increased milk production, at least among well-nourished women in industrialized countries. Nutritional supplementation of lactating women in developing countries where undernutrition may be a problem has generally been reported to have little or no impact on milk volume, but most studies have been too small to test the hypothesis adequately and lacked the design needed for causal inference. Studies of animals indicate that there may be a threshold below which energy intake is insufficient to support normal milk production, but it is likely that most studies in humans have been conducted on women with intakes well above this postulated threshold.

The weight loss ordinarily experienced by lactating women has no apparent deleterious effects on milk production. Although lactating women typically lose 0.5 to 1 kg (~1 to 2 lb) per month, some women lose as much as 2 kg (~4 lb) per month and successfully maintain milk volume. Regular exercise appears to be compatible with production of an adequate volume of milk.

The influence of maternal intake of specific nutrients on milk volume has not been investigated satisfactorily. Early studies in developing countries suggest a positive association of protein intake with milk volume, but those studies remain inconclusive. Fluids consumed in excess of thirst do not increase milk volume.

Does Maternal Nutritional Status Influence Milk Composition?

The composition of human milk is distinct from the milk of other mammals and from infant formulas ordinarily derived from them. Human milk is unique in its physical structure, types and concentrations of macronutrients (protein, fat, and carbohydrate), micronutrients (vitamins and minerals), enzymes, hormones, growth factors, host resistance factors, inducers/modulators of the immune system, and antiinflammatory agents.

A number of generalizations can be made about the effects of maternal nutrition on the composition of milk (see also Table 1-1):

• Even if the usual dietary intake of a macronutrient is less than that recommended in *Recommended Dietary Allowances* (NRC, 1989), there will be little or no effect on the total amount of that nutrient in the milk. However, the proportions of the different fatty acids in human milk vary with maternal dietary intake.

• The concentrations of major minerals (calcium, phosphorus, magnesium, sodium, and potassium) in human milk are not affected by the diet. Maternal intakes of selenium and iodine are positively related to their concentrations in human milk, but there is no convincing evidence that the concentrations of other trace elements in human milk are affected by maternal diet.

• The vitamin content of human milk is dependent upon the mother's current vitamin intake and her vitamin stores, but the strength of the relationships varies with the vitamin. Chronically low maternal intake of vitamins may result in milk that contains low amounts of these essential nutrients.

TABLE 1-1 Possible Influences of Maternal Intake on the Nutrient Composition of Human Milk and Nutrients for Which Clinical Deficiency Is Recognizable in Infants

Nutrient or Nutrient Class	Effect of Maternal Intake on Milk Composition[a]	Recognizable Nutritional Deficiency in Breastfed Infants
Macronutrients		
Proteins	+	Unknown[b]
Lipids	+[c]	Unknown
Lactose	o	Unknown
Minerals		
Calcium	o	Unknown
Phosphorus	o	Unknown
Magnesium	o	Unknown
Sodium	o	Unknown
Potassium	o	Unknown
Chlorine	o	Unknown
Iron	o	Yes[d]
Copper	o	Unknown
Zinc	+,o	Unknown
Manganese	+	Unknown
Selenium	+	Unknown
Iodine	+	Yes
Fluoride	+	Unknown
Vitamins		
Vitamin C	+	Yes
Thiamin	+	Yes
Riboflavin	+	Unknown
Niacin	+	Unknown
Pantothenic acid	+	Unknown
Vitamin B_6	+	Yes
Biotin	+	Yes
Folate	+	Yes
Vitamin B_{12}	+	Yes
Vitamin A	+	Yes
Vitamin D	+	Yes
Vitamin E	+	Yes
Vitamin K	+	Yes[e]

[a] + denotes a positive effect of intake on nutrient content of the milk. The magnitude of the effect varies widely among nutrients. o denotes no known effect of intake on nutrient content of the milk.

[b] Evidence is not sufficiently conclusive to categorize as "No."

[c] Effect appears to be on type of fatty acids present but not on total content of triglycerides or cholesterol in the milk.

[d] Deficiency is not related to maternal intake.

[e] Maternal intake is not the primary determinant of the infant's vitamin K status.

• The content of at least some nutrients in human milk may be maintained at a satisfactory level at the expense of maternal stores. This applies particularly to folate and calcium.

• Increasing the mother's intake of a nutrient to levels above the RDA ordinarily does not result in unusually high levels of the nutrient in her milk; vitamins B_6 and D, iodine, and selenium are exceptions. Studies have not been conducted to evaluate the possibility that high levels of nutrients in milk are toxic to the infant.

• Some studies suggest that poor maternal nutrition is associated with decreased concentrations of certain host resistance factors in human milk, whereas other studies do not suggest this association.

In What Ways May Breastfeeding Affect Infant Growth and Health?

Infant Nutrition

Several factors influence the nutritional status of the breastfed infant: the infant's nutrient stores (which are largely determined by the length of gestation and maternal nutrition during pregnancy), the total amount of nutrients supplied by human milk (which is influenced by the extent and duration of breastfeeding), and certain genetic and environmental factors that affect the way nutrients are absorbed and used.

Human milk is ordinarily a complete source of nutrients for the exclusively breastfed infant. However, if the infant or mother is not exposed regularly to sunlight or if the mother's intake of vitamin D is low, breastfed infants may be at risk of vitamin D deficiency. Breastfed infants are susceptible to deficiency of vitamin B_{12} if the mother is a complete vegetarian—even when the mother has no symptoms of that vitamin deficiency.

The risk of hemorrhagic disease of the newborn is relatively low. Nonetheless, all infants (regardless of feeding mode or of maternal nutritional status) are at some risk for this serious disease unless they are supplemented with a single dose of vitamin K at birth.

Full-term, exclusively breastfed infants ordinarily maintain a normal iron status for their first 6 months of life, regardless of maternal iron intake. Providing solid foods may reduce the percentage of iron absorbed by the partially breastfed infant, making it important in such cases to ensure that adequate iron is provided in the diet.

Growth and Development

Breastfed infants gain weight at about the same rate as formula-fed infants during the first 2 to 3 months post partum, although breastfed infants usually ingest less milk and thus have a lower energy intake. After the first few months post partum, healthy breastfed infants gain weight more slowly than those who are formula fed. In general, this pattern is not altered by the introduction of solid foods. Differences in linear growth between breastfed and formula-fed infants are small if statistical techniques are used to control differences in size at birth.

Infant Morbidity and Mortality

Several types of health problems occur less often or appear to have less serious consequences in breastfed than in formula-fed infants. These include certain infectious diseases (especially ones involving the intestinal and respiratory tracts), food allergies, and, perhaps, certain chronic diseases. There is suggestive evidence that severe maternal malnutrition might reduce the degree of immune protection afforded by human milk, but further studies will be required to address that issue.

Few infectious agents are commonly transmitted to the infant via human milk. The most prominent ones are cytomegalovirus in all populations that have been studied and human T lymphocytotropic virus type 1 (HTLV-1) in certain Asian populations. The transmission of cytomegalovirus by breastfeeding does not result in disease; the consequences of the transmission of HTLV-1 by breastfeeding are unknown. There are some case reports that indicate that human immunodeficiency virus (HIV) can be transmitted by breastfeeding as a result of the transfusion of HIV-contaminated blood during the immediate postpartum period. The likelihood of transmitting HIV via breastfeeding by women who tested seropositive for the agent during pregnancy has not been determined. Public policy on this issue has ranged from the Centers for Disease Control's recommendation not to breastfeed under these circumstances to the World Health Organization's encouragement to breastfeed, especially among women in developing countries.

In developing countries, mortality rates are lower among breastfed infants than among those who are formula fed. It is not known whether this advantage also holds in industrialized countries, in which death rates are lower in general. It is reasonable to believe that breastfeeding will lead to lower mortality among disadvantaged groups in industrialized countries if they have higher than usual infant and child mortality rates, but this issue has not been studied.

Medications, Drugs, and Environmental Contaminants

The few prescription drugs that are contraindicated during lactation because of potential harm to the infant can usually be avoided and replaced with safer acceptable ones. For example, there are a number of safe and effective substitutes for the antibiotic chloramphenicol, which is contraindicated for lactating women. If treatment with antimetabolites or radiotherapeutics is required by the mother, breastfeeding is contraindicated.

Cigarette smoking and alcohol consumption by lactating women in excess of 0.5 g/kg of maternal weight may be harmful to the infant, partly because of potential reduction in milk volume. Furthermore, a single report (Little et al., 1989) associates heavy alcohol use by the mother with retarded psychomotor development of the infant at 1 year of age. Infrequent cigarette smoking, occasional consumption of small amounts of alcohol, and moderate ingestion of caffeine-containing products are not considered to be contraindicated during breastfeeding. Use of illicit drugs is contraindicated because of the potential for drug transfer through the milk as well as hazards to the mother. Since the limited information on the impact of these habits upon the nutrition of women in the childbearing years is reviewed in *Nutrition During Pregnancy* (IOM, 1990), they were not considered further by this subcommittee.

In the uncommon situation of a high risk of exposure to such environmental contaminants as organochlorinated compounds (such as dichlorodiphenyl-trichloroethane [DDT] or polychlorinated biphenyls [PCBs]) or toxic metals (such as mercury), risks must be weighed against the benefits of breastfeeding for both mother and infant on a case-by-case basis. In areas of unusually high exposure, levels of the contaminant should be measured in the mother's blood and milk.

How Does Breastfeeding Affect Maternal Nutrition and Health?

Breastfeeding substantially increases the mother's requirements for most nutrients. The magnitude of the total increase is most strongly affected by the extent and duration of lactation. Adequacy of intakes of calcium, magnesium, zinc, folate, and vitamin B_6 merits special attention since average intakes may be below those recommended. The net long-term effect of lactation on bone mass is uncertain. Some data associate lactation with short-term bone loss, whereas most recent studies suggest a protective long-term effect. Those data are provocative but of such preliminary nature that no definitive conclusions may be drawn from them.

Although most lactating women lose weight gradually during lactation, some do not. The influence of lactation on long-term postpartum weight retention and maternal risk of adult-onset obesity has not been determined.

A well-documented effect of lactation is delayed return to ovulation. In addition, some recent epidemiologic evidence indicates that breastfeeding may lessen the risk that the mother will develop breast cancer, but the data are not consistent across all studies.

CONCLUSIONS AND RECOMMENDATIONS

The major conclusions of the report are as follows.

Women living under a wide variety of circumstances in the United

States and elsewhere are capable of fully nourishing their infants by breast-feeding them. Throughout its deliberations, the subcommittee was impressed by evidence that mothers are able to produce milk of sufficient quantity and quality to support growth and promote the health of infants—even when the mother's supply of nutrients and energy is limited. With few exceptions (identified later in the summary under "Infant Growth and Nutrition"), the full-term exclusively breastfed infant will be well nourished during the first 4 to 6 months after birth.

In contrast, the lactating woman is vulnerable to depletion of nutrient stores through her milk. Measures should be taken to promote food intake during lactation that will prevent net maternal losses of nutrients, especially of calcium, magnesium, zinc, folate, and vitamin B_6.

Breastfeeding is recommended for all infants in the United States under ordinary circumstances. Exclusive breastfeeding is the preferred method of feeding for normal full-term infants from birth to age 4 to 6 months. Breastfeeding complemented by the appropriate introduction of other foods is recommended for the remainder of the first year, or longer if desired. The subcommittee and advisory committee recognize that it is difficult for some women to follow these recommendations for social or occupational reasons. In these situations, appropriate formula feeding is an acceptable alternative.

Data are lacking for use in developing strategies to identify lactating women who are at risk of depleting their own nutrient stores. Although nutrient intake appears adequate for the small number of lactating women who have been studied in the United States, evidence from U.S. surveys of nonpregnant, nonlactating women suggests that usual dietary intake of certain nutrients by disadvantaged women is likely to be somewhat lower than that by women of higher socioeconomic status. Thus, if breastfeeding rates increase among less advantaged women as a result of efforts to promote breastfeeding, it will be important to examine more completely the nutrient intake of these women during lactation.

If lactating women follow eating patterns similar to those of the average U.S. woman in sufficient quantity to meet their energy requirements, they are likely to meet the recommended intakes of all nutrients except perhaps calcium and zinc. However, if they curb their energy intakes, their intakes of several nutrients are likely to be less than the RDA.

Recommendations for Women Who Wish To Breastfeed and for Their Care Providers

Because of serious gaps in information about nutrition assessment and nutrient requirements during lactation and about effects of maternal nutrition on the wide array of components in the milk, the following recommendations should be considered preliminary. Although they reflect the best judgment of the subcommittee and advisory committee, these recommendations are open to reconsideration as the knowledge base grows.

Diet and Vitamin-Mineral Supplementation

Lactating women should be encouraged to obtain their nutrients from a well-balanced, varied diet rather than from vitamin-mineral supplements.

• Provide women who plan to breastfeed or who are already doing so with nutrition information that is culturally appropriate (that is, information that is sensitive to the foodways, eating practices, and health beliefs and attitudes of the cultural group). To facilitate the acquisition of this information, health care providers are encouraged to make effective use of teaching opportunities during prenatal visits, hospitalization following delivery, and routine postpartum visits for maternal or pediatric care.

• Encourage lactating women to follow dietary guidelines that promote a generous intake of nutrients from fruits and vegetables, whole-grain breads and cereals, calcium-rich dairy products, and protein-rich foods such as meats, fish, and legumes. Such a diet would ordinarily supply a sufficient quantity of essential nutrients. The individual recommendations should be compatible with the woman's economic situation and food preferences. The evidence does not warrant routine vitamin-mineral supplementation of lactating women.

• If dietary evaluation suggests that the diet does not provide the recommended amounts of one or more nutrients, encourage the woman to select and consume foods that are rich in those nutrients.

• For women whose eating patterns lead to a very low intake of one or more nutrients, provide individualized diet counseling (preferred) or recommend nutrient supplementation (as described in Table 1-2).

• Encourage sufficient intake of fluids—especially water, juice, and milk—to alleviate natural thirst. It is not necessary to encourage fluid intakes above this level.

• The elimination of major nutrient sources (e.g., all dairy products) from the maternal diet to treat allergy or colic in the breastfed infant is not recommended unless there is evidence from oral elimination-challenge studies to determine whether the mother is sensitive or intolerant to the food or that the breastfed infant reacts to the foods ingested by the mother. If a key nutrient source is eliminated from the maternal diet, the mother should be counseled on how to achieve adequate nutrient intake by substituting other foods.

A Defined Health Care Plan for Lactating Women

There should be a well-defined plan for the health care of the lactating woman that includes screening for nutritional problems and providing dietary guidance. Since preparation for lactation should begin during the prenatal period, the physician, midwife, nutritionist, or other member of the obstetric

TABLE 1-2   Suggested Measures for Improving Nutrient Intake of Women with Restrictive Eating Patterns

Type of Restrictive Eating Pattern	Corrective Measures
Excessive restriction of food intake, i.e., ingestion of <1,800 kcal of energy per day, which ordinarily leads to unsatisfactory intake of nutrients compared with the amounts needed by lactating women	Encourage increased intake of nutrient-rich foods to achieve an energy intake of at least 1,800 kcal/day; if the mother insists on curbing food intake sharply, promote substitution of foods rich in vitamins, minerals, and protein for those lower in nutritive value; in individual cases, it may be advisable to recommend a balanced multivitamin-mineral supplement; discourage use of liquid weight loss diets and appetite suppressants
Complete vegetarianism, i.e., avoidance of all animal foods, including meat, fish, dairy products, and eggs	Advise intake of a regular source of vitamin B_{12}, such as special vitamin B_{12}-containing plant food products or a 2.6-μg vitamin B_{12} supplement daily
Avoidance of milk, cheese, or other calcium-rich dairy products	Encourage increased intake of other culturally appropriate dietary calcium sources, such as collard greens for blacks from the southeastern United States; provide information on the appropriate use of low-lactose dairy products if milk is being avoided because of lactose intolerance; if correction by diet cannot be achieved, it may be advisable to recommend 600 mg of elemental calcium per day taken with meals
Avoidance of vitamin D-fortified foods, such as fortified milk or cereal, combined with limited exposure to ultraviolet light	Recommend 10 μg of supplemental vitamin D per day

team should introduce general information about nutrition during lactation and should screen for possible problems related to nutrition. Ideally, more extensive evaluation and counseling should take place during hospitalization for childbirth. If that is precluded by the brevity of the hospital stay, an early visit to an appropriate health care professional by the mother or a visit to the mother's home is advisable.

To implement routine screening economically and practically, the subcommittee considers it sufficient to continue the practice of weighing women (using standard procedures as described in *Nutrition During Pregnancy* [IOM, 1990]) at scheduled visits and to ask a few simple questions to determine the following:

• Are calcium-rich foods eaten regularly?
• Does the diet include vitamin D-fortified milk or cereal or is there adequate exposure to ultraviolet light?

- Are fruits and vegetables eaten regularly?
- Is the mother a complete vegetarian?
- Is the mother restricting her food intake severely in an attempt to lose weight or to treat certain medical conditions?
- Are there life circumstances (e.g., poverty, or abuse of drugs or alcohol) that might interfere with an adequate diet?

It is not necessary to obtain measurements of skinfold thickness or to conduct laboratory tests as a part of the routine assessment of the nutritional status of lactating women.

The subcommittee recognizes that establishing standard health care procedures for lactating women requires expanded training of health care providers. Activities to achieve this expanded training are being initiated by the Surgeon General's workshop committee comprising representatives from the American Academy of Pediatrics, the American College of Obstetricians and Gynecologists, the American Academy of Family Physicians, and other professional organizations.

Breastfeeding Practices

Efforts to support lactation must consider breastfeeding practices.

- Because the early management of lactation has a strong influence on the establishment of an adequate milk supply, breastfeeding guidance should be provided prenatally and continued in the hospital after delivery and during the early postpartum period.
- All hospitals providing obstetric care should provide knowledgeable staff in the immediate postpartum period who have responsibility for providing support and guidance in initiating breastfeeding and measures to promote establishment of an ample supply of milk.
- Breastfeeding practices that are responsive to the infant's natural appetite should be promoted. In the first few weeks, infants should nurse at least 8 times per day, and some may nurse as often as 15 or more times per day. After the first month, infants fed on demand usually nurse 5 to 12 times per day.

Maternal Weight

Women who plan to breastfeed or who are breastfeeding should be given realistic, health-promoting advice about weight change during lactation.

- Advise women that it is normal to lose weight during the first 6 months of lactation. The average rate of weight loss is 0.5 to 1.0 kg ($\sim$ 1 to 2 lb)/month after the first month post partum. However, not all women who breastfeed lose weight; some women gain weight post partum, whether or not they breastfeed.

If a lactating woman is overweight, a weight loss of up to 2 kg (~4.5 lb) per month is unlikely to adversely affect milk volume, but such women should be alert for any indications that the infant's appetite is not being satisfied. Rapid weight loss (>2 kg/month after the first month post partum) is not advisable for breastfeeding women.

• Advise women who choose to curb their energy intake to pay special attention to eating a balanced, varied diet and to including foods rich in calcium, zinc, magnesium, vitamin B_6, and folate. Encourage energy intake of at least 1,800 kcal/day. Calcium, multivitamin-mineral supplements, or both may be advised when dietary sources are marginal and it is unlikely that appropriate dietary practices will or can be followed. Intakes below 1,500 kcal/day are not recommended at any time during lactation, although fasts lasting less than 1 day have not been shown to decrease milk volume. Liquid diets and weight loss medications are not recommended. Since the impact of curtailing maternal energy intake during the first 2 to 3 weeks post partum is unknown, dieting during this period is not recommended.

Maternal Substance Use and Abuse

The use of illicit drugs should be actively discouraged, and affected women (regardless of their mode of feeding) should be assisted to enter a rehabilitative program that makes provision for the infant. The use of certain legal substances by lactating women is also of concern, including the potential for alcohol abuse.

• There is no scientific evidence that consumption of alcoholic beverages has a beneficial impact on any aspect of lactation performance. If alcohol is used, advise the lactating woman to limit her intake to no more than 0.5 g of alcohol per kg of maternal body weight per day. Intake over this level may impair the milk ejection reflex. For a 60-kg (132-lb) woman, 0.5 g of alcohol per kg of body weight corresponds to approximately 2 to 2.5 oz of liquor, 8 oz of table wine, or 2 cans of beer.

• Actively discourage smoking among lactating women, not only because it may reduce milk volume but because of its other harmful effects on the mother and her infant.

• Discourage intake of large quantities of coffee, other caffeine-containing beverages and medications, and decaffeinated coffee. The equivalent of 1 to 2 cups of regular coffee daily is unlikely to have a deleterious effect on the nursling, although preliminary evidence suggests that maternal coffee intake may adversely influence the iron content of milk and the iron status of the infant.

Infant Growth and Nutrition

The subcommittee recommends that health care providers be informed

about the differences in growth between healthy breastfed and formula-fed infants. On average, breastfed infants gain weight more slowly than those fed formula after the first 2 to 3 months. Slower weight gain, by itself, does not justify the use of supplemental formula. When in doubt, clinicians should evaluate adequacy of growth according to the guidelines described by Lawrence (1989).

Regardless of what the mother eats, the following steps should be taken to ensure adequate nutrition of breastfed infants.

- All newborns should receive a 0.5- to 1.0-mg injection or a 1.0- to 2.0-mg oral dose of vitamin K immediately after birth regardless of the type of feeding that will be offered the infant.
- If the infant's exposure to sunlight appears to be inadequate, the infant should be given a 5- to 7.5-μg supplement of vitamin D per day.
- Fluoride supplements should be provided to breastfed infants if the fluoride content of the household drinking-water supply is low (<0.3 ppm)
- When breastfeeding is complemented by other foods, and by 6 months of age in any case, the infant should be given food rich in bioavailable iron or a daily low-dose oral iron supplement.

Infant Health

Health care providers should recognize that breastfeeding is recommended to reduce the incidence and severity of certain infectious gastrointestinal and respiratory diseases and other disorders in infancy. Breastfeeding ordinarily confers health benefits to the infant, but in certain rare cases it may pose some health risks, as indicated below.

- For mothers requiring medication and desiring to breastfeed, the clinician should select the medication least likely to pass into the milk and to the infant.
- Although medications rarely pose a problem during lactation, breastfeeding is contraindicated in the case of a few. Such drugs include antineoplastic agents, therapeutic radiopharmaceuticals, some but not all antithyroid agents, and antiprotozoan agents.
- In those rare cases when there is heavy exposure to pesticides, heavy metals, or other contaminants that may pass into the milk, breastfeeding is not recommended if maternal levels are high.

Recommendations for Nutrition Monitoring

The committee recommends that the U.S. government provide a mechanism for periodically monitoring trends in lactation and developing normative indicators of nutritional status during lactation.

• *Monitoring of trends.* Data are needed on the incidence and duration of breastfeeding among the population as a whole, and among some particularly vulnerable subpopulations. Exclusive, partial, and minimal breastfeeding should be distinguished; and data should be collected at several ages during infancy. Current or planned surveys by such agencies as the National Center for Health Statistics or the Nutrition Monitoring Division of the U.S. Department of Agriculture could be modified to serve these goals.

• *Developing normative indicators of nutritional status.* There is a need for data on dietary intakes by, and nutritional status among, lactating women and their relationship to lactation performance. Identification of groups of lactating women who are at nutritional risk is a problem of public health importance.

Research Recommendations

In its deliberations, the subcommittee was well aware that many factors (such as hospital practices, social attitudes, governmental policies, and exposure to infectious agents) may have a great influence on breastfeeding rates and lactation performance and that there is a need for studies to examine approaches that hold the most promise for improving both of these. Similarly, the subcommittee recognized the great need for studies to examine the short- and long-term benefits of breastfeeding in the United States among mothers and infants in all segments of the population, but especially among disadvantaged groups, which currently have the lowest rates of breastfeeding. Research recommendations concerning several of these issues (infant mortality, growth charts for breastfed infants, possible transmission of HIV, indicators of infant nutritional status) are contained in Chapter 10. They have been excluded from this summary, not because they are unimportant, but rather because they relate only indirectly to the nutrition of healthy U.S. women during lactation.

• **Research is needed to develop indicators of nutritional status for lactating women.** First, the identification of normative values for nutritional status should be based on observations of representative, healthy, lactating women in the United States. In addition, indicators are needed of both (1) risks of adverse outcomes related to the mother's dietary intake and (2) the potential of the mother or her nursing infant to benefit from interventions designed to improve their nutritional status or health.

• **Research is needed to identify groups of lactating women in the United States who are at nutritional risk or who could benefit from nutrition intervention programs.** In general, it has been difficult to identify groups of mothers and infants in the United States with nutritional deficits that are severe enough to have measurable functional consequences. Priority should be given to the study of lactating women in subpopulations believed to be at risk of inadequate intake of certain nutrients, such as calcium by blacks and vitamin A by low-income women. The potential influence of culture-specific food beliefs on nutrient intake of lactating women should be included in any such investigations.

• **Intervention studies of improved design and technical sophistication are needed to investigate the effects of maternal diet and nutritional status on milk volume; milk composition; infant nutritional status, growth, and health; and maternal health.** The nursing dyad (the mother and her infant) has seldom been the focus of studies. Thus, a key aspect of this recommendation is concurrent examination of the mother, the volume and composition of the milk, and the infant. The design of such research needs to be adequate for causal inference; thus, if possible, it should include random assignment of lactating subjects to treatment groups. Appropriate sampling and handling of milk for the valid assessment of energy density, nutrient concentration, and total milk volume are essential, as is accurate measurement of nutrient concentrations.

With regard to the energy balance of lactating women, the threshold below which energy intake is insufficient to support adequate milk production has not yet been identified. Resolution of this question will probably require supplementation studies of women in developing countries whose diets are chronically energy deficient. Although such deficient diets are not common in the United States, identification of the level of energy intake that is too low to support lactation will be useful in establishing guidelines for women who want to breastfeed but who also want to restrict their energy intake to lose weight. Although chronically low energy intakes by women in disadvantaged populations may not be completely analogous to acute energy restriction among otherwise well-nourished women, ethical considerations limit the kinds of investigations that could directly address the influence of energy restriction. In supplementation studies, measurements should be made of lactation performance and of any impact on the mother's nutritional status and health, including the period of lactation amenorrhea.

With regard to specific nutrients, the impact of relatively low intakes of folate, vitamin B_6, calcium, zinc, and magnesium during lactation on the mother's nutritional status and health needs to be assessed in more detail. As a part of this assessment, studies of the absorption of calcium, zinc, and magnesium during lactation will be useful. There is also a need to identify a reliable indicator of vitamin B_6 status of infants and to document the relationships between this indicator, maternal vitamin B_6 intake, and vitamin B_6 content in milk. Finally, resolution of the conflicting findings concerning the impact of maternal protein intake on milk volume would be desirable.

REFERENCES

DHHS (Department of Health and Human Services). 1980. Promoting Health/Preventing Disease: Objectives for the Nation. Public Health Service, U.S. Department of Health and Human Services, U.S. Government Printing Office, Washington, D.C. 102 pp.

DHHS (Department of Health and Human Services). 1984. Report of the Surgeon General's Workshop on Breastfeeding and Human Lactation. DHHS Publ. No. HRS-D-MC 84-2. Health Resources and Services Administration, Public Health Service, U.S. Department of Health and Human Services, Rockville, Md. 93 pp.

DHHS (Department of Health and Human Services). 1985. Followup Report: The Surgeon General's Workshop on Breastfeeding & Human Lactation. DHHS Publ. No. HRS-D-MC 85-2. Health Resources and Services Administration, Public Health Service, U.S. Department of Health and Human Services, Rockville, Md. 46 pp.

DHHS (Department of Health and Human Services). 1990. Healthy People 2000: National Health Promotion and Disease Prevention Objectives. Conference Edition. U.S. Department of Health and Human Services, Public Health Service, Office of the Assistant Secretary of Health, Washington, D.C. 672 pp.

IOM (Institute of Medicine). 1990. Nutrition During Pregnancy: Weight Gain and Nutrient Supplements. Report of the Subcommittee on Nutritional Status and Weight Gain During Pregnancy, Subcommittee on Dietary Intake and Nutrient Supplements During Pregnancy, Committee on Nutritional Status During Pregnancy and Lactation, Food and Nutrition Board. National Academy Press, Washington, D.C. 468 pp.

Lawrence, R.A. 1989. Breastfeeding: A Guide for the Medical Profession, 3rd ed. C.V. Mosby, St. Louis. 652 pp.

Little, R.E., K.W. Anderson, C.H. Ervin, B. Worthington-Roberts, and S.K. Clarren. 1989. Maternal alcohol use during breast-feeding and infant mental and motor development at one year. N. Engl. J. Med. 321:425-430.

Malone, C. 1980. Breast Feeding. Cumberland County WIC Program, People's Regional Opportunity Program, Portland, Maine. 13 pp.

NRC (National Research Council). 1989. Recommended Dietary Allowances, 10th ed. Report of the Subcommittee on the Tenth Edition of the RDAs, Food and Nutrition Board, Commission on Life Sciences. National Academy Press, Washington, D.C. 284 pp.

The Steering Committee to Promote Breastfeeding in New York City. 1986. The Art and Science of Breastfeeding. Division of Maternal and Child Health, Bureau of Health Care Delivery and Assistance, Health Resources and Services Administration, U.S. Department of Health and Human Services, Washington, D.C. 74 pp.

USDA (U.S. Department of Agriculture). 1988. Promoting Breastfeeding in WIC: A Compendium of Practical Approaches. FNS-256. Food and Nutrition Service, U.S. Department of Agriculture, Alexandria, Va. 171 pp.

2

Introduction

Lactation is a remarkable process during which the maternal body produces a secretion that provides no immediate benefit to the mother but can totally sustain the offspring. All mammals produce milks with different compositions, each one specific to the needs for growth and development of their offspring. Regardless of a woman's intention to breastfeed, her body prepares for lactation from the first moments of pregnancy: the mammary gland begins its maturational process with the development of the alveolar ductal system and the lacteal cells so that the breast is ready to produce milk upon delivery of the infant. The woman's hormonal balance during pregnancy contributes to the preparation of the breast and promotes accumulation of energy stores, but it suppresses the production of milk until the birth of the infant.

Between 1940 and 1980, there was relatively little active investigation of nutrition during lactation and of the impact of breastfeeding on the mother. Except for the 10 editions of *Recommended Dietary Allowances*, which have included specific nutrient recommendations for lactating women since they were first published (NRC, 1943), relatively few publications by the National Academy of Sciences, the government, or professional organizations have paid detailed attention to nutrition during lactation. The Academy's publications include three reports prepared by committees of the Food and Nutrition Board under the sponsorship of the Maternal and Child Health Program (Title V, Social Security Act): *Nutrition in Pregnancy and Lactation* (NRC, 1967), *A Selected Annotated Bibliography on Breast Feeding, 1970-1977* (NRC, 1978), and *Nutrition Services in Perinatal Care* (NRC, 1981). However, these reports did not include interpretive reviews of the literature.

20

The first clear evidence that the federal government was increasing its attention to breastfeeding appeared in the report *Promoting Health/Preventing Disease: Objectives for the Nation* (DHHS, 1980). That publication included an explicit objective to increase the proportion of breastfed infants. The target breastfeeding rates were 75% at hospital discharge and 35% at 6 months post partum. At that time, the Maternal and Child Health Program of the U.S. Department of Health and Human Services (DHHS) was charged with the responsibility of developing national policy related to lactation and breastfeeding and of convening a national group periodically to advise them on specific issues.

Lactation research received increased attention in 1982, when the National Institute of Child Health and Human Development (NICHD) sponsored a conference that dealt primarily with techniques for collection, analysis, and storage of human milk—prerequisites for meaningful studies as well as for milk banking. This was followed by other lactation research conferences (see, for example, FASEB [1984] and Jensen and Neville [1985]).

In 1984, before it was recognized that national rates of breastfeeding had begun to decline (see Chapter 3), Surgeon General C. Everett Koop convened a workshop on Breastfeeding and Human Lactation (DHHS, 1984) and said, "We must . . . identify and reduce those barriers which keep women from initiating or continuing to breastfeed their infants" (DHHS, 1984, p. 6). The following six recommendations were made at that workshop to facilitate progress toward the previously mentioned 1990 breastfeeding objective:

- Improve *professional education* in human lactation and breastfeeding
- Develop *public education* and promotional efforts
- Strengthen the support for breastfeeding in the *health care system*
- Develop a broad range of *support services* in the community
- Initiate a national breastfeeding promotion effort directed to women in the *world of work*
- Expand *research* on human lactation and breastfeeding (DHHS, 1985, p. 1).

The publication *Followup Report: The Surgeon General's Workshop on Breastfeeding & Human Lactation* (DHHS, 1985) summarizes many of the activities that emanated from the recommendations made at the 1984 workshop. Attention to nutrition during lactation fell primarily under the research recommendation.

Between 1985 and 1989, NICHD sponsored three additional lactation-related workshops: the first one on the effects of maternal and environmental factors on human milk (Hamosh and Goldman, 1986), the next one on the effects of milk on the recipient infant (Goldman et al., 1987), and the third one on future needs for human milk research. Statements issued from these workshops and through other forums (e.g., Goldman and Garza, 1987) have clearly indicated that there is a need for additional study of nutrition during lactation and how it may influence the health of both the mother and her infant.

Many of the studies presented at these workshops suggested that breastfeeding might have both immediate and long-lasting beneficial effects.

Despite efforts to promote breastfeeding following the Surgeon General's workshop, breastfeeding rates have declined further, probably because of a combination of social and economic forces. Social attitudes, such as the perceived low value of breastfeeding, may be partially responsible. These attitudes might be expected to continue with the recent adoption of television advertising and direct mail distribution of infant formula by formula manufacturers. Social forces that may be contributing to decreased rates of breastfeeding include the increased participation of women in the work force coupled with the scarcity of job-site day-care facilities and lack of provisions for routine postpartum maternal respite from work. Because of economic pressures on hospitals and cost-containment policies of third-party payers, mothers in many places are routinely discharged 24 hours after delivery, with no opportunity for breastfeeding instruction or support.

These social and economic forces driving the decline of breastfeeding are virtually inseparable from government policies, and current government policies offer little hope of change. The United States is one of the few industrialized countries without a national policy of maternity and parental leave. Moreover, there are few government programs supporting day care. Thus, many mothers must return to work soon after delivery or face the loss of wages or even the loss of a job. Often, they must leave their infants to be cared for at sites distant from their places of employment. The combination of fatigue, stress, and physical separation from their infants makes breastfeeding prohibitive for all but the most strongly committed.

Although nutrition during lactation has not been a priority in breastfeeding promotion efforts, there has been recognition of the need to promote adequate food intake to support milk production and the woman's health. For example, the Special Supplemental Food Program for Women, Infants, and Children (WIC) was encouraged to increase the options for food packages to be more responsive to the food preferences of adolescent mothers and mothers of various ethnic groups.

Many reasons have been given to support breastfeeding promotion (AAP, 1982; AAP/ACOG, 1988; ACOG, 1985; ADA, 1986; APHA, 1983; AAP, 1978; DHHS, 1988):

- the favorable balance and bioavailability of nutrients in human milk compared with those of nutrients in formula,
- the immunologic properties conferred by human milk that help reduce infant morbidity and mortality during breastfeeding,
- the potential for reducing the risk of early development of allergic disease,

- the psychologic benefits to both the infant and the mother resulting from the intimate relationship that is repeated throughout the day and night over an extended period,
- the facilitation of contractions and the involution of the once gravid uterus and the control of postpartum bleeding associated with oxytocin release,
- the maternal feelings of well-being associated with the changes in hormone concentrations during lactation, and
- the enhancement of mothering behaviors by the stimulus of hormones during suckling.

The accumulated evidence of the beneficial effects of breastfeeding has led many professional groups (e.g., the American Academy of Pediatrics, the American Dietetic Association, the American College of Obstetricians and Gynecologists, Academy of Family Medicine) to endorse and actively support breastfeeding.

PURPOSE AND SCOPE

In April 1987, the Office of Maternal and Child Health of DHHS asked the Food and Nutrition Board to establish a committee on nutrition during pregnancy and lactation. In response to the request, a committee was formed to oversee the work of three subcommittees: (1) nutritional status and weight gain during pregnancy, (2) dietary intake and nutritional supplementation during pregnancy, and (3) nutrition during lactation. The deliberations of the third subcommittee constitute this report.

The specific charge to the lactation subcommittee was "to evaluate and document the current scientific evidence and formulate recommendations for the nutritional needs of lactating women." Consideration was to be given to the following:

- the effect of maternal dietary intake during lactation on the volume and composition of human milk;
- the effect of maternal nutritional status during pregnancy and post partum on the volume and composition of human milk;
- the appropriateness of various anthropometric methods for assessing nutritional status during lactation; and
- the effects of lactation on the recipient infant, maternal health, and maternal nutritional status.

The subcommittee was also asked to consider justification for special recommendations for different maternal age and ethnic groups, taking particular note of the needs of lactating adolescents; women over age 35; and women of black, Hispanic, and Southeast Asian origins. Although there are data on lactation and breastfeeding derived from cultures throughout the world, this report focuses on lactating women and their infants in the United States.

The subcommittee is well aware that nutrient stores and nutrient intake are only two of the many factors that influence production of milk, growth and health of the infant, and maternal health. Other factors (such as hospital practices, the need to resume employment, anatomic adequacy, hormonal response, maternal insecurity, and exposure to infectious agents) are mentioned only briefly in the report, even though they may have great influence on milk volume and composition. The subcommittee restricted its coverage of these factors, however, because they are not directly related to its task. The subcommittee did consider it essential to discuss the components of human milk that may contribute positively or negatively to the health status of infants, even in the absence of data indicating that maternal nutrition might influence those components. Furthermore, the subcommittee also considered it important to place the role of nutrition during lactation in proper perspective relative to the many other factors that can influence the success of breastfeeding.

There remains an urgent need to reduce the many barriers to successful initiation and maintenance of breastfeeding. The reader is encouraged to obtain more information on this from publications such as the *Report of the Surgeon General's Workshop on Breastfeeding and Human Lactation* (DHHS, 1984) and *Promoting Breastfeeding in WIC: A Compendium of Practical Approaches* (USDA, 1988).

METHODS

The Subcommittee on Nutrition During Lactation conducted an extensive review of the literature to examine the impact of lactation on the mother and the infant as well as the impact of maternal diet and nutritional status on maternal stores, the milk, and the infant. Valuable assistance was provided by the Committee on Nutritional Status During Pregnancy and Lactation, which served in an advisory capacity to the subcommittee.

Methods that were used to estimate how lactation influences maternal nutrient requirements included consideration of the nutrient content of human milk and its variability, mean milk production and variations in milk production between and within women, and physiologic changes that may enhance maternal nutrient absorption or reduce nutrient losses.

Imprecise terminology in the literature complicated the subcommittee's task. For example, the terms *breastfeeding* and *breastfed* were often used indiscriminately, without definition of extent or duration. *Extent* of breastfeeding refers to the daily frequency and length of suckling sessions, while *duration* refers to the number of months or weeks over which breastfeeding occurs. In this report, the subcommittee applies the term *exclusive breastfeeding* when infants are fed only by this method; *partial breastfeeding* when breastfeeding is supplemented with limited amounts of formula, juice, water, or solid foods;

and *minimal breastfeeding* when the infant receives nearly all sustenance from formula and other foods.

Furthermore, terms such as *well nourished, malnourished*, and *undernourished* were given various definitions (or none at all) in the literature. The subcommittee uses the term *apparently well nourished* or, simply, *well nourished* to describe the healthy woman who is of appropriate weight for height and who has no notable dietary limitations.

The term *lactation performance* is broadly defined to include the quality and quantity of milk produced, duration of lactation, various indices of maternal health (such as folate status), and selected indices of child health (such as growth and morbidity). When evaluating evidence to determine whether maternal nutrition is likely to influence one or more aspects of lactation performance, careful consideration was given to the adequacy of the study for answering the specific question being addressed. In nearly all cases, the formulation of recommendations required substantial exercise of judgment because of limitations of the data.

ORGANIZATION OF THIS REPORT

This volume begins with a summary of the report and its principal conclusions and recommendations. Chapter 3 addresses the question "Who is breastfeeding?" by identifying breastfeeding rates in the United States by different demographic characteristics (such as age, ethnic background, region of the country, and employment status). It also provides a historical perspective of the incidence and duration of breastfeeding in the past century.

Chapter 4 examines anthropometric and biochemical methods for assessing the nutritional status of lactating women and points out their uses and limitations. The subcommittee tabulated and interpreted nutrient intake data from studies of lactating women.

Chapters 5 and 6 contain discussions of the volume and composition of human milk, respectively, and explain factors that must be considered when evaluating the impact of maternal nutrition on these two lactation outcomes. These chapters also provide the basis for estimating the range of the mother's increased need for nutrients resulting from breastfeeding.

Although infant growth, development, and health are key outcomes of breastfeeding, the effects of maternal nutrition during lactation on these outcomes have been largely ignored in the literature. To the extent possible, Chapter 7 reports the links between the nutrition of the mother and the nutrition and growth of the nursing infant. Since a slower than expected rate of infant weight gain may be given as a reason for discontinuing breastfeeding, the subcommittee paid special attention to the assessment of the growth of breastfed infants. It also raised the possibility that maternal nutrition may influence infant health through altered immunologic function. Links between maternal food intake while lactating and infant health are also considered in Chapter 7 as they relate to allergic diseases and environmental toxins. To provide a balanced overview of infant health, the risk of transmission of infectious agents via human milk and the presence of drugs in human milk are also covered. In addition, there is brief mention of the development of obesity and atherosclerosis in later life in relation to the method of infant feeding.

Chapter 8 explores ways that maternal health can be influenced by lactation. Topics include obesity, osteoporosis, and breast cancer. Maternal health outcomes also include the impact of lactation on ovulation and fertility. In Chapter 9, information from preceding chapters is synthesized in a discussion of ways to meet the nutrient needs of lactating women. Chapter 10 presents the subcommittee's recommendations for research based on the contents of this report.

REFERENCES

AAP (American Academy of Pediatrics). 1978. Breast-feeding: a commentary in celebration of the International Year of the Child, 1979. Pediatrics 62:591-601.

AAP (American Academy of Pediatrics). 1982. The promotion of breastfeeding: policy statement based on task force report. Pediatrics 69:654-661.

AAP/ACOG (American Academy of Pediatrics/American College of Obstetricians and Gynecologists). 1988. Guidelines for Perinatal Care, 2nd ed. American Academy of Pediatrics, Elk Grove, Ill. 356 pp.

ACOG (American College of Obstetricians and Gynecologists). 1985. Standards for Obstetric-Gynecologic Services, 6th ed. The American College of Obstetricians and Gynecologists, Washington, D.C. 109 pp.

ADA (American Dietetic Association). 1986. Position of the American Dietetic Association: promotion of breast feeding. J. Am. Diet. Assoc. 86:1580-1585.

APHA (American Public Health Association). 1983. Policy statements: breastfeeding. Am. J. Public Health 73:347-348.

DHHS (Department of Health and Human Services). 1980. Promoting Health/Preventing Disease: Objectives for the Nation. Public Health Service, U.S. Department of Health and Human Services, U.S. Government Printing Office, Washington, D.C. 102 pp.

DHHS (Department of Health and Human Services). 1984. Report of the Surgeon General's Workshop on Breastfeeding & Human Lactation. DHHS Publ. No. HRS-D-MC 84-2. Health Resources and Services Administration, Public Health Service, U.S. Department of Health and Human Services, Rockville, Md. 93 pp.

DHHS (Department of Health and Human Services). 1985. Followup Report: The Surgeon General's Workshop on Breastfeeding & Human Lactation. DHHS Publ. No. HRS-D-MC 85-2. Health Resources and Services Administration, Public Health Service, U.S. Department of Health and Human Services, Rockville, Md. 46 pp.

DHHS (Department of Health and Human Services). 1988. The Surgeon General's Report on Nutrition and Health. DHHS (PHS) Publ. No. 88-50210. Public Health Service, U.S. Department of Health and Human Services. U.S. Government Printing Office, Washington, D.C. 727 pp.

FASEB (Federation of American Societies for Experimental Biology). 1984. Proceedings of the Federation of American Societies for Experimental Biology. J. Pediatr. Gastroenterol. Nutr. 3.

Goldman, A.S., and C. Garza. 1987. Future research in human milk. Pediatr. Res. 22:493-496.

Goldman, A.S., S.A. Atkinson, and L.A. Hanson. 1987. Human Lactation 3: The Effects of Human Milk on the Recipient Infant. Plenum Press, New York. 400 pp.

Hamosh, M., and A.S. Goldman, eds. 1986. Human Lactation 2: Maternal and Environmental Factors. Plenum Press, New York. 657 pp.

Jensen, R.G., and M.C. Neville, eds. 1985. Human Lactation: Milk Components and Methodologies. Plenum Press, New York. 307 pp.

NRC (National Research Council). 1943. Recommended Dietary Allowances. Report of the Food and Nutrition Board. Reprint and Circular Series No. 115. National Academy of Sciences, Washington, D.C. 6 pp.

NRC (National Research Council). 1967. Nutrition in Pregnancy and Lactation. Report of the Committee on Maternal Nutrition, Food and Nutrition Board. For Transmittal to the Children's Bureau. National Academy of Sciences, Washington, D.C. 67 pp.

NRC (National Research Council). 1978. A Selected Annotated Bibliography on Breast Feeding, 1970-1977. Report of the Food and Nutrition Board. National Academy of Sciences, Washington, D.C. 58 pp.

NRC (National Research Council). 1981. Nutrition Services in Perinatal Care. Report of the Committee on Nutrition of the Mother and Preschool Child, Food and Nutrition Board, Assembly of Life Sciences. National Academy Press, Washington, D.C. 72 pp.

USDA (U.S. Department of Agriculture). 1988. Promoting Breastfeeding in WIC: A Compendium of Practical Approaches. FNS-256. Food and Nutrition Service, U.S. Department of Agriculture, Alexandria, Va. 171 pp.

3

Who Breastfeeds in the United States?

Although this volume focuses on the physiologic process of *lactation*, lactation occurs only in the context of the behavior *breastfeeding*. Virtually all mothers are physiologically capable of lactation, but not all of them decide to breastfeed their infants; those who breastfeed do so with varying degrees of intensity and continue for different lengths of time. The subcommittee examined the distribution of mothers who breastfeed in order to determine whether or not findings on nutrition during lactation apply equally across the population. It also examined trends over the past several decades and relationships between the demographics of breastfeeding and maternal diet (see Chapter 4) to identify those segments of the population for which information on nutrition during lactation is most crucial. These demographic data can also suggest the best ways to present information on nutrition during lactation to reach target audiences as a part of a national effort to increase rates of breastfeeding in the United States (DHHS, 1984).

In this discussion, the incidence of breastfeeding in the hospital or within the first week of life is used to indicate the percentage of women who initiated breastfeeding.

HISTORY OF BREASTFEEDING IN THE UNITED STATES

Before 1970

During the twentieth century, infant-feeding practices have undergone dramatic changes that reflect shifts in values and attitudes in the U.S. society as

28

a whole. They have tended to occur first among those women at the forefront of changes in dominant social values and among those with the resources (whether it is time, energy, or money) to permit adoption of new feeding practices.

Examples of alternative feeding practices, such as the use of wet nurses or human milk substitutes, occur throughout recorded history (Fildes, 1986). The early twentieth century was marked, however, by an unprecedented increase in formula feeding, in part because the development of nutrition science coincided with a pervasive increase in the value placed on scientific products and processes (Rosenberg, 1976; Starr, 1982). As women asserted their rights for self-determination in public life, those who were wealthy enough and sufficiently in tune with contemporary values were adopting formula feeding for their infants.

A corresponding and consistent decline in breastfeeding is evident in data from U.S. fertility surveys (Hendershot, 1980, 1981; Hirschman and Hendershot, 1979), specific studies of infant feeding (Meyer, 1958, 1968), and market research surveys conducted by Ross Laboratories,[1] a manufacturer of infant formula (Martinez and Krieger, 1985; Martinez and Nalezienski, 1979, 1981; Martinez et al., 1981). Seventy-seven percent of the infants born between 1936 and 1940 were breastfed; the incidence declined during the subsequent decades to about 25% by 1970 (Hendershot, 1980, 1981; Hirschman and Hendershot, 1979; Meyer, 1958, 1968). Duration of breastfeeding declined as well, dropping from a mean of 4.2 months in the early 1930s to 2.2 months in the late 1950s.

Because this decline in breastfeeding was not uniform in all segments of the U.S. population, the demographic characteristics of the group of mothers who breastfed changed substantially (Table 3-1). Ethnic differences in rates of decline are especially striking. Rates fell sharply among blacks; there was a less pronounced decline among whites and Hispanics (Hirschman and Hendershot,

---

[1] Although the subcommittee considers the data compiled annually by Ross Laboratories to be the best data on breastfeeding rates in the United States, these data have two limitations common to many survey data: sampling bias and response bias. The list from which the Ross sample is derived represents 85% of all new mothers in the United States. This list probably underrepresents any unregistered births and those not occurring in hospitals. Such births are more likely to be to economically disadvantaged mothers, including illegal aliens.

The response rate for the 1987 survey was 54% (Ryan and Martinez, 1989), a rate fairly typical of past surveys (Fomon, 1987). Responses are weighted before analysis to attempt to compensate for nonrespondents. Compared with all mothers in the U.S. population, the unweighted sample has a lower percentage of mothers who are black or Hispanic, unmarried, and less than age 24; have high school or lower education levels; and have family incomes of less than $25,000; but it is comparable in terms of maternal employment status and geographic region of residence.

The weighting procedures cannot correct for, and indeed may amplify, any response bias associated with breastfeeding status. If, for example, those black or Hispanic mothers who breastfeed are more likely to respond than those who do not breastfeed, the weighted data will give the false impression that a higher percentage of black and Hispanic women breastfeed than is actually the case.

The Ross Laboratories data probably are least representative of that segment of the U.S. population with the lowest income. Therefore, it is likely that the breastfeeding rates among participants in the Special Supplemental Food Program for Women, Infants, and Children (WIC), blacks, and mothers of lower socioeconomic class are even lower than the Ross data indicate.

1979). Before 1960, black mothers were more likely than white mothers to breastfeed. After 1960, the reverse was true because of the more rapid decline among black mothers.

The trends are somewhat more complex for mothers with different educational levels. In the 1950s breastfeeding rates were lower for women with a high school education than for those with more or less education, but by 1970, these rates varied directly with education (Hendershot, 1981; Hirschman and Hendershot, 1979). According to some observers (Meyer, 1968; Salber et al., 1958), the differences in trends for women with different educational levels represent the trickling down of values and behaviors from economically and socially advantaged women to less advantaged women. Those observers conclude that women with less education adopted formula feeding as the culmination of a trend initiated by better educated mothers earlier in the century.

Turnaround in the 1970s

The overall downward trend in breastfeeding incidence reached its nadir at 22% in 1972 (Hendershot, 1981) (Figure 3-1). The subsequent increase was not uniform across the population. Breastfeeding incidence rose among white and black mothers, although the increase was greater among whites (Hendershot, 1981). Although data on Hispanic mothers are incomplete, there are indications that their breastfeeding incidence remained stable or even continued to fall (Smith et al., 1982). The incidence rose in all education groups (Hendershot, 1981; Martinez and Nalezienski, 1981; Martinez et al., 1981). There are few data on the association between breastfeeding and income. Those from the National Survey of Family Growth indicate that breastfeeding rates remained unchanged among low-income mothers but increased among those with middle and higher incomes (Hendershot, 1981).

Duration of breastfeeding increased after 1972 as well. Approximately 10% of breastfeeding mothers continued the practice for at least 3 months in 1972, whereas approximately 20% did so in 1975 and 37% did so in 1984 (Hendershot, 1981; Martinez and Krieger, 1985; Martinez and Nalezienski, 1981; Martinez et al., 1981).

Ironically, this return to breastfeeding in the 1970s parallelled its decline in the early twentieth century. Once again, women of higher socioeconomic status were the first to adopt a "new" feeding method (breastfeeding), and their rationale was couched in scientific language, this time, focused on such issues as immunologic factors and maternal-infant bonding. Reflecting broader cultural values, many women adopted natural childbirth and, with it, what they considered natural infant feeding.

The upward trend in breastfeeding after 1972 appeared to peak in 1982 at about 61% for initiation and 40% for the percentage of mothers breastfeeding 3 months or longer. The exact zenith of the trend is difficult to pinpoint, because

TABLE 3-1   Percentages of First-Born Infants
Breastfed Between 1951 and 1970 in the United
States, by Ethnic Group and Education[a]

Category	1951–1955	1956–1960	1961–1965	1966–1970
Ethnic group				
White	49	43	39	29
Black	59	42	24	14
Hispanic	58	55	39	35
Education				
<9 yr	62	53	40	32
9–11 yr	50	40	29	17
12 yr	45	40	32	23
13–15 yr	57	48	50	35
>15 yr	46	50	69	57

[a]From Hirschman and Hendershot (1979).

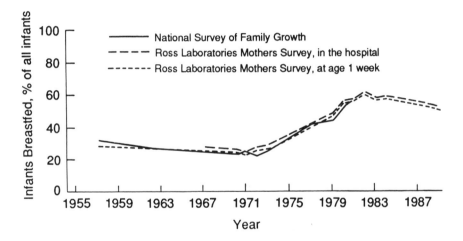

FIGURE 3-1   Percentage of infants breastfed, by survey and year, based on data from the
National Survey of Family Growth (Hendershot, 1981; Pratt et al., 1984) and A. Ryan, Ross
Laboratories, personal communication, 1990.   Both government and market survey data are
presented to show the similarity in trends found.   Government data are not available after 1981.
The subcommittee considers the Ross Laboratories data to be the more reliable source.   Those
data are collected quarterly, and annual rates are computed from a nationally representative
sample of mothers of 6-month-old infants.   The government data were derived from three surveys
of women aged 15 to 44 who were ever married or who were single with coresident children
at the time of the interview.   Data on breastfeeding were gathered for all infants born to the
respondents.   Because no women aged 45 or older were interviewed, data for the earliest years
are biased toward the practices of women who were young at the time.   Hendershot (1980)
reviews the strengths and weaknesses of these data sources in detail.

Ross Laboratories changed its weighting procedures to obtain a better reflection of the socioeconomic makeup of the U.S. population (Martinez and Krieger, 1985), and data for the 1980s from the National Survey of Family Growth were not yet available for the subcommittee's use. The evidence from Ross Laboratories suggests a gradual, persistent decline in breastfeeding during the 1980s.

CURRENT STATISTICS FOR BREASTFEEDING IN THE UNITED STATES

1989 Data

The initiation of breastfeeding by women delivering in 1989 was reported to be 52.2% (Table 3-2) (A. Ryan, Ross Laboratories, personal communication, 1990). By age 5 or 6 months,[2] only 19.6% of the infants were still breastfed. Of the three ethnic groups compared, white mothers initiated breastfeeding at the highest rates and black mothers did so at the lowest rates. Forty percent of white mothers who initiated breastfeeding were still breastfeeding at 5 or 6 months, compared with approximately 30% of black or Hispanic mothers. A breakdown of these data by parity indicates that, except among Hispanics, primiparous and multiparous women initiate breastfeeding at about the same rates, but the former breastfeed for a shorter duration. The data also show that married mothers are much more likely than unmarried mothers to breastfeed and that they experience a far lower rate of attrition by 5 to 6 months. This difference is especially pronounced among black mothers.

Higher percentages of older mothers initiate breastfeeding, and they continue for a longer duration than younger mothers do. Breastfeeding both in the hospital and at 5 or 6 months is positively associated with maternal education and family income. Mothers with any college education are especially likely to initiate breastfeeding. Black mothers with a high school education or less initiate breastfeeding only about half as often as college educated black mothers do.

A breakdown of breastfeeding by census region shows distinct regional trends. The highest rates for initiating breastfeeding (Figure 3-2 [in the hospital]) and at 5 or 6 months post partum (Figure 3-3) are found in the Mountain and Pacific regions; rates in the East South Central region are the lowest. Ethnic differences within census regions are the same as those seen in national data.

The Ross Laboratories data on participants in the Special Supplemental Program for Women, Infants, and Children (WIC) indicate that 34% breastfeed

---

[2]Mothers were surveyed when their infants were 6 months of age. They were asked to recall how their infant was fed in the hospital, at week 1, at months 1 through 5, and on the previous day. Responses labeled "5 or 6 months" are an average of the 5-month and previous-day responses.

TABLE 3-2 Percentage of Mothers Breastfeeding Newborn Infants in the Hospital and Infants at 5 or 6 Months of Age in the United States in 1989,[a] by Ethnic Background and Selected Demographic Variables[b]

Category	Total New-borns	Total 5–6 mo Infants	White New-borns	White 5–6 mo Infants	Black New-borns	Black 5–6 mo Infants	Hispanic[c] New-borns	Hispanic[c] 5–6 mo Infants
All mothers	52.2	19.6	58.5	22.7	23.0	7.0	48.4	15.0
Parity								
Primiparous	52.6	16.6	58.3	18.9	23.1	5.9	49.9	13.2
Multiparous	51.7	22.7	58.7	26.8	23.0	7.9	47.2	16.5
Marital status								
Married	59.8	24.0	61.9	25.3	35.8	12.3	55.3	18.8
Unmarried	30.8	7.7	40.3	9.8	17.2	4.6	37.5	8.6
Maternal age								
<20 yr	30.2	6.2	36.8	7.2	13.5	3.6	35.3	6.9
20–24 yr	45.2	12.7	50.8	14.5	19.4	4.7	46.9	12.6
25–29 yr	58.8	22.9	63.1	25.0	29.9	9.4	56.2	19.5
30–34 yr	65.5	31.4	70.1	34.8	35.4	13.6	57.6	23.4
≥35 yr	66.5	36.2	71.9	40.5	35.6	14.3	53.9	24.4
Maternal education								
No college	42.1	13.4	48.3	15.6	17.6	5.5	42.6	12.2
College[d]	70.7	31.1	74.7	34.1	41.1	12.2	66.5	23.4
Family income								
<$7,000	28.8	7.9	36.7	9.4	14.5	4.3	35.3	10.3
$7,000–$14,999	44.0	13.5	49.0	15.2	23.5	7.3	47.2	13.0
$15,000–$24,999	54.7	20.4	57.7	22.3	31.7	8.7	52.6	16.5
≥$25,000	66.3	27.6	67.8	28.7	42.8	14.5	65.4	23.0
Maternal employment								
Full time	50.8	10.2	54.8	10.8	30.6	6.9	50.4	9.5
Part time	59.4	23.0	63.8	25.5	26.0	6.6	59.4	17.7
Not employed	51.0	23.1	58.7	27.5	19.3	7.2	46.0	16.7
U.S. census region								
New England	52.2	20.3	53.2	21.4	35.6	5.0	47.6	14.9
Middle Atlantic	47.4	18.4	52.4	21.8	30.6	9.7	41.4	10.8
East North Central	47.6	18.1	53.2	20.7	21.0	7.2	46.2	12.6
West North Central	55.9	19.9	58.2	20.7	27.7	7.9	50.8	22.8
South Atlantic	43.8	14.8	53.8	18.7	19.6	5.7	48.0	13.8
East South Central	37.9	12.4	45.1	15.0	14.2	3.7	23.5	5.0
West South Central	46.0	14.7	56.2	18.4	14.5	3.8	39.2	11.4
Mountain	70.2	30.4	74.9	33.0	31.5	11.0	53.9	18.2
Pacific	70.3	28.7	76.7	33.4	43.9	15.0	58.5	19.7

[a]Mothers were surveyed when their infants were 6 months of age. They were asked to recall the method of feeding the infant when in the hospital, at age 1 week, at months 1 through 5, and on the day preceding completion of the survey. Numbers in the columns labeled "5–6 mo Infants" are an average of the 5-month and previous day responses.

[b]From A. Ryan, Ross Laboratories, personal communication, 1990.

[c]Hispanic is not exclusive of white or black.

[d]College includes all women who reported completing at least 1 year of college.

34

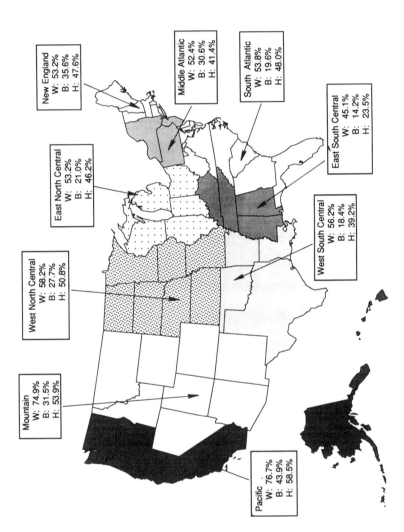

New England
W: 53.2%
B: 35.6%
H: 47.6%

Middle Atlantic
W: 52.4%
B: 30.6%
H: 41.4%

South Atlantic
W: 53.8%
B: 19.6%
H: 48.0%

East South Central
W: 45.1%
B: 14.2%
H: 23.5%

East North Central
W: 53.2%
B: 21.0%
H: 46.2%

West South Central
W: 56.2%
B: 18.4%
H: 39.2%

West North Central
W: 58.2%
B: 27.7%
H: 50.8%

Mountain
W: 74.9%
B: 31.5%
H: 53.9%

Pacific
W: 76.7%
B: 43.9%
H: 58.5%

FIGURE 3-2   Breastfeeding initiation rates, by census region and ethnic background (W, white; B, black; H, Hispanic). Data from the 1989 Ross Mothers Survey (A. Ryan, Ross Laboratories, personal communication, 1990).

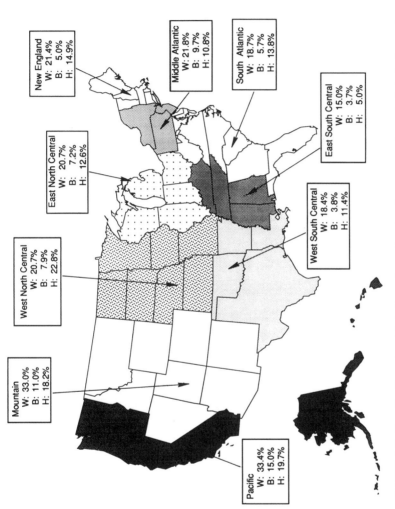

New England
W: 21.4%
B: 5.0%
H: 14.9%

Middle Atlantic
W: 21.8%
B: 9.7%
H: 10.8%

South Atlantic
W: 18.7%
B: 5.7%
H: 13.8%

East South Central
W: 15.0%
B: 3.7%
H: 5.0%

East North Central
W: 20.7%
B: 7.2%
H: 12.6%

West South Central
W: 18.4%
B: 3.8%
H: 11.4%

West North Central
W: 20.7%
B: 7.9%
H: 22.8%

Mountain
W: 33.0%
B: 11.0%
H: 18.2%

Pacific
W: 33.4%
B: 15.0%
H: 19.7%

FIGURE 3-3   Breastfeeding rates at 5 to 6 months post partum, by census region and ethnic background (W, white; B, black; H, Hispanic). Data from the 1989 Ross Mothers Survey (A. Ryan, Ross Laboratories, personal communication, 1990).

TABLE 3-3 Percentage of Mothers Breastfeeding Newborn Infants in the
Hospital and at 5 or 6 Months of Age in 1989,[a] by Participation in the
Special Supplemental Food Program for Women, Infants, and Children
(WIC) and Selected Demographic Variables[b]

Category	WIC[c] Newborns	5–6 mo Infants	Non-WIC Newborns	5–6 mo Infants
All mothers	34.2	9.2	62.9	25.7
Ethnic group				
White	41.3	11.2	65.0	27.1
Black	17.9	4.8	36.7	12.3
Hispanic	39.1	10.7	58.9	19.8
Maternal age				
<20 yr	26.2	4.2	40.8	10.9
20–24 yr	34.2	8.0	55.8	16.9
25–29 yr	40.3	13.3	64.8	25.9
30–34 yr	42.3	18.1	70.2	34.0
≥35 yr	42.5	19.2	71.5	39.6
Maternal education				
No college	31.1	7.8	52.5	18.4
College	50.7	16.5	74.6	33.9

[a]See footnote a of Table 3-2.
[b]From A. Ryan, Ross Laboratories, personal communication, 1990.
[c]Includes all mothers who reported that either they or their infant had participated in the
WIC program since the birth of that infant.

and 9% continue the practice for at least 5 or 6 months (Table 3-3). The
demographic patterns observed in this group are the same as those in the
general population: higher rates of breastfeeding are reported for white women,
older women, and those with some college education. Except for the Ross
Laboratories data, there are only sparse data on breastfeeding rates among the
national WIC population. A comparison of WIC and non-WIC respondents in
the Ross Laboratories surveys shows consistently lower rates of breastfeeding
among WIC mothers. However, these differences are likely due to differences
in income and other sociodemographic variables. Rush et al. (1988) found no
difference between WIC and non-WIC women in the rates of breastfeeding
when women with similar levels of socioeconomic status were compared.

Limitations of the Data

There are no data on the total length of breastfeeding (actual duration)
and the ages at which other milk or foods are added to the infant's diet. For
example, it is not known how much longer the 20% of women in the Ross
Laboratories survey still breastfeeding their 5- to 6-month old infants will

continue breastfeeding. Neither is it known how many of the breastfed infants are exclusively breastfed and how many are partially breastfed. The lack of these data makes it difficult to calculate the amounts of nutrients delivered to the infant in human milk as well as the nutritional cost of milk synthesis to the mother. The increased incidence of breastfeeding from 1969 to 1980 (Forman et al., 1985) appears to be accounted for primarily by women who chose exclusive breastfeeding (and not partial breastfeeding) over bottle feeding. Thus, the total amount of nutrients delivered in human milk to the infant would have been different on average for lactating women in 1969 and 1980.

At present, data are inadequate for documenting breastfeeding rates among several subgroups of the U.S. population of particular interest to health care providers. These include Hispanics, Southeast Asians, and working mothers.

Hispanic Mothers

There are no nationwide data on recent trends in breastfeeding incidence and duration among Hispanic women because, until recently, the percentage of Hispanic women in nationwide surveys has been too small for analysis. For example, Ross Laboratories first published data on Hispanic women in their 1986 survey (Ryan and Martinez, 1987). Furthermore, the Hispanic population in the United States is heterogeneous; it includes people who trace their origin or descent from Cuba, Puerto Rico, Mexico, other Latin American countries, and Spain. The incidence of breastfeeding in this population has been reported in different studies to range from 10 to 60% (Bryant, 1982; Dungy, 1989; John and Martorell, 1989; Kokinos and Dewey, 1986; Rassin et al., 1984; Romero-Gwynn and Carias, 1989; Samuels et al., 1985; Scrimshaw et al., 1987; Seger et al., 1979; Smith et al., 1982; Young and Kaufman, 1988). These large differences may reflect the ethnic heterogeneity, the area of the United States in which the women now reside, time since migration to the United States, or research design differences in the surveys.

Perhaps the best data for Hispanic women exist for Mexican-American mothers. John and Martorell (1989) analyzed data from the Mexican-American component of the Hispanic Health and Nutrition Examination Survey conducted between 1982 and 1984. The investigators noted a substantial recent increase in breastfeeding incidence—from 30.7% in 1970 to 1974, to 38.1% in 1975 to 1978, and to 47.6% in 1979 to 1982. When all years in which births were reported were combined, breastfeeding incidence was higher for those with higher annual household incomes, advanced maternal age, infants with birth weights greater than 2.5 kg, and a choice of Spanish as the interview language. Education of the household head has a curvilinear relationship to breastfeeding incidence: incidence is highest among those with more than 12 years of education, lowest for those with 9 to 12 years, and intermediate for those with less than 9 years.

Southeast Asian Mothers

With the influx of Southeast Asian immigrants into the United States, there has been increasing concern about their nutrition and their infant-feeding practices. Although the number of Southeast Asian mothers has been too small to produce definitive data in national surveys, the experience of health care professionals in areas where these mothers are highly concentrated indicates that (1) the incidence of breastfeeding has dropped in the years since the first Southeast Asian immigrants arrived and (2) rates are now lower for Southeast Asians than they are for other minority groups in the same geographic areas of the country (Fishman et al., 1988; Romero-Gwynn, 1989). Although this may reflect in part the changing composition of the Southeast Asian population in the United States over time, virtually all mothers in these studies reported breastfeeding their children born in Southeast Asia. This suggests that the apparent decline in breastfeeding is real.

Employed Mothers

There are no statistics that adequately compare the incidence and duration of breastfeeding by mothers who work outside the home and those who do not. Ryan and Martinez (1989) attempted to make this comparison by using the Ross Laboratories data for 1987, but their analysis provides only limited information about the infant-feeding practices of women in the labor force (see Table 3-4). In that study, mothers were classified as "employed full time" or "not working" based on their response to a question on employment status when their infants were 6 months of age. Mothers working part time were excluded. The investigators determined the rates of breastfeeding for these two groups both when their infants were newborns (in the hospital) and when they were 6 months old. From these data, they calculated a breastfeeding continuance rate, that is, the percentage of women who initiated breastfeeding who were still breastfeeding when their infants reached 6 months of age.

Ryan and Martinez (1989) reported that identical proportions (54.5%) of women in both employment categories initiated breastfeeding. By 6 months, however, 10% of the employed mothers were still breastfeeding compared with 24.3% of those who were not working. When these data are broken down by sociodemographic variables, trends generally follow those seen in the population as a whole. As described above, women in the Mountain and Pacific regions were more likely to initiate breastfeeding than were those living in other regions, regardless of their employment status.

One intriguing finding is that at 6 months post partum, more black mothers in the "employed full time" category than in the "not working" category had initiated breastfeeding (32.7% compared with 21.2%, respectively). This contrasts with whites, who initiated breastfeeding at similar rates (58.9 and

62.3%, respectively) whether or not they would be employed outside the home at 6 months post partum.

At 6 months after delivery, sociodemographic differences were not associated with breastfeeding continuance rates among employed mothers. At this stage, employed black mothers breastfed at the same rate as white mothers; this was higher than expected for black mothers, considering their generally shorter duration of breastfeeding.

There are no data relating breastfeeding to prenatal employment or prenatal intentions to breastfeed. Ryan and Martinez (1989) did not include the 15% of mothers employed part time in their sample; many of these women may use part-time employment as a strategy to accommodate breastfeeding.

Kurinij and colleagues (1989) examined the effect of intention to return to work outside the home on breastfeeding among mothers in Washington, D.C. Among blacks, but not whites, more mothers who intended to return to work part time initiated breastfeeding than those who intended to return full time. In examining duration of breastfeeding, they found that professional women returning to work breastfed longer than women working in other occupations did, and those employed part time breastfed longer than those in full-time work did. Among white women only, the later the return to work, the longer the duration of breastfeeding. In general, they found breastfeeding duration to be shorter among blacks than whites. This finding may differ from that of Ryan and Martinez (1989) because of the high socioeconomic status of the whites studied by Kurinij and associates (1989).

DETERMINANTS OF BREASTFEEDING DISTRIBUTION

Wide variation in research designs limits the extent to which the subcommittee could separate determinants of the types of infant feeding. As was clear from the results of Ryan and Martinez (1989) for working mothers, it is difficult to attribute causation from observed associations (Simopoulos and Grave, 1984; Winikoff, 1981). Because ethnic origin is strongly associated with income and education, it is difficult to differentiate the effects of socioeconomic status from ethnic origin. Ethnographic, marketing, and other qualitative methods can be useful for eliciting mothers' own reasons for choosing breast or formula feeding. Much of this work consists of single case studies in a particular population. Thus, there is a need to validate such results.

Ethnic Groups

Black Mothers

The reason why black mothers breastfeed less often than whites is not apparent from the results of correlation studies that relate marital status, parity, and income—variables known to be associated with infant feeding in the general

TABLE 3-4 Newborn Infants Breastfed in the Hospital and at 6 Months of Age, and Breastfeeding Continuance Rate, Among Mothers Employed Full Time and Mothers Not Employed[a,b]

Variable	Newborn Infants Breastfed in the Hospital, %		Infants Breastfed in the Hospital at Age 6 mo, %		Breastfeeding Continuance Rate, %[c]	
	Mothers Employed Full Time	Mothers Not Employed	Mothers Employed Full Time	Mothers Not Employed	Mothers Employed Full Time	Mothers Not Employed
All mothers						
Maternal age						
<20 yr	54.5	54.5	10.0	24.3	18.3	44.6
20–24 yr	38.4	33.4	4.5	7.5	11.7	22.5
25–29 yr	47.9	49.6	5.8	17.7	12.1	35.7
30–34 yr	57.5	63.2	9.7	31.0	16.9	49.1
≥35 yr	61.1	68.4	14.5	39.3	23.7	57.5
	61.1	66.1	20.0	40.4	32.7	61.1
Family income						
<$7,000	34.3	31.0	5.6	8.3	16.3	26.8
$7,000–$15,000	40.5	49.4	6.4	19.2	15.8	38.9
$15,001–$25,000	49.7	62.4	8.1	29.1	16.3	46.6
>$25,000	63.1	72.9	12.5	38.2	19.8	52.4

Maternal education						
High school or less	43.8	46.0	5.7	17.7	13.0	38.5
College	67.6	75.9	15.3	41.1	22.6	54.2
Parity						
Primiparous	58.1	54.4	10.1	20.7	17.4	38.1
Multiparous	49.1	54.7	9.8	27.6	20.0	50.5
Ethnic background						
White	58.9	62.3	10.7	28.7	18.2	46.1
Black	32.7	21.2	6.0	7.6	18.3	35.8
U.S. census region						
New England	56.5	59.0	10.6	27.1	18.8	45.9
Middle Atlantic	48.5	48.3	9.5	22.0	19.6	45.5
East North Central	50.8	48.7	8.9	22.0	17.5	45.2
West North Central	57.5	58.7	8.6	25.3	15.0	43.1
South Atlantic	47.5	45.8	7.7	20.4	16.2	44.5
East South Central	39.2	38.0	7.1	15.1	18.1	39.7
West South Central	50.1	49.9	7.4	19.5	14.8	39.1
Mountain	71.3	75.5	15.5	37.2	21.7	49.3
Pacific	73.7	72.7	16.5	33.5	22.4	46.1

[a] From Ryan and Martinez (1989) with permission.
[b] Breastfeeding included supplemental bottle feeding, i.e., formula in addition to human milk.
[c] Breastfeeding continuance rate was calculated by using the following formula: (% breastfed at 6 months/% breastfed in hospital) × 100.

U.S. population—to the breastfeeding practices of blacks (Kurinij et al., 1988; Rassin et al., 1984). Ethnic background and education are highly correlated; their independent effects on breastfeeding practices are difficult to distinguish.

In a study of economically disadvantaged women delivering in Texas, Baranowski et al. (1986) found that issues of personal convenience and benefits for infants differentiated black mothers who intended to breastfeed from those who intended to bottle feed. Breastfeeders were more likely to agree that breastfeeding is best for infant health, is more nutritious, and brings mother and infant closer together. They were more likely to disagree with statements that breastfeeding ties a mother down and that bottle feeding is more convenient.

Comparing black and white mothers, Baranowski et al. (1986) found that attitudes toward issues of social convenience predicted whether or not white but not black women breastfed. In particular, white women who breastfed disagreed with statements that breastfeeding in public is embarrassing and that it would make it difficult for the mother to see friends, while white women who bottle fed agreed with them. These statements did not differentiate the black breastfeeders and bottle feeders. Bailey (1990) obtained similar results when comparing black and white WIC clients from a variety of sites in the southeastern United States. Compared with black mothers, white mothers were more likely to identify embarrassment and offending others who might observe their breastfeeding as issues in the decision of whether or not to breastfeed.

Hispanic Mothers

Most surveys exploring the determinants of breastfeeding among Hispanic mothers have linked higher breastfeeding rates to immediate postnatal factors, such as early initiation of breastfeeding, extended maternal-infant contact, and vaginal rather than cesarean delivery (Romero-Gwynn and Carias, 1989; Scrimshaw et al., 1987). Mothers born in Mexico are more likely to breastfeed than are those born in the United States, especially those with previous infants born in Mexico (Kokinos and Dewey, 1986; Romero-Gwynn and Carias, 1989). Romero-Gwynn and Carias (1989) and Scrimshaw et al. (1987) found that mothers who did not intend to work were more likely to breastfeed than were those who intended to work.

Using qualitative ethnographic strategies to study breastfeeding determinants among Hispanic mothers, Bryant (1982) found that positive attitudes of kin and friends toward breastfeeding were associated with increased initiation of breastfeeding among mothers of Cuban and Puerto Rican descent. Using qualitative market research techniques in a study in California, Weller and Dungy (1986) reported similar responses from white and Hispanic mothers asked to characterize infant feeding practices, except that Hispanic women believed that (1) anger and other emotions can be transferred to the infant through the milk and cause damage to the infant and (2) the breastfeeding baby consumes a part of the mother, thus causing the mother to age faster and deteriorate. Mothers were asked to rank the responses they used to characterize infant feeding in order of importance. When the responses were compared within groups defined by ethnic affiliation and feeding practices (white breastfeeders, white bottle feeders, Hispanic breastfeeders, and Hispanic bottle feeders), white mothers (especially breastfeeders) were very similar to each other, indicating a strongly consistent set of values attributed to breastfeeding and bottle feeding. Hispanic mothers differed far more among themselves. These findings indicate the existence of different underlying cultural patterns. Weller and Dungy (1986) suggest that the lack of a clear preference pattern in Hispanics may be characteristic of an ethnic group in transition.

Southeast Asian Mothers

Research to explain breastfeeding rates among Southeast Asian immigrants has been limited. Romero-Gwynn (1989) reported that receiving formula samples at hospital discharge was the only one of several predictors significantly associated with the decision to breastfeed or use formula. Anthropological investigation, however, shows the complexity of the issues surrounding the decision of whether or not to breastfeed (Fishman et al., 1988). Many women of Cambodian, Chinese, and Vietnamese descent subscribe to variations of a humoral ethnomedical system, derived from a philosophy of balance between such fundamental qualities of nature as hot and cold or wet and dry. Attempts to maintain or restore the body's equilibrium in these qualities often involves regulation of both maternal diet and postpartum behaviors. Foods consumed by the mother are believed to transmit particular qualities to a vulnerable breastfed infant. In the traditional context and environment of Southeast Asia, mothers reported that they frequently consumed foods that they believed could pass on harmful properties to their infants in their breast milk. However, because such foods were usually chosen and prepared by other family members, such conflicts between food beliefs and eating behavior were not considered important threats to infant well-being. With many of the elements of traditional social support absent, some immigrants to the United States exhibit a heightened sense of the importance of particular foods and their potential impact on the infant. Their dilemma is solved by feeding formula to the infant, allowing the mother the freedom to eat whatever she wishes. In addition, Southeast Asian women were reported to perceive bottle feeding as the U.S. norm and associate it with the general good health of U.S. infants (Fishman et al., 1988; Romero-Gwynn, 1989).

Employed Mothers

Few studies have been conducted to examine the effects of working outside the home on breastfeeding. On the whole, the demographic characteristics of breastfeeding mothers employed outside the home are the same as those of breastfeeding mothers in the general population. However, the overall rate of breastfeeding is lower among employed mothers and the duration is shorter.

Mothers employed outside the home face special problems when breastfeeding their infants. A survey of employed breastfeeding mothers by Auerbach and Guss (1984) shows that excessive fatigue, the logistics of pumping and storing milk, the excessive time spent traveling to and from the baby during the workday, and concern about having an adequate milk supply were common problems in this group. These problems were compounded by lack of time to complete work duties and to eat properly.

These findings are not surprising in light of a survey of policies and practices to support breastfeeding mothers in the workplace (Moore and Jansa, 1987). The survey sought responses from 100 of the most profitable Fortune 500 companies and an additional 12 companies that were known to have breastfeeding support programs. All the Fortune 500 companies responding had maternal leave policies and guaranteed a return to an equivalent job. However, only about 33% offered flex-time or part-time work, only 14% allowed breastfeeding at work, and fewer than 5% allowed job sharing or provided day care. Most of the 12 companies known to support breastfeeding allowed flex time, part-time schedules, and job sharing. However, fewer than half provided a place for mothers to breastfeed, and none provided day care or permitted mothers breaks for breastfeeding.

In another study, Barber-Madden and colleagues (1987) reviewed published research as well as policy statements of professional groups such as the American Academy of Pediatrics (AAP, 1982) and identified six types of barriers to breastfeeding for employed mothers. They include (1) lack of child care at or near the workplace, (2) work environments that do not provide a place for pumping and storing milk, (3) restrictive employer policies that fail to provide adequate maternity leave and job security, (4) social attitudes of employers and coworkers toward breastfeeding that result in disapproval and harassment, (5) inadequate maternal knowledge about breastfeeding, and (6) lack of knowledge concerning breastfeeding on the part of health professionals, especially those in occupational health. These authors suggest both short- and long-term strategies for dealing with such barriers that would require economic commitments by employers or governments as well as the development of educational materials on breastfeeding targeted specifically at the problems of employed mothers.

Adolescent Mothers

The few small studies conducted on pregnant adolescents or adolescent mothers indicate that these adolescents may not differ substantially from older mothers in their selection of infant-feeding methods. In a survey of pregnant inner-city adolescents aged 12 to 19 years, investigators found that those intending to breastfeed were likely to perceive more benefits of breastfeeding, desired more information about it, had supportive environments, had been breastfed themselves, and perceived relatively fewer barriers to breastfeeding than those who did not intend to breastfeed (Joffee and Radius, 1987; Radius and Joffee, 1988). Overall, perceived differences in benefits differentiated the potential breastfeeders from nonbreastfeeders better than did perceived barriers.

Baisch and associates (1989) found that 13- to 20-year-old low-income adolescents intending to breastfeed had more positive attitudes about breast-feeding than those who did not intend to breastfeed, especially if they had been breastfed themselves. Prenatal intentions were highly predictive of actual postnatal feeding practices.

Neifert and associates (1988b) found that among 129 breastfeeding mothers less than 18 years of age in Denver, 35% nursed for less than 1 month, 22% nursed for 1 to 2 months, and 43% nursed for 2 months or longer. The most common reason given for weaning in the first month was the "inability of the infant to grasp the maternal nipple and nurse effectively" (Neifert et al., 1988b, p. 472). These infants were said to have had this problem in the hospital and continued to have it at home. Although 75% of these teenage mothers persevered by expressing milk and feeding it to the infant in a bottle, all weaned their infants by 1 month. None of the social and demographic variables studied (mother's age, ethnic group, intended duration of breastfeeding, social support) predicted the duration of breastfeeding. In a companion study, Neifert et al. (1988a) reported that gift packs containing formula presented upon hospital discharge had no observed effect on breastfeeding duration.

These results suggest that decisions on the timing of weaning are probably highly individual; the reasons for the decisions cannot accurately be determined from surveys.

Determinants of Breastfeeding Common to Different Subgroups

Some of the determinants of breastfeeding may be specific to selected segments of the U.S. population, whereas others are common to all. For example, maternal education is a common correlate of breastfeeding initiation and duration among blacks (Kurinij et al., 1988), whites (Rassin et al., 1984), and Hispanics (John and Martorell, 1989) and among mothers employed outside the home (Kurinij et al., 1989). Maternal education is also strongly related to attitudes toward breastfeeding (e.g., Dusdieker et al., 1985). However, the reasons for these associations are not clear. Formal education may be a measure of enculturation, since it provides exposure to, and promotes adoption of, major social values.

The studies reviewed above suggest that two categories of determinants influence the selection of the infant-feeding method: *infant-feeding ideology* and *external constraints*. Infant-feeding ideology includes beliefs about the efficacy of different feeding methods and values placed on breastfeeding as compared with bottle feeding. Such ideology has idiosyncratic components based on personal experience, but it also has more general components derived from affiliation with a particular ethnic group or membership in other subcultures. External constraints include factors such as separation from the infant resulting from commitments outside the home and the demands of household and family responsibilities. Particular combinations of these constraints may be common to groups that cut across ethnic boundaries, for example, mothers working outside the home, adolescent mothers, and economically disadvantaged mothers.

CONCLUSIONS

• Rates of breastfeeding have changed markedly during the twentieth century. Incidence and duration of breastfeeding in the United States fell during the 1950s and 1960s and then rose during the 1970s. In the early 1980s, rates peaked, and they have steadily decreased since then. Among groups who recently immigrated to the United States (such as Southeast Asians and some Hispanics), breastfeeding rates are declining even more rapidly.

• Women who choose to breastfeed are not randomly distributed across the population. Such demographic variables as ethnic group affiliation, maternal age, and maternal education can largely account for variations in breastfeeding rates at the population level. However, infant-feeding practices reflect both personal and culture-specific ideologies as well as situational constraints. Thus, some breastfeeding mothers are found even among groups where breastfeeding is uncommon.

• Clinicians may need to direct special attention to women at risk of possible nutritional problems associated with sociodemographic factors. For example, some adolescent mothers may have the same inadequate dietary status or eating disorders as other members of their age cohort. Economically disadvantaged mothers may have income levels that act as barriers to optimal nutrition during breastfeeding. Members of some ethnic groups may have culturally based restrictions on maternal diet or behavior that run counter to clinical advice. The ability of clinicians to identify and accommodate such potential obstacles may help ensure lactation that is nutritionally sound for both mothers and infants.

REFERENCES

AAP (American Academy of Pediatrics). 1982. The promotion of breastfeeding: policy statement based on task force report. Pediatrics 69:654-661.
Auerbach, K.G., and E. Guss. 1984. Maternal employment and breastfeeding. Am. J. Dis. Child. 138:958-960.

Bailey, D.F.C. 1990. Cultural Models of Infant Feeding: A Comparison of Euro- and African-American Mothers in the Southeastern United States. Thesis, M.S. University of Kentucky, Lexington, Kentucky. 156 pp.

Baisch, M.J., R.A. Fox, and B.D. Goldberg. 1989. Breast-feeding attitudes and practices among adolescents. J. Adol. Health Care 10:41-45.

Baranowski, T., D.K. Rassin, C.J. Richardson, J.P. Brown, and D.E. Bee. 1986. Attitudes toward breastfeeding. Dev. Behav. Pediatr. 7:367-372.

Barber-Madden, R., M.A. Petschek, and J. Pakter. 1987. Breastfeeding and the working mother: barriers and intervention strategies. J. Public Health Policy 8:531-541.

Bryant, C.A. 1982. The impact of kin, friend and neighbor networks on infant feeding practices. Soc. Sci. Med. 16:1757-1765.

DHHS (Department of Health and Human Services). 1984. Report of the Surgeon General's Workshop on Breastfeeding & Human Lactation. DHHS Publ. No. HRS-D-MC 84-2. Health Resources and Services Administration, Public Health Service, U.S. Department of Health and Human Services, Rockville, Md. 93 pp.

Dungy, C.I. 1989. Breast feeding preference of Hispanic and Anglo women 1978-1985. Clin. Pediatr. 28:92-94.

Dusdieker, L.B., B.M. Booth, B.F. Seals, and E.E. Ekwo. 1985. Investigation of a model for the initiation of breastfeeding in primigravida women. Soc. Sci. Med. 20:695-703.

Fildes, V. 1986. Breast, Bottles and Babies: A History of Infant Feeding. University of Edinburgh Press, Edinburgh. 200 pp.

Fishman, C., R. Evans, and E. Jenks. 1988. Warm bodies, cool milk: conflicts in post partum food choice for Indochinese women in California. Soc. Sci. Med. 26:1125-1132.

Fomon, S.J. 1987. Reflections on infant feeding in the 1970s and 1980s. Am. J. Clin. Nutr. 46:171-182.

Forman, M.R., K. Fetterly, B.I. Graubard, and K.G. Wooton. 1985. Exclusive breast-feeding of newborns among married women in the United States: the National Natality Surveys of 1969 and 1980. Am. J. Clin. Nutr. 42:864-869.

Hendershot, G.E. 1980. Trends in Breast Feeding. DHEW Publ. No. 80-1250. National Center for Health Statistics, Public Health Service, U.S. Department of Health, Education, and Welfare, Hyattsville, Md. 7 pp.

Hendershot, G.E. 1981. Trends and Differentials in Breast Feeding in the United States, 1970-75. Working Paper Series No. 5. Family Growth Survey Branch, National Center for Health Statistics, Public Health Service, U.S. Department of Health and Human Services, Hyattsville, Md. 28 pp.

Hirschman, C., and G.E. Hendershot. 1979. Trends in Breast Feeding Among American Mothers. Vital and Health Statistics, Series 23, No. 3. DHEW Publ. No. (PHS) 79-1979. National Center for Health Statistics, Public Health Service, U.S. Department of Health, Education, and Welfare, Hyattsville, Md. 39 pp.

Joffe, A., and S.M. Radius. 1987. Breast versus bottle: correlates of adolescent mothers' infant-feeding practices. Pediatrics 79:689-695.

John, A.M., and R. Martorell. 1989. Incidence and duration of breast-feeding in Mexican-American infants, 1970-1982. Am. J. Clin. Nutr. 50:868-874.

Kokinos, M., and K.G. Dewey. 1986. Infant feeding practices of migrant Mexican-American families in northern California. Ecol. Food Nutr. 18:209-220.

Kurinij, N., P.H. Shiono, and G.G. Rhoads. 1988. Breast-feeding incidence and duration in black and white women. Pediatrics 81:365-371.

Kurinij, N., P.H. Shiono, S.F. Ezrine, and G.G. Rhoads. 1989. Does maternal employment affect breast-feeding? Am. J. Public Health 79:1247-1250.

Martinez, G.A., and F.W. Krieger. 1985. 1984 Milk-feeding patterns in the United States. Pediatrics 76:1004-1008.

Martinez, G.A., and J.P. Nalezienski. 1979. The recent trend in breast-feeding. Pediatrics 64:686-692.

Martinez, G.A., and J.P. Nalezienski. 1981. 1980 Update: the recent trend in breast-feeding. Pediatrics 67:260-263.

Martinez, G.A., D.A. Dodd, and J.A. Samartgedes. 1981. Milk feeding patterns in the United States during the first 12 months of life. Pediatrics 68:863-868.

Meyer, H.F. 1958. Breast feeding in the United States: extent and possible trend. A survey of 1,904 hospitals with two and a quarter million births in 1956. Pediatrics 22:116-121.

Meyer, H.F. 1968. Breast feeding in the United States: report of a 1966 national survey with comparable 1946 and 1956 data. Clin. Pediatr. 7:708-715.

Moore, J.F., and N. Jansa. 1987. A survey of policies and practices in support of breastfeeding mothers in the workplace. Birth 14:191-195.

Neifert, M., J. Gray, N. Gary, and B. Camp. 1988a. Effect of two types of hospital feeding gift packs on duration of breast-feeding among adolescent mothers. J. Adol. Health Care 9:411-413.

Neifert, M., J. Gray, N. Gary, and B. Camp. 1988b. Factors influencing breast-feeding among adolescents. J. Adol. Health Care 9:470-473.

Radius, S.M., and A. Joffe. 1988. Understanding adolescent mothers' feelings about breast-feeding: a study of perceived benefits and barriers. J. Adol. Health Care 9:156-160.

Rassin, D.K., C.J. Richardson, T. Baranowski, P.R. Nader, N. Guenther, D.E. Bee, and J.P. Brown. 1984. Incidence of breast-feeding in a low socioeconomic group of mothers in the United States: ethnic patterns. Pediatrics 73:132-137.

Romero-Gwynn, E. 1989. Breast feeding pattern among Indochinese immigrants in northern California. Am. J. Dis. Child. 143:804-808.

Romero-Gwynn, E., and L. Carias. 1989. Breast-feeding intentions and practice among Hispanic mothers in southern California. Pediatrics 84:626-632.

Rosenberg, C.E. 1976. No Other Gods: On Science and American Social Thought. Johns Hopkins University Press, Baltimore, Md. 273 pp.

Rush, D., N.L. Sloan, J. Leighton, J.M. Alvir, D.G. Horvitz, W.B. Seaver, G.C. Garbowski, S.S. Johnson, R.A. Kulka, M. Holt, J.W. Devore, J.T. Lynch, M.B. Woodside, and D.S. Shanklin. 1988. The National WIC Evaluation: evaluation of the Special Supplemental Food Program for Women, Infants, and Children. V. Longitudinal study of pregnant women. Am. J. Clin. Nutr. 48:439-483.

Ryan, A.S., and G.A. Martinez. 1987. Incidencia de la lactancia materna en la población hispanoamericana de los Estados Unidos, 1986. Médico Interamericano 6:52-53, 57.

Ryan, A.S., and G.A. Martinez. 1989. Breast-feeding and the working mother: a profile. Pediatrics 83:524-531.

Salber, E.J., P.G. Stitt, and J.G. Babbott. 1958. Patterns of breast feeding. I. Factors affecting the frequency of breast feeding in the newborn period. N. Engl. J. Med. 259:707-713.

Samuels, S.E., S. Margen, and E.J. Schoen. 1985. Incidence and duration of breast-feeding in a health maintenance organization population. Am. J. Clin. Nutr. 44:504-510.

Scrimshaw, S.C.M., P.L. Engle, L. Arnold, and K. Haynes. 1987. Factors affecting breastfeeding among women of Mexican origin or descent in Los Angeles. Am. J. Public Health 77:467-470.

Seger, M.T., C.E. Gibbs, and E.A. Young. 1979. Attitudes about breast-feeding in a group of Mexican-American primigravidas. Tex. Med. 75:78-80.

Simopoulos, A.P., and G.D. Grave. 1984. Factors associated with the choice and duration of infant-feeding practice. Pediatrics 74:603-614.

Smith, J.S., C.G. Mhango, C.W. Warren, R.W. Rochat, and S.L. Huffman. 1982. Trends in the incidence of breastfeeding for Hispanics of Mexican origin and Anglos on the US-Mexico border. Am. J. Public Health 72:59-61.

Starr, P. 1982. The Social Transformation of American Medicine. Basic Books, New York. 514 pp.

Weller, S.C., and C.I. Dungy. 1986. Personal preferences and ethnic variations among Anglo and Hispanic breast and bottle feeders. Soc. Sci. Med. 23:539-548.

Winikoff, B. 1981. Issues in the design of breastfeeding research. Stud. Fam. Plann. 12:177-184.

Young, S.A., and M. Kaufman. 1988. Promoting breastfeeding at a migrant health center. Am. J. Public Health 78:523-525.

4
Nutritional Status and Usual Dietary Intake of Lactating Women

As a first step in the process of describing the nutritional status of lactating women in the United States, the subcommittee evaluated the methods used to assess the nutritional status of lactating women as well as anthropometric and biochemical data from apparently well-nourished lactating women. It also conducted a detailed review of the information on dietary intake by lactating women in the United States. The lack of nationally representative data on dietary intake and laboratory values of lactating women presented a substantial barrier to this effort.

Few lactating women have been included in the nutrition monitoring activities conducted by the U.S. Departments of Agriculture (USDA) and Health and Human Services (LSRO, 1989) (for example, only 59 of 2,910 women in the Continuing Survey of Food Intake by Individuals, core sample, wave 1, were lactating) (S. Krebs-Smith, USDA, Human Nutrition Information Service, personal communication, 1988). Thus, the lack of general knowledge about nutritional status in this population group is destined to continue for some time unless action is taken to obtain more data on this subject.

ASSESSMENT OF THE NUTRITIONAL STATUS OF LACTATING WOMEN

The subcommittee briefly reviewed the general reasons for assessing nutritional status, as well as the tools for doing so, and their suitability for application to lactating women. It also identified purposes for which new tools may be necessary and provided guidance on interim strategies for the assessment of nutritional status among lactating women. These are all discussed below along with a summary of the normative data that are available on the nutritional status of well-nourished lactating women.

Reasons for Assessing Nutritional Status Among Lactating Women

In general, assessments of the nutritional status of lactating women and other groups have many applications—in research, in patient management, in public policy development, and in program planning and evaluation. The selection of the indicator of nutritional status to be used should consider its intended application (Habicht and Pelletier, 1990).

To date, there have been few efforts to develop indicators specifically for the assessment of nutritional status among lactating women (Rasmussen and Habicht, 1989). Most indicators are *normative*; that is, they reveal how an individual's value for that indicator compares to some standard, usually derived from a population of normal, healthy subjects. Values outside a range defined by designated cutoff points are called abnormal, but may or may not be associated with any particular functional consequence. An example of a normative indicator is the comparison of weight for height or blood nutrient values to a reference standard. As discussed further below, no standards for anthropometric or biochemical indicators have been established for nutritional status among lactating women. The usefulness of values obtained from nonpregnant, nonlactating women as a reference standard for lactating women requires evaluation.

There are few indicators of *risk* of undesirable outcomes for lactating women. Instead, the risk is usually related to the health of the nursing infant. An example of such an indicator is an abnormally low concentration of riboflavin in milk, which is associated with the likelihood of nutritional deficiency in the nursing infant (Bates et al., 1982). Another is the classic association of low thiamin concentrations in the milk of mothers in a rice-eating population with a high incidence of infantile beriberi among breastfed babies (Kinney and Follis, 1958). In contrast, indicators of poor nutritional status with respect to certain micronutrients (e.g., iron) are well understood in lactating women and can be used for the targeting of nutrient-specific interventions.

Indicators of *benefit* (ways to identify lactating women who would benefit from a planned intervention) have yet to be developed. These would be the most useful indicators for targeting interventions. The theoretical work needed to develop indicators of benefit from interventions designed to ameliorate protein-energy malnutrition has been started in studies of young children (Rothe, 1988). It is clear from a supplementation trial conducted in The Gambia (Prentice et al., 1983; see Chapter 5) that the indicators of poor nutritional status used (residence in a low-income community characterized by seasonal decreases in milk volume or low weight for height) are inadequate for predicting who will benefit (at least in terms of increased milk volume) from a program of general nutritional supplementation.

Use of Biochemical Indicators

The few investigations in which biochemical measures have been used to assess the nutritional status of lactating women have used values for nonpregnant, nonlactating women as reference standards. This approach makes the assumption that the interpretation of levels of vitamins, minerals, hormones, and metabolites is unaffected by lactation. For this to be true, plasma volume in lactating women must be the same as that in nonlactating women and remain stable over the course of lactation. These ideas about plasma volume are difficult to evaluate with the currently available data. Unfortunately, few researchers have investigated changes in plasma volume post partum (Brown et al., 1947; Caton et al., 1951; Taylor and Lind, 1979), and it is impossible to tell whether the subjects in those studies were lactating. The results of those studies suggest that even in nonlactating women, plasma volume remains elevated for weeks to a few months after delivery. The only study that compared the plasma volume of lactating and nonlactating women post partum (Donovan et al., 1965) confirmed the decrease in plasma volume from 3 days to 6 weeks after delivery and established that the magnitude of these decreases was the same in both groups. At 6 weeks post partum, values for the lactating women (53.6 ml/kg of body weight) as well as the nonlactating women (50.1 ml/kg) remained above those reported earlier by the same authors (Donovan et al., 1964) for nonpregnant, nonlactating subjects (46.1 ml/kg). Plasma volume values were higher at both times in the lactating subjects, but this difference was not statistically significant.

Changes in plasma volume during lactation have also been reported for various other species. In cows (Reynolds, 1953), sows (Anderson et al., 1970), rabbits (Tarvydas et al., 1968), and rats (Bond, 1958), plasma volume is greater in lactating than in nonlactating animals.

The findings concerning plasma volume in lactating women and animals make it clear that plasma volume does not return rapidly to prepregnancy values. Thus, for this reason alone, it is probably inappropriate to assess the nutritional status of lactating women by comparing plasma nutrient values with reference values for a nonpregnant women, especially in the early postpartum period.

The assumption that blood values of vitamins, minerals, hormones, and metabolites are unaffected by lactation is known not to be correct. For example, insulin and glucose levels in lactating women respond quite differently to a test meal than they do in the same women after cessation of lactation (Illingworth et al., 1986). Protein metabolism also appears to change during lactation (Motil et al., 1989, 1990). Nitrogen balance among lactating women is lower than that among nonlactating postpartum and nulliparous women studied at similar levels of nitrogen intake. Differences in nitrogen balance are not accounted for by nitrogen losses in milk; urinary 3-methyl histidine excretion (a measure of muscle protein breakdown) also is lower in lactating women. Some changes in blood concentrations of vitamins and minerals over the course of lactation are unrelated to changes in plasma volume. For example, serum zinc concentration increases while serum copper decreases between weeks 1 to 2 and 19 to 21 of lactation (van der Elst et al., 1986).

In summary, evidence suggests that, in principle, it is likely to be inappropriate to compare blood values of various nutrients or metabolites of lactating women with reference values for nonpregnant women. However, the degree to which this approach misclassifies women's nutritional status depends on the degree to which levels in lactating women differ from those of their nonpregnant, nonlactating counterparts. As will be evident from the data summarized and discussed below, too few lactating women have been studied to make a meaningful evaluation of the validity of this approach at present.

Inferences about maternal nutritional status also can be made from the nutritional status of the infant. For example, infants with evidence of vitamin B_{12} deficiency (that is, those with increased concentrations of methylmalonic acid in their urine) may have mothers with poor vitamin B_{12} status (Specker et al., 1988). The reverse is not necessarily true, however. For example, the nutritional status of breastfed infants of mothers with inadequate folacin (Salmenperä et al., 1986) or vitamin C (Salmenperä, 1984) status may remain optimal. This issue is discussed further in Chapter 7.

Uses of Anthropometric Indicators

Tables developed by the Metropolitan Life Insurance Company have generally been used as normative standards for weight, height, and weight for height (MLI, 1959, 1983). For women in the United States, values derived from recent data from the National Center for Health Statistics (NCHS) (NRC, 1989) also could be used. There are drawbacks for both sets of values for studies of lactating women (Rasmussen, 1988). The use of such normative standards is fraught with all the problems discussed in Chapter 4 of *Nutrition During Pregnancy, Part I: Weight Gain* (IOM, 1990) as they relate to pregnant women. In particular, it is difficult to obtain accurate measurements without extensive training and monitoring, and comparison of a woman's values with either of these standards does not provide the information needed to make inferences about either the risk of adverse outcomes or the potential benefit from a nutritional intervention for the mother or the infant.

Many anthropometric indicators of nutritional status change continuously during lactation (Butte et al., 1984) and, even at 6 months post partum, may still differ from prepregnancy values (Sadurskis et al., 1988). The rate at which a woman (lactating or not) returns to her prepregnancy weight after delivery is affected by many factors. These include edema during pregnancy and the route of delivery (Dennis and Bytheway, 1965); prepregnancy weight, postpartum weight, parity, and maternal age (Brewer et al., 1989); and weight gained during pregnancy (Greene et al., 1988).

There is a need for research to develop indicators of nutritional status, analogous to those for weight gain during pregnancy, that make use of either the pattern or the total magnitude of the changes. Further research is also needed to investigate the use of other anthropometric indicators (e.g., various skinfold thicknesses or circumference measurements) for assessing the nutritional status of lactating women. Other approaches (e.g., bioelectrical impedance or isotope dilution [Wong et al., 1989]) for the evaluation of changes in body composition also merit study in lactating women.

Biochemical and Anthropometric Data from Well-Nourished Lactating Women

Biochemical Measures of Nutritional Status

Table 4-1 provides the biochemical measures of nutritional status from the few studies that have been conducted in lactating women and compares them with values for nonpregnant, nonlactating women. Also included are compiled values from presumably well-nourished lactating women living in industrialized countries. It is evident from Table 4-1 that data on a variety of biochemical measures of nutritional status have been collected for lactating women, but that the sample sizes range from only 3 to 36. Where comparison was possible, there was remarkably little difference between values for lactating women and those for nonpregnant, nonlactating women.

Blood Lipids

The blood lipid profiles of lactating women at 6 weeks post partum have been compared with those of parturient women who were not lactating (Knopp et al., 1985). The lactating women maintained lower total triglyceride and higher total cholesterol values than those in the nonlactating group. There also were statistically significant differences between the two groups in values for various lipoprotein lipids and apoproteins (Table 4-2). In contrast, both plasma cholesterol and triglyceride concentrations were higher at 8 weeks post partum than they were before conception among 14 lactating Swedish women (Fåhraeus et al., 1985). These studies suggest that lactation causes changes in lipoprotein metabolism.

Change in Body Weight During Lactation

Table 4-3 provides anthropometric measurements of nutritional status for lactating women and for nonpregnant, nonlactating women in the United States.

TABLE 4-1 Biochemical Measures of Nutritional Status for Healthy Nonpregnant, Nonlactating Women and for Adults Not Receiving Supplements of the Nutrient Studied

Measure of Nutritional Status	Nonpregnant, Nonlactating Adults Mean or Range[a]	Reference	Lactating Women Mean Value	Number of Subjects	Duration of Lactation	Reference
Macrominerals						
Serum calcium, total (mg/dl)	8.8–10.0	Young, 1987	8.60 ± 0.17 SEM[b]	18	3 wk	Greer et al., 1982
	8.4–10.2	Tietz, 1986	9.59 ± 0.17 SEM	14	26 wk	Greer et al., 1982
Serum magnesium (mg/dl)	1.8–3.0	Young, 1987	1.95 ± 0.06 SEM	18	3 wk	Greer et al., 1982
	1.3–2.1[c]	Tietz, 1986	2.15 ± 0.07 SEM	14	26 wk	Greer et al., 1982
Trace elements						
Plasma selenium (µg/liter)	NA[d,e]	Levander, 1988	136 ± 5 SEM	21	1 mo	Levander et al., 1987
			137 ± 5 SEM	22	3 mo	
			138 ± 5 SEM	22	6 mo	
			97 ± 6 SEM	10	4, 8 wk	Mannan and Picciano, 1987
RBC[f] selenium (ng/g of hemoglobin)	NA[e]		470 ± 33 SEM	20	1 mo	Levander et al., 1987
			450 ± 33 SEM	21	3 mo	
			501 ± 31 SEM	23	6 mo	
			173 ± 6.4 SEM	10	4, 8 wk	Mannan and Picciano, 1987
Plasma zinc (µg/dl)	88–123	NRC, 1978	79.1 ± 1.7 SEM	23	1 mo	Moser and Reynolds, 1983
	65–140	Solomons, 1988	87.6 ± 2.2 SEM	21	3 mo	
			84.4 ± 2.4 SEM	19	6 mo	Krebs et al., 1985
			70 ± 11 SD[g]	29	1 mo	
			79 ± 10 SD	27	4 mo	
Serum zinc (µg/dl)	75–120	Young, 1987	73 ± 4.8 SD	10	5–75 days	Moore et al., 1984
	70–150	Tietz, 1986				
RBC zinc (µg/g)	NA		12.9 ± 0.2 SEM	23	1 mo	Moser and Reynolds, 1983
			12.0 ± 0.2 SEM	21	3 mo	
			10.7 ± 0.4 SEM	19	6 mo	

Table 4-1 continues

TABLE 4-1—Continued

Measure of Nutritional Status	Nonpregnant, Nonlactating Adults		Lactating Women			
	Mean or Range[a]	Reference	Mean Value	Number of Subjects	Duration of Lactation	Reference
Water-soluble vitamins						
Erythrocyte transketolase activity coefficient	NA		1.07 ± 0.07 SD	10	5–10 wk	Dostálová, 1984
Urinary thiamin (mg/day)	NA		0.90 ± 0.46 SD	6	6 mo	Thomas et al., 1980
Erythrocyte glutathione reductase activity coefficient	NA		1.05 ± 0.14 SD	10	5–10 wk	Dostálová, 1984
Urinary riboflavin (mg/day)	NA		0.44 ± 0.23 SD	6	6 mo	Thomas et al., 1980
Erythrocyte oxaloacetate transaminase activity coefficient	1.69	NRC, 1978	1.75 ± 0.16 SD	10	5–10 wk	Dostálová, 1984
Plasma vitamin B_6 (ng/ml)	3.6–18	Tietz, 1986	4.9 ± 2.4 SD	11	5–10 wk	Dostálová, 1984
	5–23	McCormick, 1988	8.4 ± 3.2 SD	NR	2 mo	Andon et al., 1989
Erythrocyte glutamic pyruvic transaminase activity coefficient	1.19[h]	NRC, 1978	1.17 ± 0.19 SD	6	6 mo	Thomas et al., 1980
Serum folate (ng/ml)	4.7–8.2	NRC, 1978	13.0 ± 3.13 SD	6	6 mo	Thomas et al., 1980
	1.8–9	Tietz, 1986	3.8 ± 0.5 SEM	30	1 mo	Ek, 1983
	5–16	Herbert and Colman, 1988	4.1 ± 0.3 SEM	29	3 mo	
			4.3 ± 0.3 SEM	46	6 mo	
			4.8 ± 0.3 SEM	42	9 mo	
			4.6 ± 0.2 SEM	45	12 mo	
			8.6 ± 4.5^{i}	8	5–10 wk	Dostálová, 1984

	Range[a]		Value	n	Time	Reference
RBC folate (ng/ml)	165–250	NRC, 1978	124.4 ± 11.3 SEM[b]	39	1 mo	Ek, 1983
			128.5 ± 8.0 SEM	35	3 mo	
			130.1 ± 8.1 SEM	46	6 mo	
			136.3 ± 8.6 SEM	42	9 mo	
			136.3 ± 8.6 SEM	45	12 mo	
Serum vitamin B$_{12}$ (pg/ml)	458–498	NRC, 1978	692 ± 30 SD	6	6 mo	Thomas et al., 1980
	100–700	Tietz, 1986	565 ± 184 SEM	8	5–10 wk	Dostálová, 1984
Plasma vitamin C (mg/dl)	0.87	NRC, 1978	0.55 ± 0.32 SD	6	6 mo	Thomas et al., 1980
	0.6–2.0	Tietz, 1986	0.68 ± 0.27 SD	7	5–10 wk	Dostálová, 1984
Biotin (ng/liter)	NA		358 ± 64 SD	6	5–10 wk	Dostálová, 1984
Fat-soluble vitamins						
β-Carotene (μg/liter)	600–2,000	Tietz, 1986	516 ± 203 SD	11	5–10 wk	Dostálová, 1984
Vitamin A (μg retinol/ liter)	550	NRC, 1978	546 ± 107 SD	11	5–10 wk	Dostálová, 1984
	300–650	Tietz, 1986	408 ± 64 SD	17	20 wk	Ala-Houhala et al., 1988
	490	Young, 1987	416 ± 56 SD	15	20 wk	
Retinol-binding protein (mg/liter)	NA		57 ± 12 SD	11	5–10 wk	Dostálová, 1984
Vitamin E (mg/liter)	8.9–12.3	NRC, 1978	11.8 ± 2.6 SD	11	5–10 wk	Dostálová, 1984
	5.0–20	Tietz, 1986				

[a] Range = Reference range from all sources except NRC, 1978; in that case it represents the range of means.
[b] SEM = Standard error of the mean.
[c] Higher in females during their menses.
[d] NA = Not readily available from standard references.
[e] No suitable clinical parameters.
[f] RBC = Red blood cells.
[g] SD = Standard deviation.
[h] Originally expressed as % stimulation.
[i] Measure of variance not reported.

TABLE 4-2 Lipoprotein Lipids and Apoproteins for Lactating and Nonlactating Women 6 Weeks Post Partum[a]

	Mean Value, mg/dl ± SD[b]	
Type of Lipoprotein	Lactating Women (N = 56)	Nonlactating Women (N = 16)
Total		
Triglycerides[c]	92 ± 71	112 ± 56
Cholesterol[c]	207 ± 31	188 ± 29
Phospholipids	227 ± 29	217 ± 32
Apoprotein B	79 ± 29	69 ± 20
Very low density lipoprotein		
Triglycerides[c]	54 ± 67	78 ± 52
Cholesterol	14 ± 14	17 ± 11
Phospholipids[c]	16 ± 17	24 ± 16
Apoprotein B	3 ± 3	4 ± 2
Low-density lipoprotein		
Triglycerides	26 ± 12	24 ± 9
Cholesterol	129 ± 31	121 ± 30
Phospholipids	70 ± 21	70 ± 26
Apoprotein B	76 ± 28	66 ± 20
High-density lipoprotein		
Triglycerides	12 ± 5	10 ± 4
Cholesterol[c]	65 ± 15	51 ± 8
Phospholipids[c]	141 ± 22	123 ± 20
Apoprotein A-I[c]	142 ± 23	126 ± 19
Apoprotein A-II[c]	34 ± 6	31 ± 3

[a]From Knoop et al. (1985) with permission.
[b]SD = Standard deviation.
[c]Significant difference ($p < .05$) between lactating and nonlactating subjects.

These measurements (like those for biochemical indicators) have been reported for very few women at any stage of lactation. Two longitudinal studies (Butte and Garza, 1986; Butte et al., 1984; Manning-Dalton and Allen, 1983) and one abstract (Heinig et al., 1990) provide the data base for examining anthropometric changes during lactation. These data reveal a consistent average rate of weight loss of 0.6 to 0.8 kg/month during the first 4 to 6 months post partum, although mean weight early in lactation differed among the groups of women studied (Figure 4-1). Heinig and colleagues (1990) followed lactating women longitudinally for 12 months and found that, on average, weight loss continued between 6 and 12 months post partum, but at a slower rate than that in the first 6 months.

Not all the lactating women studied lost weight post partum; for example,

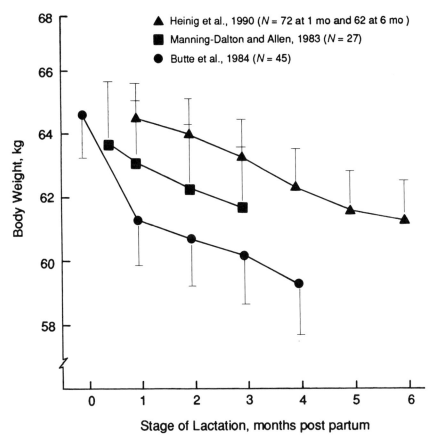

FIGURE 4-1   Change in maternal body weight during lactation. Means with standard error of the mean are illustrated.

in the study of Manning-Dalton and Allen (1983), 22% actually gained weight during breastfeeding. In an investigation of weight change in the 12 months after delivery among 1,423 Swedish women who attended maternity clinics, Öhlin and Rössner (1990) observed that lactation score (a measure of the intensity and duration of breastfeeding) was only very weakly ($R = -.09$) but significantly ($p < .01$) correlated with weight loss in this period. A stronger relationship between lactation score and weight loss was found between 2.5 and 6 months post partum. The authors concluded that "lactation has no general clinical importance for post partum weight loss for the majority of women, and cannot be practically used as a predictor for weight development after delivery" (Öhlin and Rössner, 1990, p. 172).

60

TABLE 4-3 Anthropometric Measures of Nutritional Status for Healthy Nonpregnant, Nonlactating Women and for Lactating Women in the United States

Measure of Nutritional Status	Nonpregnant, Nonlactating Women		Lactating Women			
	Mean	Reference	Mean ± SD[a]	Number of Subjects	Stage of Lactation	Reference
Overall body size						
Weight (kg)	62[b]	Frisancho, 1984	63.7 ± 10.1	27	2 wk	Manning-Dalton and Allen, 1983
			63.1 ± 10.1		4 wk	
			62.3 ± 10.3		8 wk	
			61.7 ± 9.8		12 wk[c]	
			61.3 ± 9.5	45	1 mo	Butte and Garza, 1986
			60.7 ± 10.0		2 mo	
			60.2 ± 10.4		3 mo	
			59.3 ± 10.5		4 mo	
Height (cm)	163	Najjar and Rowland, 1987	163.0 ± 6.3	45	NA	Butte and Garza, 1986
Body mass index (kg/m²)	23.1 ± 4.7 SD	Najjar and Rowland, 1987	23.0 ± 2.6	45	1 mo	Butte and Garza, 1986
			22.8 ± 2.8		2 mo	
			22.5 ± 3.0		3 mo	
			22.2 ± 3.0		4 mo	
Skinfold thickness (mm)						
Triceps	23	Frisancho, 1984	19.8 ± 6.6	27	2 wk	Manning-Dalton and Allen, 1983
			21.1 ± 6.7		12 wk[c]	
			16.9 ± 4.6	45	1 mo	Butte and Garza, 1986
			17.0 ± 4.7		2 mo	
			17.3 ± 5.3		3 mo	
			17.2 ± 5.2		4 mo	
Biceps	NA[d]		8.3 ± 5.2	27	2 wk	Manning-Dalton and Allen, 1983
			8.0 ± 4.9		12 wk[c]	
			6.9 ± 3.2	45	1 mo	Butte and Garza, 1986
			6.9 ± 3.3		2 mo	

Measurement	Reference	Value[b]	Mean ± SD[a]	n	Time	Reference
			7.3 ± 4.6		3 mo	
			6.8 ± 3.4		4 mo	
Subscapular	Frisancho, 1984	16	20.6 ± 7.4	27	2 wk	Manning-Dalton and Allen, 1983
			18.0 ± 7.2		12 wk[c]	
			16.8 ± 6.4	45	1 mo	Butte and Garza, 1986
			16.4 ± 7.4		2 mo	
			15.7 ± 7.2		3 mo	
			15.1 ± 7.3		4 mo	
Suprailiac		NA	29.4 ± 8.9	27	2 wk	Manning-Dalton and Allen, 1983
			25.3 ± 8.4		12 wk[c]	
			25.7 ± 6.9	45	1 mo	Butte and Garza, 1986
			25.2 ± 7.6		2 mo	
			23.1 ± 8.1		3 mo	
			22.2 ± 8.0		4 mo	
Umbilical		NA	25.3 ± 7.4	27	2 wk	Manning-Dalton and Allen, 1983
			21.3 ± 6.9		12 wk[c]	
Circumference (cm)						
Upper arm	Frisancho, 1981	27.7	27.4 ± 3.3	27	2 wk	Manning-Dalton and Allen, 1983
			28.1 ± 3.3		12 wk[c]	
			26.7 ± 2.6	45	1 mo	Butte et al., 1984
			26.8 ± 3.2		2 mo	
			26.6 ± 2.9		3 mo	
			26.7 ± 2.6		4 mo	
Mid-thigh		NA	52.3 ± 5.3	27	2 wk	Manning-Dalton and Allen, 1983
			52.6 ± 5.5		12 wk[c]	
Umbilical		NA	89.0 ± 8.3	27	2 wk	Manning-Dalton and Allen, 1983
			82.2 ± 9.1		12 wk[c]	

[a] SD = Standard deviation.

[b] The 50th percentile for white women with medium frames, 64-in. tall, aged 25 to 54, derived from the combined data sets from the first and second National Health and Nutrition Examination Surveys (NHANES).

[c] A total of 18% of subjects had ceased lactating at this time.

[d] NA = Nationally representative data not available.

Change in Skinfold Thickness Measurements During Lactation

In contrast to body weight, mean triceps skinfold thickness remained the same or increased only slightly in the U.S. women studied during lactation (Butte et al., 1984; Heinig et al., 1990; Manning-Dalton and Allen, 1983) (Table 4-3 and Figure 4-2) but was reported to increase dramatically in recent studies of Australian (Dugdale and Eaton-Evans, 1989) and Swedish (Forsum et al., 1989) women. The reason for this increase in triceps skinfold thickness while body weight is decreasing is not known. In Australian women, the increase was transient; it was greatest at 4 to 5 months post partum and decreased toward the 1-month post partum value thereafter. In Swedish women, the maximum had not been reached by 6 months post partum. This was not true for the other skinfold thicknesses examined in U.S. women; biceps, subscapular, and suprailiac skinfold thicknesses all decreased during the first 4 months post partum (see Figure 4-2). The relationship between the anthropometric changes that occur during lactation and long-term maternal health is discussed in Chapter 8.

USUAL DIETARY INTAKE DURING LACTATION

It is important to determine the usual dietary intake of lactating women because it is a major determinant of nutritional status and because most inter- ventions designed to improve nutritional status try to improve dietary intake. The subcommittee reviewed the nationwide data on dietary intake among lac- tating women in the United States as well as data on dietary intake among less representative groups of lactating women. Its goal was to establish a firm basis for developing recommendations about future collection of dietary intake data on lactating women.

Several limitations were considered. First, dietary intake is but one of a number of determinants of nutritional status during lactation. Second, estimates of dietary intake in all free-living subjects are difficult and, depending on the method used, may be quite imprecise. Increasing either the number of records per subject or the number of subjects may improve the accuracy of the estimate. However, the studies found by the subcommittee had small sample sizes, and most of the studies were based on single 24-hour recalls or, at most, 7-day dietary records. Third, dietary intake estimates are only as accurate as the food composition data used. For nutrients such as folate, vitamin B_6, and many trace elements, such data have often been unavailable or inaccurate. Thus, the subcommittee focused on identifying *patterns* of dietary intakes in groups of lactating women.

As is the case during pregnancy, one cannot assume a priori that dietary intake remains static during lactation. In fact, there are good reasons to assume that dietary intake changes because of various cultural beliefs, advice from

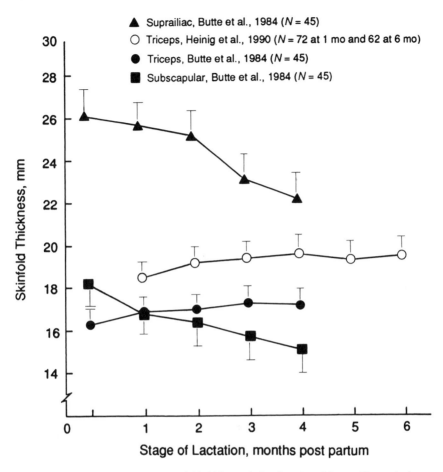

FIGURE 4-2   Change in maternal skinfold thickness during lactation. Means with standard error of the mean are illustrated.

health care providers or others, and changing energy requirements and appetite (related in part to changing needs of the infant and changes in activity patterns). Very few investigators have tried to examine the stability of dietary intake during lactation, and most such studies have lacked the statistical power to distinguish among intakes at various stages.

The extent of lactation (whether the infant is breastfed exclusively, most of the time, or only once or twice a day) may have a greater impact on dietary intake than the stage of lactation does. For example, at 4 months post partum, an exclusively breastfeeding woman has much greater energy and nutrient needs than a woman at the same stage of lactation who is only partially breastfeeding. Except for those studies expressly limited to exclusively breastfeeding women, most investigators have neither commented upon nor adjusted for differences among their subjects in the extent of breastfeeding.

Current Recommendations for Dietary Intake Among Lactating Women

Lactating women in the United States receive nutritional advice from a variety of sources. The Recommended Dietary Allowances (RDAs) may reach women through their health care providers or through publications in the lay press. Other kinds of nutritional advice may also come from the lay press, organizations interested in promoting successful breastfeeding, or from friends and family members. Although all these sources of information may have an impact on the food intake by individual women, the subcommittee chose to focus on the RDAs.

The RDAs "are the levels of intake of essential nutrients that . . . are . . . adequate to meet the known nutrient needs of practically all healthy persons" (NRC, 1989, p. 10). For some nutrients, they are based partially on body size; the reference weights used in the 1989 edition are the medians for the U.S. population of the designated age and sex. The RDAs are to be achieved over time—"at least 3 days for nutrients that turn over rapidly" (NRC, 1989, p. 22) and longer for nutrients that turn over more slowly. Separate allowances have been established for the first and second 6 months of lactation, reflecting differences in the amount of milk produced (estimated to average 750 and 600 ml, respectively) (see Table 4-4).

Extent to Which Lactating Women in the United States Meet Current Recommendations

Data from Nationally Representative Samples

Only one study of food and nutrient intake has provided data on a nationally representative sample of lactating women in the United States (Krebs-Smith and Clark, 1989). Data from the basic survey portion of USDA's 1977-1978 Nationwide Food Consumption Survey were used to validate a nutrient adequacy score for women and children. Three days of food intake information (a 24-hour recall and a 2-day food record) were obtained in four seasons from a stratified area probability sample of households in the 48 conterminous states and the District of Columbia. All 85 lactating women in the Nationwide Food Consumption Survey sample were included in this analysis; the stage of lactation of these women was not reported. Using the 1980 RDAs (NRC, 1980), the authors calculated a dietary score as well as nutrient adequacy ratios[1] for

---

[1]Nutrient adequacy ratio (NAR) = (a subject's average daily intake of a nutrient)/ (age- and sex-specific RDA for that nutrient). Nutrients included were iron; magnesium; phosphorus; thiamin; riboflavin; and vitamins B_6, B_{12}, A, and C.

selected nutrients and then used these to calculate two mean adequacy ratios,[2] one for overall nutrient adequacy and the other to represent what the authors called "problem nutrients" (calcium, iron, magnesium, and vitamins A and C). Only 19% of the lactating women had both high nutrient adequacy ratios and high mean adequacy ratios.

Data from Nonrepresentative Samples

The subcommittee identified relatively recent studies (published since 1976) that presented dietary intake data on intakes of nutrients for which there is an RDA by lactating women in the United States. The characteristics of the study groups are summarized in Table 4-4, and the observed dietary intake values are summarized in Tables 4-5 and 4-6. Energy and nutrients commonly included in tables of food composition are presented in Table 4-5. All but one of the studies covered in Table 4-5 reported intake of energy and protein in addition to that of micronutrients. In most cases, studies reported in Table 4-6 were more limited in their overall assessment of nutrient intake. The values shown in Table 4-6 represent the intake of nutrients obtained from food sources only; in many cases, these are underestimates of total nutrient intake, because many of the women were ingesting various kinds of nutrient supplements. Dietary intake usually was quantified through food records kept by the subjects for 2 to 7 days.

The subcommittee's compilation shows that a disappointingly small number (only 361) of presumably well-nourished lactating women have been studied, and nearly all of them were well-educated Caucasians. Furthermore, there has been no consistency across studies in the stages of lactation at which the women were studied, and very few investigators collected longitudinal data on dietary intake. The longitudinal data reported are generally limited to the first few months of lactation. In no studies were dietary intake values from the same women compared during the first and second 6 months of lactation.

The mean values reported for intake of all nutrients shown in Table 4-5 were at least 80% of the 1989 RDAs and, in many cases, substantially exceeded these RDAs. However, there was considerable variability of nutrient intake within studies: most standard deviations ranged from one-half of the mean to more than the mean value, indicating large differences in intake among the women. The relatively high mean reported intakes of most of these nutrients were achieved despite fairly low reported energy intakes: at their highest (early in lactation), they were about 86% of the RDA. In general, "presumably well-nourished" women in these studies do, on average, appear to be receiving adequate intakes of the nutrients shown in Table 4-5. The high degree of

---

[2]Mean adequacy ratio (MAR) = (sum of NARs for selected nutrients)/(number of nutrients being assessed).

66

TABLE 4-4 Studies of Dietary Intake Among Lactating Women in the United States

Population Group and Reference	Characteristics of Group Studied	Number of Subjects	Stage of Lactation	Dietary Intake Method
Well-nourished, adult women				
Blackburn and Calloway, 1976	Mature women, mixed ethnic backgrounds, average socioeconomic status	12	8–12 wk	3-day record
Sims, 1978	Mean age, 28 yr; 97% white; mean duration of education, 15.5 yr	61	1–26 mo	3-day record by mail survey
Thomas and Kawamoto, 1979	Healthy women	17	4–7 days and 42–45 days	Initial 24-h recall, 3-day record
Thomas et al., 1980	Permission obtained from their physician; no routine medication or recent use of oral contraceptives; no need for vitamin supplements	12	6 mo	4-day record
Manning-Dalton and Allen, 1983	Age 23 to 27 yr, white, middle income, well educated	27	2–12 wk	24-h recall at each of five interviews
Stuff et al., 1983	All married, Caucasian, non-Hispanic, nonsmoking, on no medications, healthy by history	40	3 wk–6 mo	7-day record
Levander, et al., 1987; Moser and Reynolds, 1983; Reynolds et al., 1984	Healthy, upper middle class	23	1 mo, 3 mo, 6 mo	Duplicate plate food and drink composites, 3-day record

Reference	Subjects	No.	Duration	Method
Butte et al., 1984	Mean age, 28 yr; 91% Caucasian; mean duration of education, 15.4 yr	45	1–4 mo	Four 3-day records
Song et al., 1985	Age, 20 to 35 yr; all Caucasian	26	2 wk and 3 mo	2-day record (checked with 24- and 48-h recalls)
Strode et al., 1986	Mean age, 30 yr	14	6–24 wk	Two 7-day records (1 wk apart)
Teenagers				
Lipsman et al., 1985	Age, 14 to 20 yr; mixed ethnic backgrounds; 56% WIC[a] participants; 72% receiving AFDC[b]	25	1–6 mo	24-h recall, one to nine recalls per subject
Vegetarians				
Finley et al., 1985	Mean age, 29 yr; 60% college graduates	29 (those who consumed no meat or poultry)	2–18 mo	24-h recall and 2-day record; food frequency questionnaire administered twice
American Indian				
Butte et al., 1981	Navajos on reservation; mean age, 22.4 yr; mean duration of education, 10.6 yr	23	1 mo	24-h recall, food habits and beliefs questionnaire
Low-income women				
Sneed et al., 1981	Recruited from WIC program; low socioeconomic status determined subjectively from home visits and personal information; age, 18 to 32 yr; no recent use of oral contraceptives	7	5–6 days and 43–45 days	4-day record

[a] WIC = Special Supplemental Food Program for Women, Infants and Children.
[b] AFDC = Aid to Families with Dependent Children.

68

TABLE 4-5 Reported Mean Daily Intake of Energy and Selected Nutrients by Lactating Women in the United States Compared with Recommended Dietary Allowances (RDAs)[a]

RDA, Population Group, and Reference	Months Post Partum	Sample Size	Mean Daily Intake									
			Energy, kcal ± SD[b]	Protein, g ± SD	Calcium, mg ± SD	Phosphorus, mg ± SD	Iron, mg ± SD	Vitamin A, IU[c] ± SD	Thiamin, mg ± SD	Riboflavin, mg ± SD	Niacin, mg ± SD	Ascorbic acid, mg ± SD
RDAs												
NRC, 1989	0–6	NA[d]	2,700[e,f]	65	1,200	1,200	15	1,200[g]	1.6	1.8	20	95
	6–12	NA	2,700	62	1,200	1,200	15	1,200	1.6	1.7	20	90
Well-nourished, adult women												
Blackburn and Calloway, 1976	Mixed	12	1,800 ± 454	85 NA	NR[h]	NR	NR	NR	NR	NR	NR	NR
Sims, 1978												
Group 1[i]	Mixed	50	2,141 ± 578	94 ± 23	1,298 ± 478	NA	14.4 ± 5.5	6,837 ± 5,686	1.56 ± 0.96	2.41 ± 0.86	17.6 ± 7.7	145 ± 84
Group 2[j]	Mixed	11	2,076 ± 525	86 ± 27	1,066 ± 627	NA	12.2 ± 2.8	6,319 ± 4,389	1.55 ± 0.89	2.04 ± 1.09	16.3 ± 2.6	108 ± 45
Thomas et al., 1980[j]	6	6	NR	NR	NR	NR	NR	NR	1.49 ± 0.96	1.87 ± 0.95	NR	131 ± 88
Moser and Reynolds, 1983	1	23	1,945 ± 99[k]	78 ± 4[k]	NR	NR	NR	NR	NR	NR	NR	NR
	3	20	1,919 ± 110[k]	86 ± 5[k]	NR	NR	NR	NR	NR	NR	NR	NR
	6	19	1,838 ± 106[k]	76 ± 4[k]	NR	NR	NR	NR	NR	NR	NR	NR

Study	Age	N										
Manning-Dalton and Allen 1983[l]	0.5	12	2,165 ±757	95 ±20	NR	NR	NR	NR	NR	NR	NR	NR
	1	12	2,337 ±593	87 ±20	NR	NR	NR	NR	NR	NR	NR	NR
	2	12	1,951 ±749	81 ±30	NR	NR	NR	NR	NR	NR	NR	NR
	3	12	2,171 ±749	90 ±27	NR	NR	NR	NR	NR	NR	NR	NR
Stuff et al., 1983	Mixed	40	2,028 ±357	84.5 ±22.4	1,004 ±413	1,385 ±399	13.0 ±3.0	NR	NR	NR	NR	NR
Butte et al., 1984	1	43	2,334 ±536	98 ±28	1,219 ±543	1,722 ±553	16.2 ±4.8	9,070 ±5,920	1.9 ±0.9	2.6 ±1.1	23.6 ±8.4	150 ±90
	2	44	2,125 ±582	91 ±23	1,030 ±466	1,496 ±456	14.1 ±3.7	8,532 ±5,341	1.5 ±0.6	2.1 ±0.7	20.3 ±5.8	124 ±89
	3	40	2,170 ±629	89 ±25	1,024 ±478	1,467 ±459	13.9 ±4.0	7,598 ±4,807	1.5 ±0.5	2.1 ±0.8	20.5 ±7.2	114 ±81
	4	40	2,092 ±498	87 ±20	1,009 ±460	1,465 ±434	13.5 ±2.7	7,126 ±3,775	1.5 ±0.7	2.1 ±0.8	20.2 ±5.9	115 ±56
Song et al., 1985	Mixed	26[m]	2,014 ±620	79 ±26	1,243 ±595	1,446 ±563	26 ±24	9,627 ±5,206	2.1 ±1.1	2.8 ±1.4	70 ±90	199
Strode et al., 1986	Mixed	14	2,316 ±240	108 ±21	NR	NR	NR	NR	NR	NR	NR	NR
Teenagers Lipsman et al., 1985	Mixed	25	2,897 ±699	115 ±27	1,640 ±601	2,005 ±588	15.0 ±3.8	5,995 ±2,839	1.49 ±0.44	2.88 ±0.91	20.0 ±5.0	156 ±136

Table 4-5 continues

TABLE 4-5—Continued

RDA, Population Group, and Reference	Months Post Partum	Sample Size	Mean Daily Intake									
			Energy, kcal ± SD[b]	Protein, g ± SD	Calcium, mg ± SD	Phosphorus, mg ± SD	Iron, mg ± SD	Vitamin A, IU[c] ± SD	Thiamin, mg ± SD	Riboflavin, mg ± SD	Niacin, mg ± SD	Ascorbic acid, mg ± SD
Vegetarians												
Finley, 1985	Mixed	29	2,158 ± 601	78 ± 28	1,303 ± 611	1,736 ± 605	16.8 ± 6.9	9,756 ± 6,149	1.80 ± 1.02	2.15 ± 0.91	15.4 ± 6.5	175 ± 137
American Indians												
Butte and Calloway, 1981	1	23	2,190 ± 990	87 ± 38	718 ± 458	1,270 ± 559	15.2 ± 5.9	5,467 ± 10,002	1.39 ± 0.69	1.81 ± 1.07	20.1 ± 9.1	150 ± 165

[a]Nutrients listed in this table are those most commonly included in nutrient data bases.
[b]SD = Standard deviation.
[c]IU = International units.
[d]NA. = Not applicable.
[e]Calculated as the recommended daily energy increment for lactation (500 kcal) plus the energy allowance for females 11 to 50 years of age (2,200 kcal).
[f]Standard deviation not applicable to the RDA.
[g]Units for the RDAs are micrograms of retinol equivalents (RE); this is equivalent to approximately 5 IU of vitamin A obtained from the typical U.S. diet in the form of retinol (from animal products) and carotenoids (from plants) (Olson, 1987).
[h]NR = Not reported.
[i]Women taking supplements; intake from food only.
[j]Women taking no supplements.
[k]Standard error of the mean.
[l]Women in the study who averaged 95% lactation over the entire lactation period.
[m]Given as $N = 46$ for 26 subjects studied twice.

variability is, however, of concern. Clearly, there were individuals within these samples whose dietary intake was either lower or much higher than the mean. There is much less information concerning the adequacy of dietary intake of other micronutrients, as illustrated in Table 4-6. For example, iodine and vitamins E and K were omitted from the table because no relevant studies included them. Of the micronutrients reported in Table 4-6, vitamins B_{12}, B_6, and folate were the only ones studied by more than one group of investigators. The scant data do suggest closer examination of the adequacy of intake of folate and zinc, which were well below the 1989 RDAs in two studies, and of vitamin B_6, which was consistently below the 1989 RDA. Clearly, research is needed to provide a more complete nutritional profile of lactating women.

Data from Various Population Groups

The subcommittee identified only two studies focusing on groups of lactating women defined by factors of culture, ethnic background, life-style, or religion. These were studies of American Indians (Butte and Calloway, 1981) and of vegetarians (Finley et al., 1985) (see Tables 4-5 and 4-6). Among American Indians, vitamin A intake was highly variable and intakes of calcium; magnesium; zinc; and vitamins D, E, and folate appeared to be low. Among all the studies for which results are shown in Table 4-5, mean protein intake was lowest in the vegetarian group but still exceeded the RDA. As expected, the mean vitamin A intake of the vegetarians was the highest. The subcommittee identified only one study of lactating teenagers (Lipsman et al., 1985) and none of lactating women over age 35. The teenagers were found to have mean dietary intakes that met or exceeded the 1989 RDAs (Table 4-5).

Data on the dietary intake of lactating women of low socioeconomic status were also difficult to find. The first national evaluation of the Special Supplemental Food Program for Women, Infants, and Children (WIC) included 179 postpartum women. Of these, less than 79% were breastfeeding at the time that dietary data were collected (at enrollment in WIC, approximately 12 weeks post partum; breastfeeding was a prerequisite for enrollment for most of these women); unfortunately, those maternal nutrient intake values were not presented separately by breastfeeding status (Edozien et al., 1976). In general, the dietary intakes of these women were much lower than the current RDAs. Dietary intake of vitamins B_6, B_{12}, and folate was assessed in seven low-income women recruited from a WIC program (Sneed et al., 1981) (Table 4-6). At two stages of lactation, their reported intakes of vitamin B_6 were well below the RDA but were comparable to the values for the other groups included in these tables.

TABLE 4-6 Mean Daily Dietary Intakes of Selected Micronutrients by Lactating Women in the United States Compared with the Recommended Dietary Allowances (RDAs)[a]

Population Group and Reference	Stage of Lactation	Vitamin D, μg ± SD[b]	Vitamin E, mg ± SD	B6, mg ± SD	B12, μg ± SD	Folate, μg ± SD	Magnesium, mg ± SD	Zinc, mg ± SD	Selenium, μg ± SD
RDAs									
NRC, 1989	0–6 mo	10[c]	12	2.1	2.6	280	355	19	75
	7–12 mo	10	11	2.1	2.6	260	340	16	75
Well-nourished adult women									
Thomas and Kawamoto, 1979	4–7 days	NR[d]	NR	1.69 ± 0.65	NR	NR	NR	NR	NR
	42–45 days	NR	NR	1.11 ± 0.35	NR	NR	NR	NR	NR
Thomas et al., 1980	6 mo	NR	NR	1.13 ± 0.91	2.88 ± 2.29	194 ± 151	NR	NR	NR
Levander et al., 1987; Moser and Reynolds et al., 1983; Reynolds et al., 1984	1 mo	NR	NR	1.51 ± 0.11[e]	NR	NR	NR	9.4 ± 0.5[e]	84 ± 4[e]
	3 mo	NR	NR	1.55 ± 0.08[e]	NR	NR	NR	12.8 ± 1.8[e]	84 ± 4[e]
	6 mo	NR	NR	1.51 ± 0.11[e]	NR	NR	NR	9.6 ± 0.7[e]	87 ± 4[e]

American Indians									
Butte et al., 1981	NR	136 ± 115[f]	4.5 ± 3.8	1.44[g]	7.96 ± 1.47	169 ± 139	221 ± 114	12.2 ± 5.3	NR
Low-income women									
Sneed et al., 1981[h]	5–7 days	NR	NR	1.52 ± 0.40	7.0 ± 3.1	290 ± 100	NR	NR	NR
	43–45 days	NR	NR	1.41 ± 0.56	5.2 ± 1.8	340 ± 200	NR	NR	NR

[a] From NRC (1989). Details of the studies cited are given in Table 4-4.
[b] SD = Standard deviation.
[c] Standard deviation not applicable to RDA.
[d] NR = Not reported.
[e] Standard error of the mean.
[f] Units are IU; 1 μg vitamin D = 40 IU.
[g] Reported standard deviation is not included because of a suspected error.
[h] Unsupplemented women.

CONCLUSIONS

• The nutritional status of lactating women in the United States has not been thoroughly or extensively studied; therefore, data are lacking on all aspects of this subject. The lactating subjects who have been studied (mainly Caucasian women with some college education) appear, in general, to be well nourished. Groups of U.S. women who are likely to have poor dietary intakes either tend not to breastfeed or if they do breastfeed, have not been studied extensively.

• On average, lactating women who eat to appetite lose weight at the rate of 0.6 to 0.8 kg (1.3 to 1.6 lb) per month in the first 4 to 6 months of lactation, but there is wide variation in the weight loss experience of lactating women (some women gain weight during lactation). Those who continue breastfeeding beyond 4 to 6 months ordinarily continue to lose weight, but at a slower rate than during the first 4 to 6 months. Measurements of subscapular and suprailiac—but not triceps—skinfold thickness decrease during the first 4 to 6 months of lactation.

• Until reference standards for nutritional status based on biochemical or anthropometric criteria have been developed for lactating women, there is not a sound basis for using standards derived from nonpregnant, nonlactating women in the routine care of healthy lactating women. If such standards are used in special situations, there is a risk of misclassification. To reduce misclassification, it would be appropriate to consider other factors (such as low socioeconomic status) that might increase the risk of an adverse outcome or factors (such as low weight for height) that might predict the likelihood of a benefit.

RECOMMENDATIONS FOR CLINICAL PRACTICE

• Women who plan to breastfeed or who are breastfeeding should be given realistic, health-promoting advice about weight change during lactation (see also Chapters 5 and 9).

• In the opinion of the subcommittee, it is not necessary to obtain measurements of skinfold thickness or to conduct laboratory tests as a part of the routine assessment of the nutritional status of lactating women because of the difficulty of obtaining accurate skinfold thickness measurements and the high expense of both types of measurements relative to the likelihood of identifying nutritional problems.

REFERENCES

Ala-Houhala, M., T. Koskinen, R. Mäki, and S. Rinkari. 1988. Serum vitamin A levels in mothers and their breast-fed term infants with or without supplemental vitamin A. Acta Paediatr. Scand. 77:198-201.

Anderson, D.M., F.W.H. Elsley, and I. McDonald. 1970. Blood volume changes during pregnancy and lactation of sows. Q. J. Exp. Physiol. 55:293-300.

Andon, M.B., R.D. Reynolds, P.B. Moser-Veillon, and M.P. Howard. 1989. Dietary intake of total and glycosylated vitamin B_6 and the vitamin B_6 nutritional status of unsupplemented lactating women and their infants. Am. J. Clin. Nutr. 50:1050-1058.

Bates, C.J., A.M. Prentice, M. Watkinson, P. Morrell, B.A. Sutcliffe, F.A. Foord, and R.G. Whitehead. 1982. Riboflavin requirements of lactating Gambian women: a controlled supplementation trial. Am. J. Clin. Nutr. 35:701-709.

Blackburn, M.W., and D.H. Calloway. 1976. Energy expenditure and consumption of mature, pregnant and lactating women. J. Am. Diet. Assoc. 69:29-37.

Bond, C.F. 1958. Blood volume changes in the lactating rat. Endocrinology 63:285-289.

Brewer, M.M., M.R. Bates, and L.P. Vannoy. 1989. Postpartum changes in maternal weight and body fat depots in lactating vs nonlactating women. Am. J. Clin. Nutr. 49:259-265.

Brown, E., J.J. Sampson, E.O. Wheeler, B.F. Gundelfinger, and J.E. Giansiracusa. 1947. Physiologic changes in the circulation during and after obstetric labor. Am. Heart J. 34:311-333.

Butte, N.F., and D.H. Calloway. 1981. Evaluation of lactational performance of Navajo women. Am. J. Clin. Nutr. 34:2210-2215.

Butte, N.F., and C. Garza. 1986. Anthropometry in the appraisal of lactation performance among well-nourished women. Pp. 61-67 in M. Hamosh and A.S. Goldman, eds. Human Lactation 2: Maternal and Environmental Factors. Plenum Press, New York.

Butte, N.F., D.H. Calloway, and J.L. Van Duzen. 1981. Nutritional assessment of pregnant and lactating Navajo women. Am. J. Clin. Nutr. 34:2216-2228.

Butte, N.F., C. Garza, J.E. Stuff, E.O. Smith, and B.L. Nichols. 1984. Effect of maternal diet and body composition on lactational performance. Am. J. Clin. Nutr. 39:296-306.

Caton, W.L., C.C. Roby, D.E. Reid, R. Caswell, C.J. Maletskos, R.G. Fluharty, and J.G. Gibson II. 1951. The circulating red cell volume and body hematocrit in normal pregnancy and the puerperium: by direct measurement, using radioactive red cells. Am. J. Obstet. Gynecol. 61:1207-1217.

Dennis, K.J., and W.R. Bytheway. 1965. Changes in body weight after delivery. J. Obstet. Gynaecol. Br. Commonw. 72:94-102.

Donovan, J.C., C.J. Lund, and L. Whalen. 1964. Simultaneous determinations of blood volumes using Evans blue and sodium radiochromate. Surg. Gynecol. Obstet. 119:1031-1036.

Donovan, J.C., C.J. Lund, and E.L. Hicks. 1965. Effect of lactation on blood volume in the human female. Am. J. Obstet. Gynecol. 93:588-589.

Dostálová, L. 1984. Vitamin status during puerperium and lactation. Ann. Nutr. Metab. 28:385-408.

Dugdale, A.E., and J. Eaton-Evans. 1989. The effect of lactation and other factors on post-partum changes in body-weight and triceps skinfold thickness. Br. J. Nutr. 61:149-153.

Edozien, J.C., B.R. Switzer, and R.B. Bryan. 1976. Medical Evaluation of the Special Supplemental Food Program for Women, Infants, and Children (WIC), Vol. II: Results. Department of Nutrition, School of Public Health, University of North Carolina, Chapel Hill, N.C. 436 pp.

Ek, J. 1983. Plasma, red cell, and breast milk folacin concentrations in lactating women. Am. J. Clin. Nutr. 38:929-935.

Fåhraeus, L., U. Larsson-Cohn, and L. Wallentin. 1985. Plasma lipoproteins including high density lipoprotein subfractions during normal pregnancy. Obstet. Gynecol. 66:468-472.

Finley, D.A., K.G. Dewey, B. Lönnerdal, and L.E. Grivetti. 1985. Food choices of vegetarians and nonvegetarians during pregnancy and lactation. J. Am. Diet. Assoc. 85:678-685.

Forsum, E., A. Sadurskis, and J. Wager. 1989. Estimation of body fat in healthy Swedish women during pregnancy and lactation. Am. J. Clin. Nutr. 50:465-473.

Frisancho, A.R. 1981. New norms of upper limb fat and muscle areas for assessment of nutritional status. Am. J. Clin. Nutr. 34:2540-2545.

Frisancho, A.R. 1984. New standards of weight and body composition by frame size and height for assessment of nutritional status of adults and the elderly. Am. J. Clin. Nutr. 40:808-819.

Greene, G.W., H. Smiciklas-Wright, T.O. Scholl, and R.J. Karp. 1988. Postpartum weight change: how much of the weight gained in pregnancy will be lost after delivery? Obstet. Gynecol. 71:701-707.

Greer, F.R., R.C. Tsang, R.S. Levin, J.E. Searcy, R. Wu, and J.J. Steichen. 1982. Increasing serum calcium and magnesium concentrations in breast-fed infants: longitudinal studies of minerals in human milk and in sera of nursing mothers and their infants. J. Pediatr. 100:59-64.

Habicht, J.-P., and D.L. Pelletier. 1990. The importance of context in choosing nutritional indicators. J. Nutr. 120:1519-1524.

Heinig, M.J., L.A. Nommsen, and K.G. Dewey. 1990. Lactation and postpartum weight loss. FASEB J. 4:362 (abstract).

Herbert, V.D., and N. Colman. 1988. Folic acid and vitamin B_{12}. Pp. 388-416 in M.E. Shils and V.R. Young, eds. Modern Nutrition in Health and Disease. Lea & Febiger, Philadelphia.

Illingworth, P.J., R.T. Jung, P.W. Howie, P. Leslie, and T.E. Isles. 1986. Diminution in energy expenditure during lactation. Br. Med. J. 292:437-441.

IOM (Institute of Medicine). 1990. Nutrition During Pregnancy: Weight Gain and Nutrient Supplements. Report of the Subcommittee on Nutritional Status and Weight Gain During Pregnancy, Subcommittee on Dietary Intake and Nutrient Supplements During Pregnancy, Committee on Nutritional Status During Pregnancy and Lactation, Food and Nutrition Board. National Academy Press, Washington, D.C. 468 pp.

Kinney, T.D., and R.H. Follis, Jr., eds. 1958. Nutritional disease. Fed. Proc., Fed. Am. Soc. Exp. Biol. 17 Suppl. 2:1-56.

Knopp, R.H., C.W. Walden, P.W. Wahl, R. Bergelin, M. Chapman, S. Irvine, and J.J. Albers. 1985. Effect of postpartum lactation on lipoprotein lipids and apoproteins. J. Clin. Endocrinol. Metab. 60:542-547.

Krebs, N.F., K.M. Hambidge, M.A. Jacobs, and J.O. Rasbach. 1985. The effects of a dietary zinc supplement during lactation on longitudinal changes in maternal zinc status and milk zinc concentrations. Am. J. Clin. Nutr. 41:560-570.

Krebs-Smith, S.M., and L.D. Clark. 1989. Validation of a nutrient adequacy score for use with women and children. J. Am. Diet. Assoc. 89:775-783.

Levander, O.A. 1988. Selenium, chromium, and manganese. (A) Selenium. Pp. 263-267 in M.E. Shils and V.R. Young, eds. Modern Nutrition in Health and Disease. Lea & Febiger, Philadelphia.

Levander, O.A., P.B. Moser, and V.C. Morris. 1987. Dietary selenium intake and selenium concentrations of plasma, erythrocytes, and breast milk in pregnant and postpartum lactating and nonlacting women. Am. J. Clin. Nutr. 46:694-698.

Lipsman, S., K.G. Dewey, and B. Lönnerdal. 1985. Breast-feeding among teenage mothers: milk composition, infant growth, and maternal dietary intake. J. Pediatr. Gastroenterol. Nutr. 4:426-434.

LSRO (Life Sciences Research Office). 1989. Nutrition Monitoring in the United States: An Update Report on Nutrition Monitoring. Prepared for the U.S. Department of Agriculture and the U.S. Department of Health and Human Services. DHHS Publ. No. (PHS) 89-1225. U.S. Government Printing Office, Washington, D.C.

MLI (Metropolitan Life Insurance). 1959. New weight standards for men and women. Stat. Bull. Metrop. Life Insur. Co. 40:1-4.

MLI (Metropolitan Life Insurance). 1983. 1983 Metropolitan height and weight tables. Stat. Bull. Metrop. Life Found. 64:3-9.

Mannan, S., and M.F. Picciano. 1987. Influence of maternal selenium status on human milk selenium concentration and glutathione peroxidase activity. Am. J. Clin. Nutr 46:95-100.

Manning-Dalton, C., and L.H. Allen. 1983. The effects of lactation on energy and protein consumption, postpartum weight change and body composition of well nourished North American women. Nutr. Res. 3:293-308.

McCormick, D.B. 1988. Vitamin B$_6$. Pp. 376-382 in M.E. Shils and V.R. Young, eds. Modern Nutrition in Health and Disease. Lea & Febiger, Philadelphia.

Moore, M.E.C., J.R. Moran, and H.L. Greene. 1984. Zinc supplementation in lactating women: evidence for mammary control of zinc secretion. J. Pediatr. 105:600-602.

Moser, P.B., and R.D. Reynolds. 1983. Dietary zinc intake and zinc concentrations of plasma, erythrocytes, and breast milk in antepartum and postpartum lactating and nonlactating women: a longitudinal study. Am. J. Clin. Nutr. 38:101-108.

Motil, K.J., C.M. Montandon, D.L. Hachey, T.W. Boutton, P.D. Klein, and C. Garza. 1989. Whole-body protein metabolism in lactating and nonlactating women. J. Appl. Physiol. 66:370-376.

Motil, K.J., C.M. Montandon, M. Thotathuchery, and C. Garza. 1990. Dietary protein and nitrogen balance in lactating and nonlactating women. Am. J. Clin. Nutr. 51:378-384.

Najjar, M.F., and Rowland, M. 1987. Anthropometric Reference Data and Prevalence of Overweight, United States, 1976-80. Vital and Health Statistics. Series 11, No. 238. DHHS Pub. No. (PHS) 87-1688. Public Health Service. U.S. Department of Health and Human Service, Government Printing Office, Washington, D.C.

NRC (National Research Council). 1978. Laboratory Indices of Nutritional Status in Pregnancy. Report of the Committee on Nutrition of the Mother and Preschool Child, Food and Nutrition Board. National Academy of Sciences, Washington, D.C. 195 pp.

NRC (National Research Council). 1980. Recommended Dietary Allowances, 9th ed. Report of the Committee on Dietary Allowances, Food and Nutrition Board, Division of Biological Sciences, Assembly of Life Sciences. National Academy Press, Washington, D.C. 185 pp.

NRC (National Research Council). 1989. Recommended Dietary Allowances, 10th ed. Report of the Subcommittee on the Tenth Edition of the RDAs, Food and Nutrition Board, Commission on Life Sciences. National Academy Press, Washington, D.C. 284 pp.

Öhlin, A., and S. Rössner. 1990. Maternal body weight development after pregnancy. Int J. Obes. 14:159-173.

Olson, J.A. 1987. Recommended dietary intakes (RDI) of vitamin A in humans. Am. J. Clin. Nutr. 45:704-716.

Prentice, A.M., S.B. Roberts, A. Prentice, A.A. Paul, M. Watkinson, A.A. Watkinson, and R.G. Whitehead. 1983. Dietary supplementation of lactating Gambian women. I. Effect on breast-milk volume and quality. Hum. Nutr.: Clin. Nutr. 37C:53-64.

Rasmussen, K.M. 1988. Maternal nutritional status and lactational performance. Clin. Nutr. 7:147-155.

Rasmussen, K.M., and J.P. Habicht. 1989. Malnutrition among women: indicators to estimate prevalence. Food Nutr. Bull. 11:29-37.

Reynolds, M. 1953. Measurement of bovine plasma and blood volume during pregnancy and lactation. Am. J. Physiol. 175:118-122.

Reynolds, R.D., M. Polansky, and P.B. Moser. 1984. Analyzed vitamin B-6 intakes of pregnant and postpartum lactating and nonlactating women. J. Am. Diet. Assoc. 84:1339-1344.

Rothe, G.E. 1988. Determinants of response to supplementation in malnourished Guatemalan children. M.S. Thesis. Cornell University, Ithaca, N.Y. 178 pp.

Sadurskis, A., N. Kabir, J. Wager, and E. Forsum. 1988. Energy metabolism, body composition, and milk production in healthy Swedish women during lactation. Am. J. Clin. Nutr. 48:44-49.

Salmenperä, L. 1984. Vitamin C nutrition during prolonged lactation: optimal in infants while marginal in some mothers. Am. J. Clin. Nutr. 40:1050-1056.

Salmenperä, L., J. Perheentupa, and M.A. Siimes. 1986. Folate nutrition is optimal in exclusively breast-fed infants but inadequate in some of their mothers and in formula-fed infants. J. Pediatr. Gastroenterol. Nutr. 5:283-289.

Sims, L. 1978. Dietary status of lactating women. I. Nutrient intake from food and from supplements. J. Am. Diet. Assoc. 73:139-146.

Sneed, S.M., C. Zane, and M.R. Thomas. 1981. The effects of ascorbic acid, vitamin B_6, vitamin B_{12}, and folic acid supplementation on the breast milk and maternal nutritional status of low socioeconomic lactating women. Am. J. Clin. Nutr. 34:1338-1346.

Solomons, N.W. 1988. Zinc and copper. Pp. 238-262 in M.E. Shils and V.R. Young, eds. Modern Nutrition in Health and Disease. Lea & Febiger, Philadelphia.

Song, W.O., B.W. Wyse, and R.G. Hansen. 1985. Pantothenic acid status of pregnant and lactating women. J. Am. Diet. Assoc. 85:192-198.

Specker, B.L., D. Miller, E.J. Norman, H. Greene, and K.C. Hayes. 1988. Increased urinary methylmalonic acid excretion in breast-fed infants of vegetarian mothers and identification of an acceptable dietary source of vitamin B_{12}. Am. J. Clin. Nutr. 47:89-92.

Strode, M.A., K.G. Dewey, and B. Lönnerdal. 1986. Effects of short-term caloric restriction on lactational performance of well-nourished women. Acta Paediatr. Scand. 75:222-229.

Stuff, J.E., C. Garza, E.O. Smith, B.L. Nichols, and C.M. Montandon. 1983. A comparison of dietary methods in nutritional studies. Am. J. Clin. Nutr. 37:300-306.

Tarvydas, H., S.M. Jordan, and E.H. Morgan. 1968. Iron metabolism during lactation in the rabbit. Br. J. Nutr. 22:565-573.

Taylor, D.J., and T. Lind. 1979. Red cell mass during and after normal pregnancy. Br. J. Obstet. Gynaecol. 86:364-370.

Thomas, M.R., and J. Kawamoto. 1979. Dietary evaluation of lactating women with or without vitamin and mineral supplementation. J. Am. Diet. Assoc. 74:669-672.

Thomas, M.R., S.M. Sneed, C. Wei, P.A. Nail, M. Wilson, and E.E. Sprinkle III. 1980. The effects of vitamin C, vitamin B_6, vitamin B_{12}, folic acid, riboflavin, and thiamin on the breast milk and maternal status of well-nourished women at 6 months postpartum. Am. J. Clin. Nutr. 33:2151-2156.

Tietz, N.W. 1986. Textbook of Clinical Chemistry. W.B. Saunders Company. Philadelphia. 1919 pp.

van der Elst, C.W., W.S. Dempster, D.L. Woods, and H. de V. Heese. 1986. Serum zinc and copper in thin mothers, their breast milk and their infants. J. Trop. Pediatr. 32:111-114.

Wong, W.W., N.F. Butte, E.O. Smith, C.Garza, and P.D. Klein. 1989. Body composition of lactating women determined by anthropometry and deuterium dilution. Br. J. Nutr. 61:25-33.

Young, D.S. 1987. Implementation of SI units for clinical laboratory data. Style specifications and conversion tables. Published errata appear in Ann. Intern. Med. 1987 Aug;107(2):265 and 1989 Feb 15;110(4):328. Ann. Intern. Med. 106:114-129.

5

Milk Volume

(The nutritional demands imposed by breastfeeding depend primarily on the absolute quantities of nutrients transferred from the mother to the infant through the milk. Thus, in considering recommendations for maternal nutrition during lactation, it is essential to carefully examine both the volume and composition of human milk. Milk volume is the focus of this chapter; Chapter 6 covers composition.)

The subcommittee addressed the following questions in its review of milk volume:

- Is the volume or energy content of human milk compromised when intake of energy or other nutrients is restricted during lactation? Do maternal body fat or other nutrient stores modify this relationship?
- Does energy supplementation or increased intake of protein or fluid increase milk volume?
- What other factors must be considered when examining the effects of maternal nutrition on milk volume?

These questions can be examined only in the context of a clear under-standing of the regulation of milk production in humans. For this reason, this chapter includes consideration of the physiologic control of lactation and of the infant's role in this process, in addition to maternal factors such as age, parity, stress, substance use, and nutrition.

MEASUREMENT OF MILK VOLUME

A key element defining lactation performance is the total amount of milk produced. The amount of milk transferred to the infant affects the infant's nutrient intake and the mother's nutrient requirements. In this report, the subcommittee distinguishes between milk *intake* by the infant (also referred to as milk *volume*) and milk *production* by the mother. Ordinarily, production is measured as intake, but it may exceed intake if extra milk is removed from the breast and is not consumed by the infant or the infant regurgitates milk.

The most widely accepted method for measuring milk intake is test weighing, a procedure in which the infant is weighed before and after each feeding, preferably using a balance scale accurate to ±1 g. In this method, milk intake is usually underestimated by approximately 1 to 5% (Brown et al., 1982; Woolridge et al., 1985) because of evaporative water loss from the infant between weighings. The procedure is potentially disruptive to the nursing patterns of the mother and infant, especially if nursing is very frequent or the infant nurses occasionally during the night while sleeping with the mother. Under conditions typical of breastfeeding mothers in the United States, the method is generally well accepted (Dewey and Heinig, 1987). Intake is usually reported in grams because they are the unit of measurement used in test weighing; the density of human milk is approximately 1.03 g/ml (Neville et al., 1988; Woolridge et al., 1985). Newer techniques for measuring breast milk intake based on the use of stable isotopes have been developed, but few data obtained with them have been published (Butte et al., 1988; Coward et al., 1982; Fjeld et al., 1988; Wong et al., 1990). Maternal milk production can be measured mechanically by extracting all the milk or by using a combination of test weighing and extraction of residual milk.

NORMAL RANGE OF MILK INTAKE AND PRODUCTION

There is a very wide range in milk intake among healthy, exclusively breastfed infants. Figure 5-1 illustrates variability in infant milk intake during established lactation. In industrialized countries, milk intakes average approximately 750 to 800 g/day in the first 4 to 5 months, but range from approximately 450 to 1,200 g/day (Butte et al., 1984b; Chandra, 1981; Dewey and Lönnerdal, 1983; Hofvander et al., 1982; Lönnerdal et al., 1976; Neville et al., 1988; Pao et al., 1980; Picciano et al., 1981; Rattigan et al., 1981; Wallgren, 1944/1945; Whitehead and Paul, 1981). Recent data from developing countries indicate a similar mean level of intake when a rigorous methodology for measuring milk volume is used (Brown et al., 1986b; Prentice et al., 1986) (see Figure 5-2).

Milk intake after the first 4 to 5 months varies even more widely. In U.S. infants who were breastfed for at least 12 months and were given solid foods beginning at 4 to 7 months, milk intake averaged 769 g/day (range, 335 to

82

NUTRITION DURING LACTATION

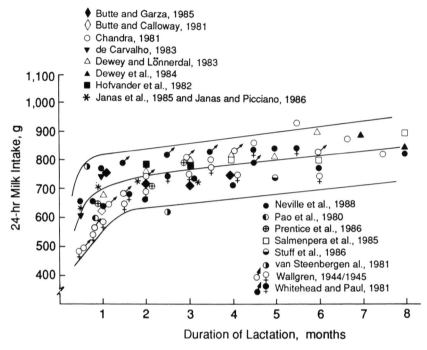

FIGURE 5-1 Milk intakes during established lactation from studies meeting defined criteria, from Neville et al. (1988) with permission. The lines show the smoothed mean ± standard deviation, from Neville et al. (1988). The points represent average intakes from studies that obtained data from test weighing, validated exclusive breastfeeding, studied three or more subjects, and reported milk transfer by monthly intervals.

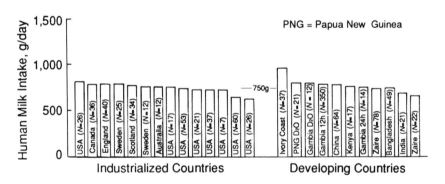

FIGURE 5-2 Average intake of human milk by infants at age 3 months in industrialized and developing countries. Data were compiled from studies later than the year 1975. Adapted from Prentice et al. (1986) with permission.

1,144 g/day) at 6 months (N = 56), 637 g/day (range, 205 to 1,185 g/day) at 9 months (N = 46), and 445 g/day (range, 27 to 1,154 g/day) at 12 months (N = 40) (Dewey et al., in press).

Several studies indicate that potential milk production in humans is considerably higher than the average intake by single infants. Kaucher and colleagues (1945) measured maximum milk output with intrusive and tedious mechanical methods to extract all the mother's milk and reported that production averaged almost 1,200 g/day at 6 to 10 days post partum. This level is much higher than the 500 to 700 g/day consumed by breastfed infants at the same age (Casey et al., 1986; Saint et al., 1984). In two separate studies, milk production increased by 15 to 40% when a breast pump was used to remove additional milk after feedings (Dewey and Lönnerdal, 1986; Neville and Oliva-Rasbach, 1987). Mothers who exclusively breastfeed twins or triplets can produce 2,000 to 3,000 g/day, although this involves nursing an average of 15 or more times per day (Saint et al., 1986). Women who express surplus milk for a milk bank have been shown to produce as much as 3,000 g/day (Macy et al., 1930).

BREAST DEVELOPMENT AND PHYSIOLOGY

The data discussed above illustrate that lactation is a physiologic process with a great deal of plasticity—that is, milk production can be regulated up or down, depending on the degree of stimulation to the mammary gland. The processes leading to a woman's ability to secrete milk start long before lactation commences.

Mammary development begins in early fetal life and extends through puberty; it resumes early in pregnancy. The process is influenced by several hormones, including estrogens, progesterone, and lactogenic hormones (Neville and Neifert, 1983). Mammary gland enlargement is especially pronounced during the first half of pregnancy, when lobuloalveolar growth is accompanied by differentiation of the epithelial cells. Both prolactin and placental lactogen may initiate this enlargement, although either one alone may provide sufficient stimulus for mammary development. Insufficient development before or during pregnancy may contribute to lactation failure (Neifert and Seacat, 1986). The prevalence of this problem has not been studied but is likely to be very low.

Lactogenesis, defined as "the onset of copious milk secretion around parturition" (Neville and Neifert, 1983, p. 108), is believed to be triggered by the decrease in progesterone following parturition. Incomplete delivery of the placenta has been shown to delay lactogenesis, presumably because it is accompanied by continued high levels of progesterone (Neifert et al., 1981). Prolactin is believed to be essential for normal lactogenesis, but the mechanism or mechanisms for its influence are not clearly understood. Once milk production has begun, the hormonal mechanisms maintaining milk secretion are believed to depend primarily on the actions of prolactin and oxytocin.

Prolactin is generally understood to promote milk synthesis and secretion into the alveolar spaces. Its metabolic effects include promotion of fat synthesis in mammary tissue, increased fat mobilization at other body sites, enhancement of casein synthesis and casein messenger RNA formation in the rat and rabbit, and stimulation of milk α-lactalbumin and lactose levels in cows (Horrobin, 1979). Prolactin levels are influenced by the amount and frequency of suckling, but vary considerably among women producing comparable volumes of milk (Martin, 1983; Noel et al., 1974; Strode et al., 1986; Tyson et al., 1978).

Oxytocin is secreted by the maternal pituitary in response to suckling and in turn stimulates contraction of the myoepithelial cells, leading to milk ejection. This milk-ejection reflex, or *let-down*, moves milk from the storage alveoli to the lacteal sinuses, allowing the milk to be easily removed by the infant (Woolridge and Baum, 1988).

Milk production may also be governed by local negative feedback within each breast, referred to by Wilde et al. (1988) as "autocrine" control. These investigators reported that a constituent of milk whey protein inhibits milk secretion in a dose-dependent manner in goats. As milk builds up in the mammary gland between feedings, the concentration of this inhibitor presumably increases and thus retards and eventually stops milk production. Removal of milk eliminates the inhibitory effect and milk production resumes or increases. This inhibitory mechanism could explain why two breasts of the same woman with different milk removal rates can produce very different quantities of milk.

Breast engorgement and the resulting increased pressure in and distension of the mammary gland also lead to decreased milk production. Studies in animals suggest that when milking ceases, distension of the alveoli caused by pooling of the milk brings about a decrease in milk secretion within 6 hours (Neville and Neifert, 1983).

INFANT FACTORS INFLUENCING MILK
PRODUCTION AND TRANSFER

Management of lactation during the first few weeks is critical to the establishment of an adequate milk supply. Successful lactation depends on several factors, such as proper positioning of the infant at the breast, precautions to avoid sore nipples, frequent feedings, avoidance of formula feeding, and timing of feedings to coincide with the infant's desire to suck. These factors are discussed in detail in breastfeeding guides (e.g., Goldfarb and Tibbetts, 1989, Lawrence, 1989). For the purposes of this report, the subcommittee restricted its discussion to infant characteristics that may influence milk volume, such as birth weight, sucking strength, gestational age at delivery, and illness, and to maternal characteristics, such as age, parity, stress, substance use, and nutritional status. These characteristics appear to be those that are most likely to affect milk volume if they influence the frequency, intensity, or duration of sucking by the infant.

Nursing Frequency

During the early postpartum period, when the milk supply is being established (Lawrence, 1985), there is a positive association between nursing frequency and milk production (de Carvalho et al., 1983, 1985; Hopkinson et al., 1988; Salariya et al., 1978). In a study of 32 mothers of preterm infants, optimal milk production was achieved when milk was pumped five or more times per day during the first month post partum (Hopkinson et al., 1988). Among women breastfeeding full-term infants, mean nursing frequency of 10 ± 3 times per day during the first 2 weeks post partum was associated with adequate milk production (de Carvalho et al., 1982). Although there is considerable interindividual variability in infants' need to suck, nursing on demand (at least eight times per day in the early postpartum period) is recommended to provide the necessary degree of hormonal stimulation to the mammary gland.

Once lactation is established, cross-sectional studies of well-nourished, exclusively breastfeeding women nursing 4 to 16 times per day indicate that there is little, if any, relationship between nursing frequency and infant milk intake (Butte et al., 1984a; de Carvalho et al., 1982; Dewey et al., 1986) or between basal serum prolactin levels and milk volume (Lunn et al., 1984; Noel et al., 1974; Strode et al., 1986; Tyson et al., 1978). These findings do not imply, however, that the milk output of individual mothers cannot be altered by changing nursing frequency. At least one report illustrates that limiting the number of feedings can reduce milk production (Egli et al., 1961), and during gradual weaning, it is obvious that mothers are able to decrease their infant's intake of human milk by nursing less often. Thus, although some infants are capable of consuming adequate amounts of milk by feeding only four to five times a day, women who are concerned about the adequacy of their milk supply are well advised to nurse more often.

Birth Weight

Prentice et al. (1986) and Dewey et al. (1986) observed an association between infant birth weight and volume of milk intake. This appears to be related to the greater sucking strength, frequency, or feeding duration among larger infants—all of which could increase milk volume. Pollitt and colleagues (1978) demonstrated that infant weight at 2 days and at 1 month of age was strongly correlated with sucking strength, which appeared to be responsible for the large variations in intake per feeding among formula-fed infants. Among breastfed infants, de Carvalho et al. (1982) found a positive relationship between infant birth weight and frequency and duration of feeding during the first 14 days post partum.

Gestational Age at Delivery

The interaction of gestational age and birth weight may have a stronger influence on milk intake than does either one alone, because preterm infants (especially those born at <34 weeks of gestation) may be too weak or immature to suck effectively. Studies of the volume of milk produced by mothers of preterm infants are complicated by the fact that many mothers must pump milk for several days or weeks before the infant can suck directly from the breast. The degree of maternal motivation to breastfeed plays a large role in the success of this phase.

Self-Regulation

Self-regulation of milk intake was studied among 18 exclusively breastfed infants of mothers who increased their milk supply by expressing extra milk daily for 2 weeks (Dewey and Lönnerdal, 1986). On average, these infants took in more milk immediately following this 2-week period, but about half of them returned to near baseline levels of milk intake after another 1 to 2 weeks. Net change in milk intake at the end of the study was greater among heavier infants and was not associated with baseline milk volume. This indicates that milk intake was influenced more by infant demand than by maternal capacity for milk production. In a subsequent study, Dewey et al. (in press) showed that *residual* milk volume (the difference between the amount that can be extracted by pump compared with usual infant intake) averages about 100 g/day, even among mothers whose infants consume relatively low amounts of milk (<650 g/day). Likewise, Woolridge and Baum (1988) demonstrated that when 29 mothers randomly selected the breast from which to feed the baby first, intake from the second breast was only about 60% of the amount taken from the first breast. These results illustrate that infants ordinarily do not take all the available milk and therefore govern their own intake to a considerable extent.

Self-regulation of milk intake by infants was also demonstrated by Stuff and Nichols (1989), who studied 45 breastfed infants before and after they began consuming solid foods. Energy intake per kilogram of body weight of these infants during exclusive breastfeeding was considerably lower than the Recommended Dietary Allowance (NRC, 1989) and did not increase after solid foods were introduced. Instead, the infants responded to solid foods by reducing breast milk intake, thereby maintaining constant levels of energy intake. Similarly, Nommsen and colleagues (1989) found that solid foods displaced energy intake from human milk in 6-month-old infants even though they were breastfed on demand.

Factors influencing the infant's demand for milk have not been studied thoroughly. When the milk supply is ample, the infant's milk intake is positively associated with infant weight. Because the mean weight of boys is heavier than that of girls of the same age, intake is also associated with the sex of the infant. Illness of the infant may reduce appetite and therefore milk intake. In The Gambia, Prentice et al. (1986) observed that decreases in milk intake by infants during the wet season (a period of food scarcity) were usually associated with gastrointestinal or respiratory infections. As described later in this chapter, maternal supplementation did not prevent the seasonal decline in milk volume, indicating that this pattern was probably not due to maternal nutritional limitations but to either altered feeding practices or illness-induced anorexia among the infants. From the Gambian data, it is difficult to separate the influence of these factors. In contrast, Brown et al. (in press) found that milk intake among breastfed infants in Peru remained constant, whereas intake of other foods was reduced during illness.

MATERNAL FACTORS

Age and Parity

Maternal variables such as age and parity have little or no relationship to milk production in most populations (as measured by the infant's intake of human milk). There have been few studies of the volume of milk produced by adolescent mothers. In one study, Lipsman et al. (1985) found that milk intake appeared adequate (based on measures of infant growth) for 22 of the 25 infants of well-nourished, lactating teenagers. Among women aged 21 to 37, no association was observed between maternal age and infant milk intake (Butte et al., 1984b; Dewey et al., 1986), despite Hytten's (1954) concerns that milk yield may decrease because of "disuse atrophy" after age 24.

There is some evidence that milk production on the fourth day post partum is higher among multiparous than it is among primiparous women (Zuppa et al., 1988); however, once lactation is established, there is no statistically significant association between parity and infant milk intake in well-nourished populations (Butte et al., 1984a; Dewey et al., 1986; Rattigan et al., 1981). In The Gambia, infants of mothers who had borne 10 or more children had low milk intakes (Prentice, 1986), but this level of parity is rarely seen in industrialized countries.

Stress and Acute Illness

Maternal anxiety and stress, which may be exacerbated by poor lactation management, are believed to influence milk production by inhibiting the milk-ejection reflex. This reflex usually operates well in women who are relaxed and confident of their ability to breastfeed. In tense women, however, the reflex may be impaired. Limited documentation of the effects of stress or relaxation on let-down is provided by Newton and Newton (1948, 1950) and Feher et al. (1989), but further studies are needed to explore the effects of various types of maternal stress, especially chronic anxiety and tension, on milk production. There are also few data concerning the potential influence of common short-term maternal illnesses on breastfeeding. It is known, however, that mothers can and should continue to nurse when they have mastitis (Lawrence, 1989).

Substance Use

Maternal behavior such as cigarette smoking and alcohol consumption may influence both milk production and milk composition. Potential consequences to the infant are discussed in Chapter 7; this section is restricted to effects on milk volume.

Cigarette Smoking

Smoking may reduce milk volume through an inhibitory effect on prolactin or oxytocin levels. Studies in rats have shown decreased release of prolactin in response to suckling and decreases in both milk output and pup growth upon exposure to nicotine or tobacco fumes (Blake and Sawyer, 1972; Ferry et al., 1974; Hamosh et al., 1979; Terkel et al., 1973). Smoking is also known to stimulate release of adrenaline, which in turn can inhibit oxytocin release (Cross, 1955). Studies in humans show a consistent association between smoking and early weaning (Lyon, 1983; Matheson and Rivrud, 1989; Whichelow and King, 1979), but milk volume was not measured directly in those studies. Since smoking is usually more common among women of lower socioeconomic status and educational level than among more advantaged women, it is possible that the smoking itself is not the factor that contributes to early weaning. However, both Lyon (1983) and Matheson and Rivrud (1989) reported a lower prevalence of breastfeeding at 6 to 12 weeks post partum among smokers compared with nonsmokers even within the same socioeconomic group. Furthermore, Matheson and Rivrud (1989) found a greater incidence of colic among infants of breastfeeding mothers who smoked.

Andersen and coworkers (1982) demonstrated that women who smoked 15 or more cigarettes per day had 30 to 50% lower basal prolactin levels on days 1 and 21 post partum than did nonsmokers, although the suckling-induced rise in prolactin was not different between groups. Oxytocin levels were not influenced by smoking. Since the infants of smokers tend to have average birth weights that are approximately 200 g lower than those of the infants of nonsmokers (IOM, 1990) (which is the case in the study by Andersen et al. [1982]), and since lower birth weight may decrease infant demand for milk and thus both prolactin levels and milk volume, it is difficult to separate cause and effect in these studies. Nonetheless, the evidence from investigations in both animals and humans strongly suggests that smoking has an adverse effect on milk volume.

Alcohol Consumption

The influence of alcohol consumption on milk production is less straight-forward than that of smoking. It has long been maintained that small amounts of alcoholic beverages can help breastfeeding mothers to relax and thus foster effective functioning of the milk-ejection reflex (Lawrence, 1989). On the other hand, ethanol is a known inhibitor of oxytocin release (Fuchs and Wagner, 1963).

Two studies have demonstrated that the milk-ejection reflex can be at least partially blocked by maternal alcohol intake and that this effect is dose dependent (Cobo, 1973; Wagner and Fuchs, 1968). Wagner and Fuchs (1968) measured uterine contractions during suckling as an indicator of oxytocin release. At ethanol doses of 0.5 to 0.8 g/kg of maternal body weight, uterine activity was 62% of normal; at 0.9 to 1.1 g/kg, it was 32% of normal. Cobo (1973) measured the milk-ejection reflex by recording intraductal pressure in the mammary gland. He observed no effect of ethanol intake at doses below 0.5 g/kg; but the milk-ejection response was inhibited by 18.2, 63.2, and 80.4% at doses of 0.5 to 0.99, 1.0 to 1.49, and 1.5 to 1.99 g/kg, respectively. At 0.5 to 0.99 g/kg, this effect was not statistically significant, but at 1.0 to 1.49 g/kg, the milk-ejection reflex was completely blocked in 6 of the 14 subjects. The effect of alcohol on this reflex was not apparent when oxytocin was injected, indicating that the inhibition involved the release rather than the activity of oxytocin.

For an average woman weighing 60 kg (132 lb), an ethanol dose of 0.5 g/kg of body weight corresponds to approximately 2 to 2.5 oz of liquor, 8 oz of wine, or 2 cans of beer. Thus, these studies indicate that the adverse effects of alcohol consumption on the milk-ejection reflex are apparent only at relatively high intakes.

Oral Contraceptive Agents

The impact of oral contraceptive agents on lactation performance has been the subject of numerous studies (see reviews by Koetsawang [1987] and Lönnerdal [1986]). In the United States, 12.6% of lactating women who participated in the 1982 National Survey of Family Growth reported that they used oral contraceptives; this proportion was much higher among blacks (26.9%) than among whites (11.7%) (Ford and Labbok, 1987).

In providing guidance to women planning to use oral contraceptives, it is important to consider the composition and dosage of the pill and the intended duration of exclusive breastfeeding. In most studies conducted on the subject, the use of combined estrogen and progestin pills has been associated with reduced milk volume and duration of breastfeeding (Koetsawang, 1987; Lönnerdal, 1986). A recent multi-center, randomized double-blind trial in Hungary and Thailand demonstrated that even low-dose combined oral contraceptives (150 μg of levonorgestrel and 30 μg of ethinyl estradiol) have this effect: between 6 and 24 weeks post partum, the rate of milk volume decrease in women taking these pills was about twice the rate observed in control women (WHO Task Force on Oral Contraceptives, 1988). The nitrogen content of milk also was lower in those taking the combined pills, but there was no consistent effect on lactose or fat concentrations.

In contrast, no effect on milk volume or composition has been associated with progestin-only pills (Koestsawang, 1987; Lönnerdal, 1986; WHO Task Force on Oral Contraceptives, 1988). Although progesterone is known to inhibit lactogenesis, once lactation has been established it has no known inhibitory effect on milk production, possibly because progesterone binding sites are apparently not present in lactating tissues (Neville and Neifert, 1983). Further, there are substantial chemical differences between natural progesterone and synthetic progestins. Progestin-only pills have been found to be slightly less effective contraceptives than combined pills in studies of nonlactating women (Winikoff et al., 1988), but it is not known if this difference in effectiveness applies to lactating women as well. Progestin-only pills are also associated with altered menstrual cycles in nonlactating women, but the prevalence of this dysfunction is unknown in lactating women, who are likely to have a longer period of postpartum amenorrhea. For lactating women who wish to use oral contraceptives and maintain milk production, the World Health Organization states that progestin-only pills are the preferred choice (WHO Task Force on Oral Contraceptives, 1988).

Maternal Nutrition and Energy Balance

This section begins with consideration of maternal energy balance during lactation; this is followed by discussions of protein and fluid intakes. Studies on the influence of other nutrients have dealt primarily with milk composition, rather than volume, and are discussed in Chapter 6.

In its review, the subcommittee gave greatest weight to evidence with the greatest relevance to making causal inferences to human populations. Causal relationships can be most definitively demonstrated in intervention studies with randomized designs; however, very few studies of the effects of maternal nutrition on milk volume meet this criterion. Thus, the subcommittee also reviewed observational studies in humans, which are useful in establishing associations between factors, and studies in animals, which can suggest hypotheses to be tested in humans. The following sections begin with discussions of data on animals and progress to studies in humans, reflecting the chain in which evidence is usually accumulated.

In examining the evidence relating energy balance to milk volume, the subcommittee addressed three major questions:

• Is the volume of human milk affected if energy intake is curbed or supplemented during lactation?

• Do maternal fat stores or weight relative to height affect the relationship between energy deficit and milk volume?

• Are the mechanisms of energy utilization during lactation relevant to the volume of milk produced by lactating women?

Energy Restriction and Milk Volume

Several investigators have developed animal models of malnutrition during lactation, primarily in rats. Studies by Warman and Rasmussen (1983), Young and Rasmussen (1985), and Kliewer and Rasmussen (1987) illustrate that milk yield is decreased by dietary restriction and that the decrease is more pronounced in rats restricted before and during lactation than it is in those restricted only during lactation. Milk yield was reduced only 12.5% in dams fed 75% of ad libitum intake by controls, suggesting that the underfed animals compensated for dietary restriction in some way. In contrast, there was a dramatic (52%) decrease in milk yield in rats restricted to 50% of ad libitum intake (Young and Rasmussen, 1985). These results suggest that there may be a threshold below which lactation can no longer be protected when food intake is restricted. Similar findings have been reported by Roberts et al. (1985) in studies of baboons. Among animals restricted to 80% of ad libitum intake, milk output was not significantly reduced, whereas milk output decreased 20% in those restricted to 60% of ad libitum intake. Reduced physical activity may protect milk output at moderate levels of energy restriction but not at high levels, when body stores were shown to be mobilized at a rapid rate in the baboons. However, this possible effect of physical activity has not been studied.

The relative energy costs of lactation are much lower for humans than for most other species, and it is not known whether there is an energy threshold for humans. Prentice and Prentice (1988) report that energy costs at peak milk output, as a function of maternal body weight, are 4- to 15-fold lower for humans than for either laboratory or domesticated animals. For example, the energy requirements of lactation in humans can be met by increasing energy intake by approximately 25%, whereas in rats, energy intake must increase by

300% or more. Thus, a similar reduction in energy intake as a percentage of total intake is likely to result in a smaller decrease in milk volume of humans and other primates than of litter-bearing animals.

Observational studies of the relationship between maternal energy intake and milk volume in human populations have yielded mixed results. Despite much lower reported energy intakes among women in developing countries compared with their counterparts in industrialized countries, average milk volumes of both groups at 3 months post partum are similar (Prentice et al., 1986, see Figure 5-2). In industrialized countries, Strode et al. (1986) found no association between maternal energy intake and infant milk intake, whereas Butte et al. (1984a) and Prentice et al. (1986) reported a weak correlation in early lactation. Such an association may reflect reverse causation: women who produce more milk might consume more food because of greater appetite. (In rats, food intake is stimulated by lactation [Roberts and Coward, 1985] or by experimentally manipulating levels of serum prolactin [Moore et al., 1986].) In The Gambia, Prentice and colleagues (1986) found a striking association between seasonal patterns of maternal energy intake and infant milk intake but concluded that this association reflected changes in breastfeeding patterns and infant illnesses rather than maternal undernutrition.

There have been several attempts to document the effects of famine on milk volume, but quantitative data are generally lacking. Historical accounts of mothers breastfeeding during wartime sieges in Europe provide mostly anecdotal evidence of insufficient milk production among some women (Gunther, 1968). Dean (1951) reported that milk volume measured at a maternity clinic in Wuppertal, Germany, on the seventh day post partum was about 60 g lower during the war (1945-1946) than before it (1938). Severe undernutrition is widely regarded as detrimental to milk production, but there are very few supporting data.

Short-term fasting has been the subject of a few investigations. In The Gambia, Prentice et al. (1983c, 1984) reported that milk volume was unaffected in women during Ramadan, when no food or fluid is consumed from 5 a.m. to 7:30 p.m. (although intake after 7:30 p.m. may be considerable). Similarly, Neville and Oliva-Rasbach (1987) found that the rate of milk secretion was no different from the baseline among five lactating women who ate no food for 20 hours.

Strode and colleagues (1986) examined the effects of energy restriction among presumably well-nourished mothers. The experimental group reduced their energy intake by an average of 32% (range, 19 to 53%) below baseline intakes for 1 week; the control group maintained their usual intake. Among the eight mothers who restricted their intake to no less than 1,500 kcal/day, there was no reduction in milk intake by their infants, but levels of plasma prolactin tended to increase relative to those of control mothers. However, milk intakes by infants of the six mothers who decreased their energy intake below

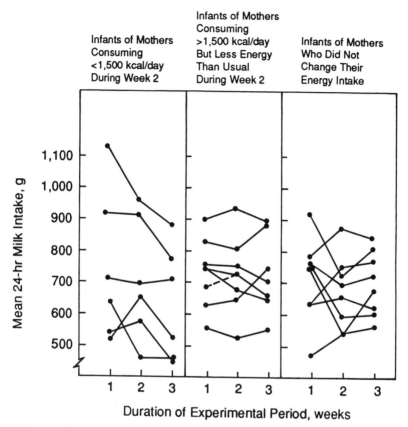

FIGURE 5-3   Change in mean milk intakes by individual infants (ages 6 to 24 weeks at week 1 of the experimental period) with change in maternal energy intake. The period of energy restriction for the mothers in the experimental group was week 2 of the 3-week experimental period. From Strode et al. (1986) with permission.

1,500 kcal/day were reduced by an average of 15% (109 g/day) during the week after restriction had ceased (Figure 5-3). Although prolactin levels before maternal energy restriction were not correlated with milk volume, there was a correlation between change in prolactin concentration after energy restriction and subsequent milk volume. The authors concluded that the impact of longer periods of energy restriction requires further investigation.

In a subsequent study (Dewey et al., in press), no relationship was found between maternal weight loss[1] from months 1 to 3 of lactation and milk volume at 3 months post partum; this confirmed the work of Butte et al. (1984a).

---

[1] Mean, 1 kg (∼2 lb); range, 0 to 6 kg (∼13 lb).

Although most of the women in these studies were not deliberately restricting their energy intake, they lost weight gradually during early lactation.

An energy deficit can also occur when energy expenditure is unusually high (in excess of energy intake). Lovelady and colleagues (1990) compared the lactation performance of eight physically fit, exercising women and eight sedentary controls. There were no significant differences in milk volume or composition despite wide group differences in energy intake and expenditure. Exercising subjects compensated for higher energy expenditure by increasing their energy intake,[2] so there was no net difference in energy deficit between groups.

Energy Supplementation During Lactation and Milk Volume

Studies in rats have been conducted to investigate the effects of dietary supplementation on milk production. Rolls et al. (1980) fed rats a high-energy, low-protein supplement in addition to their usual diet during lactation. They found that although maternal food intake increased among the supplemented compared with the control animals, litter growth rate was reduced, indicating a reduction in milk output. In contrast, Roberts and Coward (1985) provided adequately fed rats with a supplement with the same protein-to-energy ratio as that of their usual diet and observed a mean increase of 31% in milk output. On average, the rats in the latter study increased both their protein and energy intakes by 20%; therefore, it is not possible to distinguish between the effects of energy and those of protein on milk volume. In a study that is more analogous to energy supplementation trials in humans, Kliewer and Rasmussen (1987) restricted rats to 50% of usual energy intake before and during pregnancy and then allowed them to feed ad libitum during lactation. Milk volume and litter growth in this group were equivalent to those of control animals.

Findings from energy supplementation studies in humans are not conclusive. Many efforts have been made over the years to "feed the nursing mother, thereby the infant" (Sosa et al., 1976, p. 668) with mixed success. In a review of such studies up to 1980, Whitehead (1983) concludes that the results "have not been inspiring" (p. 44-45). The studies presented here are in chronologic order.

Rural Mexico. Several major investigations were conducted in Latin America and Asia during the 1960s and 1970s, but only one—a 2-year longitudinal study in a rural area of Mexico—included actual measurements of milk volume (Chávez and Martinez, 1980). In the first year of the study, one group of 17 mothers consuming their usual diet was followed throughout lactation. Milk

---

[2] Mean total energy intake was 2,739 kcal/day for the exercising subjects compared with 2,051 kcal/day for the sedentary controls.

volume was measured by the test-weighing technique in the mothers' homes for 72 consecutive hours on each of eight predetermined occasions.

In the second year of the study, another group of 17 women was followed in the same manner; however, these mothers received a food supplement providing 300 kcal and 20 g of protein per day during both pregnancy and lactation. Total mean energy intake was 2,365 kcal/day in the supplemented group, compared with the mean of 2,040 kcal/day in the unsupplemented group. (Infants in this second group were also given food supplements beginning at 3 months of age.) During the first 3 to 4 months, milk volume was 15% higher in the supplemented group than in the unsupplemented group, but the concentrations of energy, protein, and total solids in the milk were reportedly lower. Therefore, the supply of these nutrients was similar in the two groups. However, the milk sampling methods used by Chávez and Martinez (1980) were not described well enough to indicate whether the samples were representative of 24-hour production (see Chapter 6) and, thus, whether the milk energy density values were valid. Although maternal food supplementation began during pregnancy, infant weights at birth and afterward in the two groups were not compared.

The Gambia. A comprehensive food supplementation study was conducted in The Gambia between 1976 and 1982 (Prentice et al., 1983a,b). In the first phase, baseline dietary, anthropometric, and milk volume data were collected from 120 women throughout lactation. Milk volume was measured by 12-hour test weighing in the mothers's home at monthly intervals and validated against 24-hour measurements for a subsample of women. In the second phase, a food supplement was provided daily to 130 women at various stages of lactation, and the same measurements were taken. The supplement provided a net increase of 723 kcal daily and approximately 57 g of protein.

Although recent findings suggest that the absolute dietary intakes were underreported in the Gambian study (Singh et al., 1989), the estimated increase in energy intake provided by the food supplementation is likely to be reasonably accurate, and it is considerably higher than that provided by most other supplementation trials. Nevertheless, Prentice et al. (1983a) found no effect of food supplementation on milk volume at any stage of lactation. Milk volume declined during the wet season despite supplementation. Although supplemented women weighed 1.8 kg (4 lb) more than unsupplemented women, averaged over the whole year, the supplemented women still lost weight during the wet season (Prentice et al., 1983b). The range of variation (standard deviation) in milk volume was the same before and after supplementation, suggesting that energy supplementation did not even increase the milk volume of women with low milk volumes. The authors concluded, in hindsight, that the nutritional status of the Gambian women prior to food supplementation was not as poor as initially believed and, therefore, that the negative results are not surprising.

In the Gambian study, levels of maternal plasma hormones (prolactin, insulin, cortisol, and triiodothyronine) decreased significantly after supplementation, suggesting a decrease in metabolic efficiency in these mothers (Prentice et al., 1983b). The women also reported fewer gastrointestinal and respiratory illnesses after food supplementation. Lack of data on energy expenditure prevent estimation of energy balance in the Gambian women. However, prolonged high prolactin levels in marginally undernourished mothers may ensure milk synthesis by channeling nutrients to the breast (Lunn et al., 1980).

Although the Gambian study indicates that milk production tends to be maintained despite a limited food supply, it did not adequately test the hypothesis that maternal food supplementation can improve milk volume because of the following limitations in study design:

• For ethical reasons, the women could not be randomized into supplemented and control groups; the entire community was included in the project both before and after the initiation of supplementation. Thus, if changes occurred over time during the study, they may have obscured any effect of the supplement.

• The sample size was relatively small at any given time post partum and at any month of the year.

• The duration of supplementation varied because supplementation was begun all at once in the entire community, and women were at different stages of reproduction.

• Milk volume was measured for only 12 hours at each sampling point; a longer period would provide a more accurate estimate.

• Infants were also supplemented from age 3 to 12 months, which may have reduced milk volume (Prentice et al., 1986).

These limitations would generally reduce the chance of finding a statistically significant effect of food supplementation on milk volume. In addition, milk sampling methods were inadequate for estimating total milk energy output. Since there is evidence of an inverse relationship between milk volume and milk energy density (Nommsen et al., in press), total milk energy output is a more useful outcome measure than milk volume alone and may produce different results.

India. A small-scale study of dietary supplementation was conducted by Girija et al. (1984) on 20 low-income lactating women in India. The subjects were provided with a supplement contributing 417 kcal of energy and 30 g of protein per day beginning 10 days or less after delivery; another 20 women served as controls. Daytime breast milk volume measured by the test-weighing procedure was no different between the groups at 1 month post partum but was higher in the supplemented group at 3 months post partum (475 g/day compared with 328 g/day). However, feeding frequency averaged seven times per day for supplemented women compared with five times per day for controls. This difference suggests that weaning may have been initiated earlier in the control group. Thus, it is difficult to interpret the results of this study.

Burma. Results of a short-term study in Burma of 21 lactating women whose weight for height was less than 80% of standard (Naing and Oo, 1987) conflict with those found in the Gambian study. The Burmese women were randomly divided into food-supplemented ($N = 12$) and control ($N = 9$) groups. The food supplement was provided twice daily for 14 days and reportedly resulted in a large net increase of approximately 900 kcal and 39 g of protein per day—even though baseline intakes (2,425 kcal/day) were not low. Average milk volume, which was measured by the test-weighing method for 12 hours on 3 consecutive days before and after supplementation, increased significantly in the supplemented group (from 662 to 787 g/day) but not in the control group. The energy content of the milk was not measured.

The differences between the findings of the Burmese and Gambian projects may reflect short-term rather than long-term effects of changes in maternal nutrition on milk volume and the selection of low weight-for-height women in the Burmese study. The randomization design of the study by Naing and Oo does permit causal inference; however, the data they present are puzzling in two respects:

• The reported 900-kcal/day increase in maternal energy intake is much larger than most other supplementation studies have been able to achieve.

• Although a large difference in milk volume was reported after supplementation, there was no difference in the mean weight gain of supplemented and control infants (perhaps because the 14-day measurement period was too short to detect this).

For these reasons, further studies should be conducted in an attempt to replicate these findings.

Energy Supplementation During Pregnancy Only

To the subcommittee's knowledge, just one study has been conducted to examine the effect of supplementation only during pregnancy on subsequent milk volume. In this study, conducted in Indonesia, 53 women provided with a high-level energy supplement (465 kcal/day) during the last trimester of pregnancy did not produce any more milk than did 55 women given a low-level energy supplement (52 kcal/day). The findings are based on test weighings of milk intake for 48 consecutive hours at 8-week intervals from 2 to 7 weeks post partum (van Steenbergen et al., 1981). The birth weights of infants in the two groups were similar (3,010 ± 291 and 3,056 ± 298 g, respectively), as were maternal weight and body mass index prior to pregnancy and at 4 weeks post partum.

The authors concluded that short-term energy supplementation was ineffective, probably because the women included in the study were not at nutritional risk. (Their reported energy intakes of 1,570 to 1,617 kcal/day were suggestive of undernutrition, but their body mass index at 4 weeks post partum averaged 19, which is considered to be at the low end of the normal range.) Mean milk intakes of the exclusively breastfed infants in this population (686 to 830 g/day) were very similar to those of infants in industrialized countries.

Maternal Energy Reserves and Milk Volume

In theory, the energy stored as fat deposits during pregnancy is used to support milk production post partum, but there are few data with which to evaluate this relationship. Studies in animals have provided no consistent evidence of poor lactation performance resulting from poor prenatal nutrition alone (Kliewer and Rasmussen, 1987). Compared with controls, there was no statistically significant decrease in milk yield or litter weight at day 14 among rats fed 50% of ad libitum intakes before and during pregnancy but allowed to eat ad libitum during lactation. In cross-sectional studies of relatively well-nourished women in the United States, correlations between infant milk intake during the first 5 months post partum and maternal prepregnancy weight or pregnancy weight gain were not statistically significant (Butte et al., 1984a; Dewey et al., 1986). Although the range in prepregnancy weight for height was relatively wide (76 to 153% of desirable body weight) in these studies, very few of the women gained less than 11 kg (24 lb) during pregnancy.

In Indonesia, prepregnancy maternal body mass index was positively associated with milk intake of breastfed infants at 18 to 22 weeks post partum but not at 2 to 6, 10 to 14, or 26 to 30 weeks (controlling for infant birth weight did not change this association) (van Steenbergen et al., 1989). Few data have been reported in developing countries on the potential influence of pregnancy weight gain. Because maternal nutritional status (as indicated by weight for height) during pregnancy is strongly associated with nutritional status post partum, it is not possible to examine separately the influence of prenatal maternal body composition.

Mixed results have been obtained from observational studies of associations between indices of relative weight (such as body mass index) during lactation and milk volume in human populations. In industrialized countries, milk volume and maternal anthropometric variables have not been associated (Butte et al., 1984a; Dewey et al., 1986; Prentice et al., 1986). In developing countries, the situation is more complex. In an apparently undernourished population in Bangladesh, Brown et al. (1986b) found no statistically significant association between infant milk intake and maternal anthropometric variables, but they did report that milk energy output (the total energy value of the milk produced) was higher in women with greater arm circumference and triceps skinfold measurements. In that analysis, no adjustments were made for the potential influence of infant weight. However, in an analysis of data collected at different times for the same individuals, there was a significant association between increase in maternal body weight and increased milk volume even when the analysis was controlled for infant weight. Curiously, these mothers tended to gain weight during the first 3 months post partum, despite producing an average milk volume of 550 to 690 g/day.

In The Gambia, milk volume during the baseline period (before food supplementation) was positively correlated with maternal weight and height, but not when infant weight was included in the analysis (Prentice et al., 1986). In an earlier study of 16 lactating women in The Gambia, milk volume measured by 12-hour test weighing was inversely related to increases in maternal triceps and subscapular skinfold thicknesses during weeks 6 to 12 of lactation (Paul et al., 1979). This surprising finding was interpreted by the authors to indicate that there is competition between milk synthesis and replenishment of maternal fat stores during lactation.

The findings of other observational studies of maternal weight for height and milk volume are often difficult to interpret because they include infants who are not exclusively breastfed. For example, van Steenbergen et al. (1983) compared lactation performance of low weight-for-height women (70 to 80% of expected) in Kenya with the performance of normal-weight women (90 to 115% of expected) during the first 6 months post partum. In the low weight-for-height group, milk volume was found to be lower (695 compared with 790 g/day), but milk energy density was approximately 12% higher. In both groups, most infants were given supplementary foods, usually beginning in the third month. No data comparing only the exclusively breastfed infants were provided. In studies of mixed-fed infants, one cannot determine retrospectively whether low milk volume leads mothers to supplement early or whether early supplementation leads to low milk volumes.

The complaint of having an insufficient supply of milk for the baby is heard in both well-nourished and poorly nourished populations, but the incidence of this complaint was not related to maternal nutritional status in cross-cultural studies conducted by Tully and Dewey (1985).

Energy Utilization During Lactation

There are several potential mechanisms of energy conservation during lactation in addition to the mobilization and utilization of fat. Prentice and Prentice (1988) described three such "energy-sparing adaptations" that may permit lactation to proceed normally when energy intake is limited, including decreases in basal metabolic rate (BMR), thermogenesis, and physical activity. Whether these types of decreases should be considered adaptations is a matter of considerable debate.

There is conflicting evidence regarding whether BMR increases, decreases, or stays constant during lactation. Since the energy cost of milk synthesis is included within the BMR, one might predict BMR to increase slightly during lactation. Sadurskis et al. (1988) calculated an approximately 5.6% increase in BMR over prepregnancy values in the same women at 2 months of lactation, correcting for changes in body composition. Earlier studies in India also showed higher BMRs among lactating women than among nonlactating, "normal" Indian women (Khan and Belavady, 1973; Venkatachalam and Gopalan, 1960). In contrast, other investigators found lower BMRs during lactation than expected on the basis of weight and height (Blackburn and Calloway, 1985; Lovelady et al., 1990; Prentice and Whitehead, 1987; van Raaij et al., 1987) or no difference between lactating and nonlactating women (Illingworth et al., 1986; Schutz et al., 1980).

A 30% reduction in postprandial thermogenesis during lactation was observed in one study (Illingworth et al., 1986). This has little overall impact, however, since postprandial thermogenesis represents only about 10% of total energy expenditure, and thus, only about 60 kcal is saved per day.

There is considerable variation in the degree to which energy expenditure for activity could be reduced during lactation. During the postpartum period, the demands of feeding and caring for an infant take up considerable time but may require either more or less energy than the woman's former activities. Total activity levels of lactating mothers may be constrained by being housebound with a new baby. Data from small samples of relatively sedentary lactating women in the United States indicate that total energy expenditure (not including milk production) averages only 1,800 to 1,900 kcal/day (Blackburn and Calloway, 1976; Lovelady et al., 1990); the estimated expenditure for nonlactating women, assuming light to moderate activity, is 2,200 kcal/day (NRC, 1989). In contrast, lactating women exercising on a regular basis expended an average of 2,631 kcal/day, not including energy output in milk (Lovelady et al., 1990). Women who must care for several children or who are employed in physically demanding jobs may also have high activity levels. Mothers who do not have access to adequate food cannot always decrease their workload to reduce their energy deficit (Singh et al., 1989). If these mothers decrease other day-to-day activities as an energy-sparing mechanism, there may be adverse effects on their quality of life.

Maternal Protein Intake

Studies in lactating rats (Jansen and Monte, 1977; Naismith et al., 1982; Sampson and Jansen, 1985) and in swine (Mahan, 1977) indicate that protein intake can increase milk volume independently of total energy intake. Early studies in humans by Gopalan (1958) and Edozien et al. (1976) suggest the same relationship: milk output of women in India and Nigeria increased when protein intake was increased from 50 to 60 g/day to approximately 100 g/day. Increasing protein above 100 g/day caused no further change in milk volume. In both studies, however, the samples were very small (N = 6 and 8, respectively), there were no control groups, and their designs may have biased the results. In the Indian study, protein intake was increased in stages from 61 to 99 to 114 g/day in three successive 10-day periods, and milk samples were obtained by complete expression of both breasts at the 10 a.m. feeding during the last 3 days of each period. Because milk intake may increase with the age of the infants and repeated expression of extra milk may stimulate greater milk production (Dewey and Lönnerdal, 1986), milk volumes may have increased during the study for these reasons rather than in response to increased maternal protein intake. In the Nigerian study, total milk volume was calculated by measuring infant intake and by pumping residual milk after each feeding for each of the 7-day measurement periods. The extra stimulation provided by removing residual milk may have increased milk production.

In two small-scale studies of well-nourished women whose usual protein intake ranged from approximately 80 to 100 g/day, no statistically significant changes in milk volume were observed when protein intake was reduced to 8% of total calories or increased to 20% of total calories for 4 days (Forsum and Lönnerdal, 1980) or when daily protein intake was either 1.0 or 1.5 g/kg of body weight for 7 to 10 days (Motil et al., 1986). However, the very small sample sizes (N = 3 and 15, respectively) and short duration of these studies preclude any definitive conclusions regarding the impact of varying protein intake.

Fluid Intake

It is widely assumed that milk production requires a high fluid intake on the part of the mother, yet the evidence suggests that lactating women can tolerate a considerable amount of water restriction and that supplemental fluids have little effect on milk volume. Lactating women who consumed no food or fluids from 5:00 a.m. to 7:30 p.m. during Ramadan lost 7.6% of their total body water and experienced increases in serum indices of dehydration, although values remained within the normal range (Prentice et al., 1984). Milk volume was unaffected, but changes in milk composition (lower lactose concentrations; increased osmolality due to higher electrolyte concentrations) indicated alterations in mammary cell permeability. Water turnover was very high, in part because the women apparently superhydrated themselves overnight prior to the fasting period.

Two early studies from Germany (Olsen, 1941) and France (Lelong et al., 1949) also showed no influence on milk output when fluid intake ranged from 600 to 2,775 ml/day during 3- to 4-day periods or when total fluid intake from all sources was restricted to 1,765 ml/day for 10 days. Dusdieker et al. (1985) examined the effect produced by increasing fluid intake by at least 25% for 3

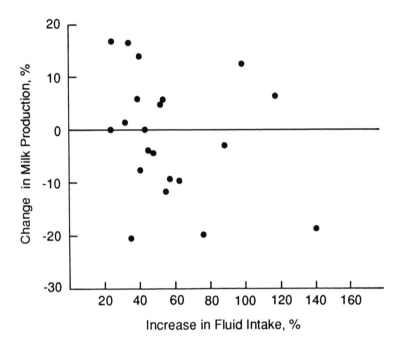

FIGURE 5-4   Relationship between increase in maternal fluid intake for 3 days and percent change in milk production. From Dusdieker et al. (1985) with permission.

days among 21 lactating women in the United States and found no change in milk volume and no correlation between fluid intake and milk volume (Figure 5-4).

In an earlier study, Illingworth and Kilpatrick (1953) asked 104 lactating women to drink at least 2,880 ml of liquid per day (high-fluids group) and 106 control women to drink as much as desired. In the first 9 days post partum, actual fluid intake averaged approximately 3,200 ml/day in the high-fluids group and about 2,100 ml/day in the control group. Neither infant growth in the first month nor duration of breastfeeding differed between groups. Milk intake at a test feed on the eighth day post partum tended to be lower in the high-fluids group. The authors thus cautioned against drinking fluids in excess of natural thirst inclination. However, thirst may sometimes function too slowly to prevention dehydration among women with high fluid losses resulting from exercise or high ambient temperature (experienced by many women without air conditioning in the summer). Thus, careful attention to adequacy of fluid intake is warranted in such situations, but under most conditions there appears to be no justification for emphasizing high fluid intake as a way to improve milk production.

CONCLUSIONS

- Studies conducted in the United States, other developed countries, and developing countries indicate that the average level of milk production is approximately 750 to 800 ml/day in women with widely varying dietary intakes and with varying nutritional status, as measured by weight and skinfold thickness.

- Potential production of milk by lactating women appears to be considerably higher than actual intakes by single infants, as indicated by the high milk volumes produced by women nursing twins or even triplets.

- Factors other than maternal nutrition affect milk volume and should be considered in any evaluation of lactation performance. Maternal age and parity appear to have little, if any, influence, but variables such as maternal stress and the nursing behavior of both mother and infant are potentially important.

- Maternal nutritional status, as measured by anthropometric indices prenatally or post partum, is not related to milk volume in studies conducted in industrialized countries such as the United States. In other words, infants of thin women generally consume as much breast milk as infants of normal-weight or overweight women. In less developed countries, the results are mixed; some studies show a positive association between maternal body composition (adiposity) and milk volume.

- Average milk volumes of lactating women are comparable in industrialized and developing countries, despite substantial differences in energy and nutrient intake. This suggests that maternal energy intake is not strongly associated with milk volume. Studies in animals indicate that there may be a threshold below which energy intake is insufficient to support normal milk production; it is likely that most studies in humans have been conducted in groups with intakes above this hypothesized threshold.

- Food supplementation of lactating women in areas where malnutrition is prevalent has generally had little, if any, impact on milk volume. However, such supplementation may improve maternal health and therefore is more likely to benefit the mother than the infant, except in cases in which milk composition is affected (see Chapter 6).

- It is customary to lose weight gradually during lactation. In the United States, lactating women tend to be heavier than their ideal body weight immediately post partum, and some successfully lose up to 2 kg (~4.5 lb) per month with no apparent deleterious effects on milk production.

- Women who exercise regularly appear to produce an adequate volume of milk.

- The influence of maternal intake of specific nutrients on milk volume has not been investigated thoroughly. Early studies in developing countries show an association of protein intake with milk volume, but limitations of the study designs prohibit definitive conclusions.

- Adequate fluid intake during lactation is desirable to maintain maternal health, but supplemental fluids consumed in excess of natural thirst have no effect on milk volume.

RECOMMENDATIONS FOR CLINICAL PRACTICE

- Advise women that the average rate of weight loss post partum (0.5 to 1.0 kg, or 1 to 2 lb, per month after the first month) appears to be consistent with maintaining adequate milk volume. If a lactating woman is overweight, a weight loss of up to 2 kg (~4.5 lb) per month is unlikely to adversely affect milk volume, but such women should be alert for any indications that the infant's appetite is not being satisfied. Rapid weight loss (>2 kg/month after the first month post partum) is not advisable for breastfeeding women.
- The level of physical activity needs to be considered when advising women about adequacy of energy intake during lactation. Intakes below 1,500 kcal/day are not recommended at any time during lactation, although brief fasts (lasting less than 1 day) are unlikely to decrease milk volume. Liquid diets and weight loss medications are not recommended.
- Since the impact of curtailing maternal energy intake during the first 2 to 3 weeks post partum is unknown, dieting during this period is not recommended.
- If alcohol is used, advise the lactating woman to limit her intake to no more than 0.5 g of alcohol per kg of maternal body weight per day. Intake over this level may impair the milk ejection reflex. For a 60-kg (132-lb) woman, 0.5 g of alcohol per kg of body weight corresponds to approximately 2 to 2.5 oz of liquor, 8 oz of table wine, or 2 cans of beer.
- Actively discourage cigarette smoking among lactating women, not only because it may reduce milk volume but because of its other harmful effects on the mother and her infant.
- Discourage intake of large quantities of coffee, other caffeine-containing beverages and medications, and decaffeinated coffee.
- Because the early management of lactation has a strong influence on the establishment of an adequate milk supply, breastfeeding guidance should be provided prenatally and continued in the hospital after delivery and during the early postpartum period.
- Promote breastfeeding practices that are responsive to the infant's natural appetite. In the first few weeks, infants should nurse at least 8 times per day, and some may nurse as often as 15 or more times per day. After the first month, infants fed on demand usually nurse 5 to 12 times per day.

REFERENCES

Andersen, A.N., C. Lund-Andersen, J.F. Larsen, N.J. Christensen, J.J. Legros, F. Louis, H. Angelo, and J. Molin. 1982. Suppressed prolactin but normal neurophysin levels in cigarette smoking breast-feeding women. Clin. Endocrinol. 17:363-368.

Blackburn, M.W., and D.H. Calloway. 1976. Energy expenditure and consumption of mature, pregnant and lactating women. J. Am. Diet. Assoc. 69:29-37.

Blackburn, M.W., and D.H. Calloway. 1985. Heart rate and energy expenditure of pregnant and lactating women. Am. J. Clin. Nutr. 42:1161-1169.

Blake, C.A., and C.H. Sawyer. 1972. Nicotine blocks the suckling-induced rise in circulating prolactin in lactating rats. Science 177:619-621.

Brown, K.H., R.E. Black, A.D. Robertson, N.A. Akhtar, G. Ahmed, and S. Becker. 1982. Clinical and field studies of human lactation: methodological considerations. Am. J. Clin. Nutr. 35:745-756.

Brown, K.H., A.D. Robertson, and N.A. Akhtar. 1986a. Lactational capacity of marginally nourished mothers: infants' milk nutrient consumption and patterns of growth. Pediatrics 78:920-927.

Brown, K.H., N.A. Akhtar, A.D. Robertson, and M.G. Ahmed. 1986b. Lactational capacity of marginally nourished mothers: relationships between maternal nutritional status and quantity and proximate composition of milk. Pediatrics 78:909-919.

Brown, K.H., R.Y. Stallings, H. Creed de Kanashiro, G. Lopez de Romaña, and R.E. Black. In press. Effects of common illnesses on infants' energy intakes from breast milk and other foods during longitudinal community-based studies in Huascar (Lima), Peru. Am. J. Clin. Nutr.

Butte, N.F., and D.H. Calloway. 1981. Evaluation of lactational performance of Navajo women. Am. J. Clin. Nutr. 34:2210-2215.

Butte, N.F., and C. Garza. 1985. Energy and protein intakes of exclusively breastfed infants during the first four months of life. Pp. 63-83 in M. Gracey and F. Falkner, eds. Nutritional Needs and Assessment of Normal Growth. Raven Press, New York.

Butte, N.F., C. Garza, J.E. Stuff, E.O. Smith, and B.L. Nichols. 1984a. Effect of maternal diet and body composition on lactational performance. Am. J. Clin. Nutr. 39:296-306.

Butte, N.F., C. Garza, E.O. Smith, and B.L. Nichols. 1984b. Human milk intake and growth in exclusively breast-fed infants. J. Pediatr. 104:187-195.

Butte, N.F., W.W. Wong, B.W. Patterson, C. Garza, and P.D. Klein. 1988. Human-milk intake measured by administration of deuterium oxide to the mother: a comparison with the test-weighing technique. Am. J. Clin. Nutr. 47:815-821.

Casey, C.E., M.R. Neifert, J.M. Seacat, and M.C. Neville. 1986. Nutrient intake by breast-fed infants during the first five days after birth. Am. J. Dis. Child. 140:933-936.

Chandra, R.K. 1981. Breast feeding, growth and morbidity. Nutr. Res. 1:25-31.

Chávez, A., and C. Martinez. 1980. Effects of maternal undernutrition and dietary supplementation on milk production. Pp. 274-284 in H. Aebi and R. Whitehead, eds. Maternal Nutrition During Pregnancy and Lactation. Hans Huber, Bern.

Cobo, E. 1973. Effect of different doses of ethanol on the milk-ejecting reflex in lactating women. Am. J. Obstet. Gynecol. 115:817-821.

Coward, W.A., T.J. Cole, H. Guber, S.B. Roberts, and I. Fleet. 1982. Water turnover and measurement of milk intake. Pflugers. Arch. 393:344-347.

Coward, W.A., A.A. Paul, and A.M. Prentice. 1984. The impact of malnutrition on human lactation: observations from community studies. Fed. Proc., Fed. Am. Soc. Exp. Biol. 43:2432-2437.

Cross, B.A. 1955. The hypothalamus and the mechanism of sympathetico-adrenal inhibition of milk ejection. J. Endocrinol. 12:15-28.

Dean, R.F.A. 1951. The size of the baby at birth and the yield of breast milk. Med. Res. Counc. (G. B.), Spec. Rep. Ser. 275:346-378.

de Carvalho, M., S. Robertson, R. Merkatz, and M. Klaus. 1982. Milk intake and frequency of feeding in breast fed infants. Early Hum. Dev. 7:155-163.

de Carvalho, M., S. Robertson, A. Friedman, and M. Klaus. 1983. Effect of frequent breast-feeding on early milk production and infant weight gain. Pediatrics 72:307-311.

de Carvalho, M., D.M. Anderson, A. Giangreco, and W.B. Pittard III. 1985. Frequency of milk expression and milk production by mothers of nonnursing premature neonates. Am. J. Dis. Child. 139:483-485.

Dewey, K.G., and M.J. Heinig. 1987. Does 4-day test-weighing to determine breast milk intake affect nursing frequency? Fed. Proc., Fed. Am. Soc. Exp. Biol. 46:571.

Dewey, K.G., and B. Lönnerdal. 1983. Milk and nutrient intake of breast-fed infants from 1 to 6 months: Relation to growth and fatness. J. Pediatr. Gastroenterol. Nutr. 2:497-506.

Dewey, K.G., and B. Lönnerdal. 1986. Infant self-regulation of breast milk intake. Acta Paediatr. Scand. 75:893-898.

Dewey, K.G., D.A. Finley, and B. Lönnerdal. 1984. Breast milk volume and composition during late lactation (7-20 months). J. Ped. Gastroenterol. Nutr. 3:713-720.

Dewey, K.G., D.A. Finley, M.A. Strode, and B. Lönnerdal. 1986. Relationship of maternal age to breast milk volume and composition. Pp. 263-273 in M. Hamosh and A.S. Goldman, eds. Human Lactation 2: Maternal and Environmental Factors. Plenum Press, New York.

Dewey, K.G., M.J. Heinig, L.A. Nommsen, and B. Lönnerdal. In press. Maternal vs. infant factors related to breast milk intake and residual milk volume: the DARLING study. Pediatrics.

Dusdieker, L.B., B.M. Booth, P.J. Stumbo, and J.M. Eichenberger. 1985. Effect of supplemental fluids on human milk production. J. Pediatr. 106:207-211.

Edozien, J.C., M.A.R. Khan, and C.I. Waslien. 1976. Human protein deficiency: results of a Nigerian village study. J. Nutr. 106:312-328.

Egli, G.E., N.S. Egli, and M. Newton. 1961. The influence of the number of breast feedings on milk production. Pediatrics 27:314-317.

Feher, S.D.K., L.R. Berger, J.D. Johnson, and J.B. Wilde. 1989. Increasing breast milk production for premature infants with a relaxation/imagery audiotape. Pediatrics 83:57-60.

Ferry, J.D., B.K. McLean, and M.B. Nikitovitch-Winer. 1974. Tobacco-smoke inhalation delays suckling-induced prolactin release in the rat. Proc. Soc. Exp. Biol. Med. 147:110-113.

Fjeld, C.R., K.H. Brown, and D.A. Schoeller. 1988. Validation of the deuterium oxide method for measuring average daily milk intake in infants. Am. J. Clin. Nutr. 48:671-679.

Ford, K., and M. Labbok. 1987. Contraceptive usage during lactation in the United States: an update. Am. J. Public Health 77:79-81.

Forsum, E., and B. Lönnerdal. 1980. Effect of protein intake on protein and nitrogen composition of breast milk. Am. J. Clin. Nutr. 33:1809-1813.

Fuchs, A., and G. Wagner. 1963. The effect of ethyl alcohol on the release of oxytocin in rabbits. Acta Endocrinol. 44:593-605.

Girija, A., P. Geervani, and R.G. Rao. 1984. Influence of dietary supplementation during lactation on lactation performance. J. Trop. Pediatr. 30:140-144.

Goldfarb, J., and E. Tibbetts. 1989. Breastfeeding Handbook: A Practical Reference for Physicians, Nurses, and Other Health Professionals. Enslow, Hillside, N.J. 256 pp.

Gopalan, C. 1958. Studies on lactation in poor Indian communities. J. Trop. Pediatr. 4:87-97.

Gunther, M. 1968. Diet and milk secretion in women. Proc. Nutr. Soc. 27:77-82.

Hamosh, M., M.R. Simon, and P. Hamosh. 1979. Effect of nicotine on the development of fetal and suckling rats. Biol. Neonate 35:290-297.

Hofvander, Y., U. Hagman, C. Hillervik, and S. Sjölin. 1982. The amount of milk consumed by 1-3 months old breast- or bottle-fed infants. Acta Paediatr. Scand. 71:953-958.

Hopkinson, J.M., R.J. Schanler, and C. Garza. 1988. Milk production by mothers of premature infants. Pediatrics 81:815-820.

Horrobin, D. 1979. Prolactin. Annual Research Reviews, X. Vol. 7. Eden Press, St. Albans, Vt. 126 pp.

Hytten, F.E. 1954. Clinical and chemical studies in human lactation. VIII. Relationship of the age, physique, and nutritional status of the mother to the yield and composition of her milk. Br. Med. J. 2:844-845.

Hytten, F.E., and A.M. Thomson. 1961. Nutrition of the lactating woman. Pp. 3-46 in Kon, S.K., and A.T. Cowie, eds. Milk: the Mammary Gland and Its Secretion. Academic Press, New York.

Illingworth, R.S., and B. Kilpatrick. 1953. Lactation and fluid intake. Lancet 2:1175-1177.

Illingworth, P.J., R.T. Jung, P.W. Howie, P. Leslie, and T.E. Isles. 1986. Diminution in energy expenditure during lactation. Br. Med. J. 292:437-441.

IOM (Institute of Medicine). 1990. Nutrition During Pregnancy: Weight Gain and Nutrient Supplements. Report of the Subcommittee on Nutritional Status and Weight Gain During Pregnancy, Subcommittee on Dietary Intake and Nutrient Supplements During Pregnancy, Committee on Nutritional Status During Pregnancy and Lactation, Food and Nutrition Board. National Academy Press, Washington, D.C. 468 pp.

Janas, L.M., and M.F. Picciano. 1986. Quantities of amino acids ingested by human milk-fed infants. J. Pediatr. 109:802-807.

Janas, L.M., M.F. Picciano, and T.F. Hatch. 1985. Indices of protein metabolism in term infants fed human milk, whey-predominant formula, or cow's milk formula. Pediatrics 75:775-784.

Jansen, G.R., and W.C. Monte. 1977. Amino acid fortification of bread fed at varying levels during gestation and lactation in rats. J. Nutr. 107:300-309.

Jansen, A.A.J., R. Luyken, S.H. Malcom, and J.J.L. Willems. 1960. Quantity and composition of breast milk in Baik Island (Neth. New Quinea). Trop. Geog. Med. 2:138-144.

Kaucher, M., E.Z. Moyer, A.J. Richards, H.H. Williams, A.L. Wertz, and I.G. Macy. 1945. Human milk studies. XX. The diet of lactating women and the collection and preparation of food and human milk for analysis. Am. J. Dis. Child. 70:142-147.

Khan, L., and B. Belavady. 1973. Basal metabolism in pregnant and nursing women and children. Indian J. Med. Res. 61:1853-1860.

Kliewer, R.L., and K.M. Rasmussen. 1987. Malnutrition during the reproductive cycle: effects on galactopoietic hormones and lactational performance in the rat. Am. J. Clin. Nutr. 46:926-935.

Koetsawang, S. 1987. The effects of contraceptive methods on the quality and quantity of breast milk. Int. J. Gynaecol. Obstet. 25 Suppl.:115-127.

Lawrence, R.A. 1985. Breastfeeding: A Guide for the Medical Profession, 2nd ed. C.V. Mosby, St. Louis. 601 pp.

Lawrence, R.A. 1989. Breastfeeding: A Guide for the Medical Profession, 3rd ed. C.V. Mosby, St. Louis. 652 pp.

Lelong, M., F. Alison, and J. Vinceneux. 1949. Secretion lactee humaine et alimentation hydrique. Lait 29:237-246.

Lipsman, S., K.G. Dewey, and B. Lönnerdal. 1985. Breast-feeding among teenage mothers: milk composition, infant growth, and maternal dietary intake. J. Pediatr. Gastroenterol. Nutr. 4:426-434.

Lönnerdal, B. 1986. Effect of oral contraceptives on lactation. Pp. 453-465 in M. Hamosh and A.S. Goldman, eds. Human Lactation 2: Maternal and Environmental Factors. Plenum Press, New York.

Lönnerdal, B., E. Forsum, M. Gebre-Medhin, and L. Hambraeus. 1976. Breast milk composition in Ethiopian and Swedish mothers. II. Lactose, nitrogen. and protein contents. Am. J. Clin. Nutr. 29:1134-1141.

Lovelady, C.A., B. Lönnerdal, and K.G. Dewey. 1990. Lactation performance of exercising women. Am. J. Clin. Nutr. 52:103-109.

Lunn, P.G., A.M. Prentice, S. Austin, and R.G. Whitehead. 1980. Influence of maternal diet on plasma-prolactin levels during lactation. Lancet 1:623-625.

Lunn, P.G., S. Austin, A.M. Prentice, and R.G. Whitehead. 1984. The effect of improved nutrition on plasma prolactin concentrations and postpartum infertility in lactating Gambian women. Am. J. Clin. Nutr. 39:227-235.

Lyon, A.J. 1983. Effects of smoking on breast feeding. Arch. Dis. Child. 58:378-380.

Macy, I.G., H.A. Hunscher, E. Donelson, and B. Nims. 1930. Human milk flow. Am. J. Dis. Child. 39:1186-1204.

Mahan, D.C. 1977. Effect of feeding various gestation and lactation dietary protein sequences on long-term reproductive performance in swine. J. Anim. Sci. 45:1061-1072.

Martin, R.H. 1983. The place of PRL in human lactation. Clin. Endocrinol. 18:295-299.

Matheson, I., and G.N. Rivrud. 1989. The effect of smoking on lactation and infantile colic. J. Am. Med. Assoc. 26:42-43.

Moore, B.J., T. Gerardo-Gettens, B.A. Horwitz, and J.S. Stern. 1986. Hyperprolactine-mia stimulates food intake in the female rat. Brain Res. Bull. 17:563-569.

Motil, K.J., C.M. Montandon, and C. Garza. 1986. Effect of dietary protein intake on milk production in lactating women. Am. J. Clin. Nutr. 43:677.

NRC (National Research Council). 1989. Recommended Dietary Allowances, 10th ed. Report of the Subcommittee on the Tenth Edition of the RDAs, Food and Nutrition Board, Commission on Life Sciences. National Academy Press, Washington, D.C. 284 pp.

Naing, K.M., and T.T. Oo. 1987. Effect of dietary supplementation on lactation performance of undernourished Burmese mothers. Food Nutr. Bull. 9:59-61.

Naismith, D.J., D.P. Richardson, and A.E. Pritchard. 1982. The utilization of protein and energy during lactation in the rat, with particular regard to the use of fat accumulated in pregnancy. Br. J. Nutr. 48:433-441.

Neifert, M.R., and J.M. Seacat. 1986. Mammary gland anomalies and lactation failure. Pp. 293-299 in M. Hamosh and A.S. Goldman, eds. Human Lactation 2: Maternal and Environmental Factors. Plenum Press, New York.

Neifert, M.R., S.L. McDonough, and M.C. Neville. 1981. Failure of lactogenesis associated with placental retention. Am. J. Obstet. Gynecol. 140:477-478.

Neville, M.C., and M.R. Neifert, eds. 1983. Lactation: Physiology, Nutrition, and Breast-Feeding. Plenum Press, New York. 466 pp.

Neville, M., and J. Oliva-Rasbach. 1987. Is maternal milk production limiting for infant growth during the first year of life in breast-fed infants? Pp. 123-133 in A.S. Goldman, S.A. Atkinson, and L.A. Hanson, eds. Human Lactation 3: The Effects of Human Milk on the Recipient Infant. Plenum Press, New York.

Neville, M.C., R. Keller, J. Seacat, V. Lutes, M. Neifert, C. Casey, J. Allen, and P. Archer. 1988. Studies in human lactation: milk volumes in lactating women during the onset of lactation and full lactation. Am. J. Clin. Nutr. 48:1375-1386.

Newton, M., and N.R. Newton. 1948. The let-down reflex in human lactation. J. Pediatr. 33:698-704.

Newton, N.R., and M. Newton. 1950. Relation of the let-down reflex to the ability to breast feed. Pediatrics 5:726-733.

Noel, G.L., H.K. Suh, and A.G. Frantz. 1974. Prolactin release during nursing and breast stimulation in postpartum and nonpostpartum subjects. J. Clin. Endocrinol. Metab. 38:413-423.

Nommsen, L.A., M.J. Heinig, B. Lönnerdal, and K.G. Dewey. 1989. Appropriate timing of complementary feeding of breast-fed infants. FASEB J. 3:A1054 (abstract).

Nommsen, L.A., C.A. Lovelady, M.J. Heinig, B. Lönnerdal, and K.G. Dewey. In press. Determinants of energy, protein, lipid and lactose concentrations in human milk during the first 12 mo of lactation: The DARLING Study. Am. J. Clin. Nutr.

Olsen, A. 1941. Om diegivningsevnen under torst og under extradrikning. Ugeskr. Laeg. 103:897-905.

Pao, E.M., J.M. Himes, and A.F. Roche. 1980. Milk intakes and feeding patterns of breast-fed infants. J. Am. Diet. Assoc. 77:540-545.

Paul, A.A., E.M. Muller, and R.G. Whitehead. 1979. The quantitative effects of maternal dietary energy intake on pregnancy and lactation in rural Gambian women. Trans. R. Soc. Trop. Med. Hyg. 73:686-692.

Picciano, M.F., E.J. Calkins, J.R. Garrick, and R.H. Deering. 1981. Milk and mineral intakes of breastfed infants. Acta Paediatr. Scand. 70:189-194.

Pollitt, E., M. Gilmore, and M. Valcarcel. 1978. The stability of sucking behavior and its relationship to intake during the first month of life. Infant Behav. Dev. 1:347-357.

Prentice, A.M. 1980. Variations in maternal dietary intake, birthweight and breast-milk output in The Gambia. Pp. 167-183 in Aebi, H. and R.G. Whitehead, eds. Maternal Nutrition During Pregnancy and Lactation. Hans Huber Publishers, Bern, Switzerland.

Prentice, A. 1986. The effect of maternal parity on lactational performance in a rural African community. Pp. 165-173 in M. Hamosh and A.S. Goldman, eds. Human Lactation 2: Maternal and Environmental Factors. Plenum Press, New York.

Prentice, A.M., and A. Prentice. 1988. Energy costs of lactation. Annu. Rev. Nutr. 8:63-79.

Prentice, A.M., and R.G. Whitehead. 1987. The energetics of human reproduction. Symp. Zool. Soc. London 57:275-304.

Prentice, A.M., S.B. Roberts, A. Prentice, A.A. Paul, M. Watkinson, A.A. Watkinson, and R.G. Whitehead. 1983a. Dietary supplementation of lactating Gambian women. I. Effect on breast-milk volume and quality. Hum. Nutr.: Clin. Nutr. 37C:53-64.

Prentice, A.M., P.G. Lunn, M. Watkinson, and R.G. Whitehead. 1983b. Dietary supplementation of lactating Gambian women. II. Effect on maternal health, nutritional status and biochemistry. Hum. Nutr.: Clin. Nutr. 37C:65-74.

Prentice, A.M., A. Prentice, W.H. Lamb, P.G. Lunn, and S. Austin. 1983c. Metabolic consequences of fasting during Ramadan in pregnant and lactating women. Hum. Nutr.: Clin. Nutr. 37C:283-294.

Prentice, A.M., W.H. Lamb, A. Prentice, and W.A. Coward. 1984. The effect of water abstention on milk synthesis in lactating women. Clin. Sci. 66:291-298.

Prentice, A., A. Paul, A. Prentice, A. Black, T. Cole, and R. Whitehead. 1986. Cross-cultural differences in lactational performance. Pp. 13-44 in M. Hamosh and A.S. Goldman, eds. Human Lactation 2: Maternal and Environmental Factors. Plenum Press, New York.

Rattigan, S., A.V. Ghisalberti, and P.E. Hartmann. 1981. Breast-milk production in Australian women. Br. J. Nutr. 45:243-249.

Roberts, S.B., and W.A. Coward. 1985. Dietary supplementation increases milk output in the rat. Br. J. Nutr. 53:1-9.

Roberts, S.B., T.J. Cole, and W.A. Coward. 1985. Lactational performance in relation to energy intake in the baboon. Am. J. Clin. Nutr. 41:1270-1276.

Rolls, B.J., E.A. Rowe, S.E. Fahrbach, L. Agius, and D.H. Williamson. 1980. Obesity and high energy diets reduce survival and growth rates of rat pups. Proc. Nutr. Soc. 39:51A.

Sadurskis, A., N. Kabir, J. Wager, and E. Forsum. 1988. Energy metabolism, body composition, and milk production in healthy Swedish women during lactation. Am. J. Clin. Nutr. 48:44-49.

Saint, L., M. Smith, and P.E. Hartmann. 1984. The yield and nutrient content of colostrum and milk of women giving birth to 1 month post-partum. Br. J. Nutr. 52:87-95.

Saint, L., P. Maggiore, and P.E. Hartmann. 1986. Yield and nutrient content of milk in eight women breast-feeding twins and one woman breast-feeding triplets. Br. J. Nutr. 56:49-58.

Salariya, E.M., P.M. Easton, and J.I. Cater. 1978. Duration of breast-feeding after early initiation and frequent feeding. Lancet 2:1141-1143.

Salmenperä, L., J. Perheentupa, and M. Siimes. 1985. Exclusively breast-fed healthy infants grow slower than reference infants. Pediatr. Res. 19:307-312.

Sampson, D.A., and G.R. Jansen. 1985. The effect of dietary protein quality and feeding level on milk secretion and mammary protein synthesis in the rat. J. Pediatr. Gastroenterol. Nutr. 4:274-283.

Schutz, Y., A. Lechtig, and R. Bradfield. 1980. Energy expenditures and food intakes of lactating women in Guatemala. Am. J. Clin. Nutr. 33:892-902.

Singh, J., A.M. Prentice, E. Diaz, W.A. Coward, J. Ashford, M. Sawyer, and R.G. Whitehead. 1989. Energy expenditure of Gambian women during peak agricultural activity measured by the doubly-labelled water method. Br. J. Nutr. 62:315-329.

Sosa, R., M. Klaus, and J.J. Urrutia. 1976. Feed the nursing mother, thereby the infant. J. Pediatr. 88:668-670.

Strode, M.A., K.G. Dewey, and B. Lönnerdal. 1986. Effects of short-term caloric restriction on lactational performance of well-nourished women. Acta Paediatr. Scand. 75:222-229.

Stuff, J.E., and B.L. Nichols. 1989. Nutrient intake and growth performance of older infants fed human milk. J. Pediatr. 115:959-968.

Stuff, J.E., C. Garza, C. Boutte, J.K. Fraley, E.O. Smith, E.R. Klein, and B.L. Nichols. 1986. Sources of variance in milk and calorie intakes in breast-fed infants: implications for lactation study design and interpretation. Am. J. Clin. Nutr. 43:361-366.

Terkel, J., C.A. Blake, V. Hoover, and C.H. Sawyer. 1973. Pup survival and prolactin levels in nicotine-treated lactating rats. Proc. Soc. Exp. Biol. Med. 143:1131-1135.

Tully, J., and K.G. Dewey. 1985. Private fears, global loss: a cross-cultural study of the insufficient milk syndrome. Med. Anthropol. 9:225-243.

Tyson, J.E., J.N. Carter, B. Andreassen, J. Huth, and B. Smith. 1978. Nursing-mediated prolactin and luteinizing hormone secretion during puerperal lactation. Fertil. Steril. 30:154-162.

van Raaij, J.M.A., M.E.M. Peek, S.H. Vermaat-Miedema, C.M. Schonk, and J.G.A.J. Hautvast. 1987. Energy requirements of lactating Dutch women. Pp. 113-123 in Infant Growth and Nutrition. Proceedings of a Workshop. Foundation for the Advancement of the Knowledge of the Nutrition of Mother and Child in Developing Countries. Ede, The Netherlands.

van Steenbergen, W.M., J.A. Kusin, and M.M. Van Rens. 1981. Lactation performance of Akamba mothers, Kenya. Breast feeding behavior, breast milk yield and composition. J. Trop. Pediatr. 27:155-61.

van Steenbergen, W.M., J.A. Kusin, C. de With, E. Lacko, and A.A.J. Jansen. 1983. Lactation performance of mothers with contrasting nutritional status in rural Kenya. Acta Paediatr. Scand. 72:805-810.

van Steenbergen, W.M., J.A. Kusin, S. Kardjati, and C. de With. 1989. Energy supplementation in the last trimester of pregnancy in East Java, Indonesia: effect on breast-milk output. Am. J. Clin. Nutr. 50:274-279.

Venkatachalam, P.S., and C. Gopalan. 1960. Basal metabolism and total body water in nursing women. Indian J. Med. Res. 48:507-510.

WHO (World Health Organization) Task Force on Oral Contraceptives. 1988. Effects of hormonal contraceptives on breast milk composition and infant growth. Stud. Fam. Plann. 19:361-369.

Wagner, G., and A.R. Fuchs. 1968. Effect of ethanol on uterine activity during suckling in post-partum women. Acta Endocrinol. 58:133-141.

Wallgren, A. 1944/1945. Breast milk consumption of healthy full-term infants. Acta Paediatr. 32:778-790.

Warman, N.L., and K.M. Rasmussen. 1983. Effects of malnutrition during the reproductive cycle on nutritional status and lactational performance of rat dams. Nutr. Res. 3:527-545.

Whichelow, M.J., and B.E. King. 1979. Breast feeding and smoking. Arch. Dis. Child. 54:240-241.

Whitehead, R.G. ed. 1983. Maternal Diet, Breast-Feeding Capacity, and Lactational Infertility. Report of a joint UNU/WHO workshop held in Cambridge, United Kingdom, 9-11 March 1981. Food and Nutrition Bulletin, Suppl. 6. United Nations University, World Health Organization, Tokyo. 107 pp.

Whitehead, R.G., and A.A. Paul. 1981. Infant growth and human milk requirements: a fresh approach. Lancet 2:161-163.

Wilde, C.J., C.V.P. Addey, M.J. Casey, D.R. Blatchford, and M. Peaker. 1988. Feedback inhibition of milk secretion: the effect of a fraction of goat milk on milk yield and composition. Q. J. Exp. Physiol. 73:391-397.

Winikoff, B., P. Semeraro, M. Zimmerman. 1988. Contraception During Breastfeeding—
    A Clinician's Source Book. The Population Council, New York. 36 pp.
Wong, W.W., N.F. Butte, C. Garza, and P.D. Klein. 1990. Estimation of milk intake
    by deuterium dilution. Pp. 359-367 in S.A. Atkinson, L.A. Hanson, and R.K.
    Chandra, eds. Human Lactation 4: Breastfeeding, Nutrition, Infection and Infant
    Growth in Developed and Emerging Countries. ARTS Biomedical Publishers and
    Distributors, St John's, Newfoundland, Canada.
Woolridge, M.W., and J.D. Baum. 1988. The regulation of human milk flow. Pp. 243-
    257 in B.S. Lindblad, ed. Perinatal Nutrition. Bristol-Myers Nutrition Symposia,
    Vol. 6. Academic Press, San Diego.
Woolridge, M.W., N. Butte, K.G. Dewey, A.M. Ferris, C. Garza, and R.P. Keller. 1985.
    Methods for the measurement of milk volume intake of the breast-fed infant. Pp.
    5-21 in R.G. Jensen and M.C. Neville, eds. Human Lactation: Milk Components
    and Methodologies. Plenum Press, New York.
Young, M.C., and K.M. Rasmussen. 1985. Effects of varying degrees of chronic
    dietary restriction in rat dams on reproductive and lactational performance and
    body composition in dams and their pups. Am. J. Clin. Nutr. 41:979-987.
Zuppa, A.A., A. Tornesello, P. Papacci, G. Tortorolo, G. Segni, G. Lafuenti, E. Moneta,
    A. Diodato, M. Sorcini, and S. Carta. 1988. Relationship between maternal parity,
    basal prolactin levels and neonatal breast milk intake. Biol. Neonate 53:144-147.

6

Milk Composition

In examining the evidence concerning the influence of maternal nutrition on human milk composition, the subcommittee considered the broad spectrum of constituents of milk, the normal variation in their concentrations, and factors in addition to maternal nutrition that influence those variations. This discussion of the subcommittee's findings is not meant to be exhaustive. Rather, this chapter provides a framework for understanding how maternal nutrition can have an impact on the composition of human milk, as well as when and in what context nutritional factors are likely to be operational. Furthermore, it provides the information needed to estimate maternal nutrient requirements—the subject of Chapter 9—and provides a basis for considering some of the effects of maternal nutrition on the nursing infant's health (Chapter 7) and the effects of lactation on the mother's longer-term health and nutrient stores (Chapters 8 and 9).

CHARACTERISTICS OF HUMAN MILK

Human milk is a complex fluid that contains more than 200 recognized constituents (see Blanc, 1981). The number of recognized constituents has increased as analytic techniques have been improved. Milk consists of several compartments, including true solutions, colloids (casein micelles), membranes, membrane-bound globules, and live cells (Ruegg and Blanc, 1982). Its constituents can be broadly divided into categories; for example, aqueous and lipid fractions (see box) or nutritive and nonnutritive constituents. Many milk constituents serve dual roles (see later section "Constituents of Human Milk with Other Biologic Functions"). Detailed discussions of human milk constituents

113

Classes of Constituents in Human Milk

Protein and Nonprotein Nitrogen Compounds
  Proteins
    Caseins
    α-Lactalbumin
    Lactoferrin
    Secretory IgA and other immunoglobulins
    β-Lactoglobulin
    Lysozyme
    Enzymes
    Hormones
    Growth factors
  Nonprotein Nitrogen Compounds
    Urea
    Creatine
    Creatinine
    Uric acid
    Glucosamine
    α-Amino nitrogen
    Nucleic acids
    Nucleotides
    Polyamines
Water-Soluble Vitamins
  Thiamin
  Riboflavin
  Niacin
  Pantothenic acid
  Biotin
  Folate
  Vitamin B_6
  Vitamin B_{12}
  Vitamin C
  Inositol
  Choline
Cells
  Leukocytes
  Epithelial cells

Carbohydrates
  Lactose
  Oligosaccharides
  Bifidus factors
  Glycopeptides
Lipids
  Triglycerides
  Fatty acids
  Phospholipids
  Sterols and hydrocarbons
  Fat-soluble vitamins
    A and carotene
    D
    E
    K
Minerals
  Macronutrient Elements
    Calcium
    Phosphorus
    Magnesium
    Potassium
    Sodium
    Chlorine
    Sulfur
  Trace Elements
    Iodine
    Iron
    Copper
    Zinc
    Manganese
    Selenium
    Chromium
    Cobalt

and properties can be found in several recent review articles and books (e.g., Blanc, 1981; Carlson, 1985; Gaull et al., 1982; Goldman et al., 1987; Goldman and Goldblum, 1990; Hamosh and Goldman, 1986; Jensen, 1989; Jensen and Neville, 1985; Koldovskỳ, 1989; Lönnerdal, 1985a, 1986a; Picciano, 1984a, 1985; Ruegg and Blanc, 1982).

METHODOLOGIC ISSUES

Types of Variation

The concentration of the individual constituents of mature human milk have been shown to vary considerably (see Table 6-1), even when they are collected and analyzed under controlled, defined conditions. The greatest variations have been observed from woman to woman, although variations are also found in different samples obtained from the same woman (Picciano, 1984b). Milk composition changes from the beginning of a feeding to the end, diurnally, from day to day, and with the onset and progression of lactation. Examples are given later in this section.

Early investigators recognized the importance of sampling techniques in obtaining valid data on the composition of human milk and recommended collection of a total 24-hour specimen at different stages of lactation (Hytten, 1954a; Macy et al., 1945). Although such a recommendation represents the ideal approach, it is seldom feasible without interfering with the normal lactation process.

No one sampling scheme can be endorsed universally for all milk constituents. Each scheme must be designed to accommodate the variation pattern of the constituents to be measured. Failure to do this will often result in an under- or overestimation of daily secretion rates, masking possible influences of maternal nutrition.

Variation in the First Weeks Post Partum

Changes in milk composition over the course of lactation are most marked during the first weeks of lactation (see examples in Figure 6-1). *Colostrum* is the fluid secreted by the mammary gland immediately following parturition. It differs from mature human milk in physical characteristics and composition. The intense yellow color of colostrum is indicative of the high concentration of carotenoids, including α-carotene, β-carotene, β-crytoxanthin, lutein, and xeaxanthin. The carotene content of colostrum is about 10-fold higher than that of mature milk (0.34 to 7.57 mg/liter compared with 0.1 to 0.3 mg/liter, respectively [Patton et al., 1990]). During the colostral period, which lasts 4 to 7 days, rapid changes occur in milk composition: concentrations of fat and lactose increase while those of protein and minerals decrease.

The term *transitional milk* is sometimes used to describe the postcolostral period (7 to 21 days post partum), when changes in milk composition occur less rapidly than in the first few days following parturition. *Mature human milk* ($\geq$21 days post partum) also exhibits variability, but to a much smaller extent than in early lactation. Data for selected nutrients (Appendix C) illustrate this point and indicate variations among studies arising from differences in analytic techniques and other experimental circumstances.

TABLE 6-1   Estimates of the Concentrations of Nutrients in Mature
Human Milk

Nutrient	Amount in Human Milk[a]	Nutrient	Amount in Human Milk[a]
	$g/liter \pm SD^b$		$\mu g/liter \pm SD$
Lactose	72.0 ± 2.5	Vitamin A, RE[d]	670 ± 200
Protein	10.5 ± 2.0		(2,230 IU[e])
Fat	39.0 ± 4.0	Vitamin D	0.55 ± 0.10
	$mg/liter \pm SD$	Vitamin K	2.1 ± 0.1
Calcium	280 ± 26	Folate	85 ± 37[f]
Phosphorus	140 ± 22	Vitamin B$_{12}$	0.97[g,h]
Magnesium	35 ± 2	Biotin	4 ± 1
Sodium	180 ± 40	Iodine	110 ± 40
Potassium	525 ± 35	Selenium	20 ± 5
Chloride	420 ± 60	Manganese	6 ± 2
Iron	0.3 ± 0.1	Fluoride	16 ± 5
Zinc	1.2 ± 0.2	Chromium	50 ± 5
Copper	0.25 ± 0.03	Molybdenum	NR[i]
Vitamin E	2.3 ± 1.0		
Vitamin C	40 ± 10		
Thiamin	0.210 ± 0.035		
Riboflavin	0.350 ± 0.025		
Niacin	1.500 ± 0.200		
Vitamin B$_6$	93 ± 8[c]		
Pantothenic acid	1.800 ± 0.200		

[a]Data taken from the Committee on Nutrition (1985), unless otherwise indicated. The
values are representative of amounts of nutrients present in human milk; some of them may
differ slightly from those reported by investigators cited in the text.
[b]SD = Standard deviation.
[c]From Styslinger and Kirksey (1985), a study of unsupplemented women.
[d]RE = Retinol equivalents.
[e]IU = International units.
[f]From Brown et al. (1986a).
[g]From Sandberg et al. (1981).
[h]Standard deviation not reported; range 0.33 to 3.20.
[i]NR = Not reported.

Variation with Length of Gestation

There are substantial differences between the milk of mothers who deliver
preterm and those who deliver at full term. The subcommittee has focused
on lactating mothers of full-term infants; therefore, these differences are only
briefly summarized here. During the first 3 to 4 days of lactation, *preterm milk*
(the milk secreted by mothers who delivered prematurely) has higher protein,
sodium, and chloride concentrations and lower lactose concentrations than milk
secreted by mothers of full-term infants. While some investigators report higher
fat concentrations in preterm milk (Anderson et al., 1981; Guerrini et al., 1981),

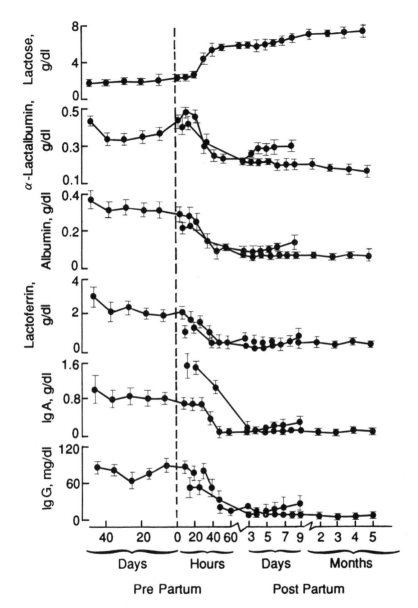

FIGURE 6-1 Changes in the concentrations of lactose and whey proteins in human milk during the progression of lactation in four women during late pregnancy and the first 5 months of lactation. Values obtained for the right and left breast of each woman were averaged and used to calculate the mean plus or minus the standard error of the mean at each period. The zero on the horizontal axis indicated the time of delivery. From Kulski and Hartmann (1981) with permission.

others do not (Bitman et al., 1983; Sann, 1981). Calcium, magnesium, and phosphorus concentrations are similar in preterm and full-term milk, as are concentrations of copper, iron, and zinc (Hamosh and Hamosh, 1987). During early lactation the milk produced by women who deliver prematurely undergoes the same changes in composition that occur after full-term pregnancies. The change occurs, however, over a longer period in mothers who deliver prematurely than in mothers of full-term infants (that is, 3 to 5 weeks compared with 3 to 5 days, respectively). The bioactive and immunologic properties of human milk also differ between preterm and full-term milk; this is discussed in detail elsewhere (Goldman, 1989b).

Variation in Content of Macronutrients (Fat, Carbohydrate, and Protein)

Lipids are among the most variable and difficult nutrients to measure accurately in human milk: among women, the total fat content of 24-hour milk samples may vary from less than 20 g/liter to more than 50 g/liter. However, Hytten (1954b) reports that the average fat content of milk secreted on the seventh day of lactation by any one woman was predictive of the average concentration in later lactation. Within one woman, the fat content of milk increases from the beginning to the end of a single nursing; it differs by as much as 20 g/liter in 24-hour collections on subsequent days, it differs from lactation to lactation in a nonconsistent manner, and it is influenced by the length of time between sample collection (the longest interval yielding the lowest fat values). These large variations complicate the measurement of total fat secreted by lactating women and, in turn, affect calculations of the energy value of milk, which are determined mainly by milk fat content.

Among the macronutrients in human milk, lactose appears to be the least variable and thus the least influenced by improper sampling. The coefficient of variation (standard deviation divided by the mean) for human milk lactose content is 7.2% compared with 13% for the total nitrogen content (which is indicative of protein content) and 25% for the fat content in total 24-hour samples (Hytten, 1954c).

Precision and Validity of Methods

There are adequate methods for quantifying many human milk constituents. Unfortunately, methods designed to study bovine milk or other biologic fluids have been inappropriately applied in the analysis of human milk, thereby providing inaccurate and unreliable information, even in some recent studies. To obtain accurate results, one must apply proper sampling, extraction, handling, and storage procedures as well as a sensitive and selective detection system. A few examples of the many problems that must be addressed are presented below:

• *Bioactive constituents.* Enzymes and other bioactive constituents of human milk may alter the composition of expressed milk (Greenberg and Graves (1984), even at temperatures well below 0° C. (Berkow et al., 1984; Bitman et al., 1983).

• *Bound forms.* Several of the vitamins (such as vitamin D, folate, and pantothenic acid) are secreted bound to other compounds, and they must be released before they can be completely extracted or detected. For example, accurate measurement of the total content of pantothenic acid in human milk requires double enzyme hydrolysis (Song et al., 1984).

• *Distribution in aqueous and lipid fractions.* Vitamin D and its metabolites are secreted in the aqueous fraction of human milk and are attached to binding proteins (Hollis et al., 1982), but on standing they diffuse to the lipid fraction of milk. Thus, whether aqueous or lipid solvents are used should be determined by the handling procedure.

• *Other sources of measurement errors.* Commercial sources of reagents such as enzymes may be contaminated with vitamins and be responsible for falsely elevated levels in milk (Song et al., 1984). Many of the water-soluble vitamins are measured by microbiological assays. Care must be taken to ensure that the vitamin to be measured is stable under the extraction method employed and that the vitamin is converted to a form that can be utilized by the test organism. For example, the folate content of human milk is likely to be underestimated unless an antioxidant is used to prevent it from being oxidized, conjugase pretreatment is performed to cleave the long-chain forms of the vitamin, heat treatment is applied to release the folate from its binding proteins before microbiological analysis, and test organisms are selected that are able to use all the forms of folate in the samples (O'Connor et al., 1990a).

The reproducibility and validity of techniques used in different studies could not always be ascertained by the subcommittee. Thus, the data on the nutrient content of human milk must be interpreted with caution. Large variations reported for many milk constituents may reflect improper sampling or analytic inaccuracies or both rather than true biologic variance.

In addition to the methodologic concerns just described, there are problems of measurement and detection specific to nonnutrient constituents, as follows:

• The leukocytes in human milk are difficult to identify because their morphology is altered by the presence of many intracytoplasmic lipid bodies.

• Certain constituents, such as secretory immunoglobulin A (IgA), exist in a different physical form than they do in other tissues, such as blood, and therefore require discrete detection procedures.

• The titer of specific antibodies in human milk depends on whether the woman has recently been exposed to the relevant immunogen via the intestinal or respiratory tract.

TABLE 6-2   Origins of Nutrients in Human Milk[a]

Origin	Proteins	Carbohydrates	Lipids	Vitamins	Minerals
Synthesis in mammary gland	x	x	x	o	o
Transfer from plasma to milk	x	x	x	x	x

[a]x indicates that the nutrient has this origin; o indicates that it does not.

• Nonspecific blocking factors in human milk may interfere with the detection of certain components by solid-phase immunoassays.

Clearly, considerable effort is required to reliably detect and quantify many of the constituents in human milk and, therefore, to determine whether changes in maternal nutrition influence the content of such constituents in milk.

There are other methodologic issues that are likely to hamper investigations of the influence of maternal nutrition on milk composition. Most recently, nutrient-nutrient interrelations have emerged as possible confounding variables. For example, a study of preterm infants indicates that zinc undernutrition could be responsible for low vitamin A levels in serum (Hustead et al., 1988). If this is also true for lactating women, supplemental vitamin A would have no effect on the vitamin A level in milk. Similarly, maternal iron deficiency in rats can cause an impairment of milk folic acid secretion that is not corrected with supplemental folic acid (O'Connor et al., 1990a).

ORIGIN OF MILK CONSTITUENTS

There are three sources of the milk constituents: some are synthesized in the mammary secretory cell from precursors in the plasma, some are produced by other cells in the mammary gland, and others are transferred directly from plasma to milk (see Table 6-2). All physiologic and biochemical phenomena that influence the composition of plasma may also affect the composition of milk. Milk composition can be modified further by hormones or other bioactive factors that are capable of influencing biosynthetic processes in the mammary gland. Metabolic changes and their relationships with milk production and composition have been well documented in studies in animals, especially cows, goats, and rats.

The mixed origin of milk constituents is well illustrated by considering the lipid components of milk. Milk triglycerides (which account for 98% of the total lipid content) are synthesized in the mammary alveolar cell. Fatty acids may be derived from the plasma (transported there from either the intestine or fat deposits), or they may be synthesized from glucose within the mammary gland. The origins of the fatty acids can be distinguished: fatty acids synthesized within the mammary gland have chain lengths of 16 carbons or less; those derived from dietary sources (other than dairy products) and from adipose tissue tend to have longer carbon chains. The increase in prolactin level preceding and during lactation (Zinder et al., 1974) has two important effects on lipids. (1) Lipoprotein lipase activity in the mammary gland increases sharply (Hamosh et al., 1970). This enzyme hydrolyzes triglycerides and thus frees their fatty acids for transport into the cell, where they are reesterified. (2) Lipoprotein lipase activity in adipose tissue decreases (Hamosh et al., 1970). Both of these channel fat to the lactating mammary gland, where it is incorporated in the milk.

MATERNAL NUTRITION AND
THE COMPOSITION OF HUMAN MILK

Three aspects of maternal nutrition could have an impact on human milk composition: current dietary intake, nutrient stores, and alterations in nutrient utilization as influenced by the hormonal milieu characteristic of lactation. Alterations in maternal nutrition that change the composition of human milk may have positive, neutral, or negative consequences to the nursing infant (see Chapter 7). When maternal nutrition is continuously compromised but the concentrations of nutrients in milk and the milk volume remain unchanged, the nutrients for milk synthesis are being furnished by maternal stores or body tissues. It has not been determined when this situation has a negative impact on the mother. Chapter 9 considers this in more detail.

As explained in the preceding section, investigators must carefully control for stage of lactation in studies to determine the effects of maternal nutrition on milk composition. Other factors that must be considered in such studies include frequency of nursing, environmental conditions (e.g., the specificity of secreted antibodies in human milk after exposure to infectious agents), and length of gestation.

Macronutrients: Protein, Fat, and Carbohydrate

Protein

Milk proteins are broadly classified as caseins and whey proteins. Caseins are phosphoproteins that occur only in milk. Molecules of casein associate in combination with calcium, phosphate, and magnesium ions in structures known as micelles. These micelles enable milk to carry a much larger quantity of calcium, phosphate, and magnesium than could be carried in a simple aqueous solution. The whey proteins, such as α-lactalbumin and lactoferrin, are synthesized in the mammary gland; other proteins (including serum albumin and several bioactive enzymes and protein hormones) are transported to the milk from plasma. In addition, dimeric IgA is produced by plasma cells in the mammary gland and is transported into the milk by specific receptors. Human milk also contains a variety of nonprotein nitrogen-containing compounds, including amino acids, peptides, N-acetyl sugars, urea, and nucleotides.

Commonly used methods for measuring the protein content of human milk are nonspecific but often produce approximately the same results (Lönnerdal, 1985b). However, if the protein content of human milk is measured colorimetrically, an overestimation of approximately 25 to 40% is possible (Lönnerdal et al., 1987).

Using amino acid analysis, Lönnerdal and coworkers (1976c) found that the protein content of mature human milk was approximately 8 to 9 g/liter. Similar values were found using nitrogen analysis of precipitated proteins, among diverse populations, i.e., disadvantaged Ethiopian women and privileged Swedish women (Lönnerdal et al., 1976a,b) and privileged U.S. women (Butte, 1984b). The nitrogen analysis method was used in a World Health Organization collaborative study, in which mature milk was found to contain 8.8, 8.3, 8.3, 7.6, and 12 g/liter in Hungary, Sweden, Guatemala, the Philippines, and Zaire, respectively (WHO, 1985). The reasons for the much higher results from Zaire are not clear.

Methods based on amino acid analysis should yield results that reflect the sum of free and protein-bound amino acids. Nitrogen analyses of precipitated proteins exclude free amino acids and small peptides which may account for approximately 7 to 10% of the total amino acids found in human milk (Svanberg et al., 1977).

There is no convincing evidence that diet or body composition influence the total concentration of milk protein, even in communities of undernourished women (Lönnerdal, 1986b); however, the interpretation of some studies is hampered by the use of total nitrogen as a proxy measure for the total amino acid content of milk (Deb and Cama, 1962) or by the short diet periods used in metabolic studies (Forsum and Lönnerdal, 1980).

In a study of three well-nourished Swedish women, Forsum and Lönnerdal (1980) demonstrated that an increased maternal intake of protein (20% compared with 8% of energy from protein) increased total nitrogen, protein, and nonprotein nitrogen contents of mature human milk and 24-hour milk protein output. There have been reports of low concentrations of protein and altered free and total amino acid nitrogen profiles in milk of women from countries with limited food supplies: India (Deb and Cama, 1962), Pakistan (Lindblad and Rahimtoola, 1974), and Guatemala (Wurtman and Fernstrom, 1979).

The nonprotein nitrogen content of human milk is higher than that in milk of other species; the importance of this to infant nutrition and health is unknown (Carlson, 1985). Taurine, an amino acid found only in animal products, is the second most abundant free amino acid in human milk (Rassin et al., 1978). Even the milk secreted by women who ingest no animal foods contains taurine concentrations of approximately 35 mg/dl—lower than concentrations in milk secreted by omnivores (54 mg/dl) but 30 times greater than levels in bovine milk (Rana and Sanders, 1986). Taurine functions in bile acid conjugation and may also function as an inhibitory neurotransmitter and as a membrane stabilizer.

A broad spectrum of nucleotides occurs in human milk (Janas and Picciano, 1982), but the effects of maternal nutrition on the concentrations of these nucleotides have not yet been reported.

Lipids

The lipids in milk are contained within membrane-enclosed milk fat globules, the core of which consists of triglycerides—the major energy source in milk. The globule membrane is composed mainly of phospholipids, cholesterol, and proteins.

Although there is no compelling evidence that changes in maternal fat intake influence the total quantity of milk fat, it has been shown repeatedly that the nature of the fat consumed by the mother will influence the fatty acid composition of milk (Jensen, 1989). For example, milk from four complete vegetarian women in Great Britain was found to contain five times as much $C_{18:2}$ fatty acids as milk from four nonvegetarian women (31.9 and 6.9%, respectively) (Sanders et al., 1978). Finley et al. (1985) noted that, as lactation progressed, milk from both vegetarian and nonvegetarian women contained more fatty acids principally synthesized in the mammary gland ($C_{8:0}$, $C_{10:0}$, $C_{12:0}$, $C_{14:0}$) and less from the diet and adipose tissue. Chappell et al. (1985a) reported that the *trans* fatty acid content of human milk was directly related to maternal intake of partially hydrogenated fats and oils; in women experiencing postpartum weight loss, fat mobilized from adipose tissue also contributed *trans* fatty acids to human milk fat independently of current dietary intake.

In the classic study of a single subject by Insull and colleagues (1959), both the total energy and fat contents of the diet were altered. Their results demonstrated that mammary lipid synthesis was influenced by energy balance as well as by the type and amount of fat in the diet. When the subject was fed excess energy as a low-fat, high-carbohydrate diet, the investigators found that 40 to 60% of the fatty acids in milk fat had carbon chain lengths of less than 16. On a very high fat diet (70% of kilocalories as corn oil) that was adequate in energy, the combined linoleic and linolenic acid content of the milk fatty acids increased from approximately 2 to 45%, and there was a corresponding drop in the content of shorter-chain saturated fatty acids. When a low-fat, calorie-restricted diet was fed, C_{16} or longer-chain saturated fatty acids predominated in the milk, indicating that stored body fat was utilized for milk fat synthesis. Effects of such changes on infant health have not been studied.

Using stable isotope methodology, Hachey and colleagues (1987, 1989) confirmed the results of the study of Insull et al. (1959) showing that diet composition affects milk fat synthesis. Hachey et al. estimate that when the mother is in energy balance, fatty acids derived directly from the diet account for approximately 30% of the fatty acids found in the milk.

There is no evidence that the concentrations of cholesterol and phospholipid in human milk can be altered by changes in the maternal diet. Indeed, milk cholesterol remains at 100 to 150 mg/liter even in hypercholesterolemic women and increases only in severe cases of pathologic hypercholesterolemia (Jensen, 1989). Since both cholesterol and phospholipids are integral components of the milk fat globule membrane, their secretion rates relate to the total quantity of fat secreted in milk, which is apparently not influenced by diet.

Studies conducted in communities where maternal undernutrition is prevalent have furnished evidence indicating that the percentage of maternal body fat may influence the concentration of fat in milk. Milk fat concentrations in The Gambia (Prentice et al., 1981) and Bangladesh (Brown et al., 1986b) were positively correlated with maternal skinfold thickness and decreased over the course of lactation. This positive relationship ($R = .46$) between milk fat concentration and body fat (as a percentage of ideal body weight) was likewise noted in U.S. women in late (6 to 12 months) lactation but not in early lactation (Nommsen et al., in press). Prentice and associates (1989) report that high- (>10) parity Gambian women had a decreased capacity for total milk fat synthesis and, thus, lower milk fat concentrations.

Carbohydrates

The principal carbohydrate in human milk is lactose, a disaccharide that consists of galactose joined by a β linkage to glucose. In human milk, lactose is present in an average concentration of 70 g/liter and is second only to water as a major constituent. In all species of mammals studied, milk is isotonic with plasma, which helps keep the energy cost of milk secretion low. Lactose exerts 60 to 70% of the total osmotic pressure of milk. Compared with glucose, lactose provides nearly twice the energy value per molecule (per unit of osmotic pressure). The concentrations of lactose in human milk are remarkably similar among women, and there is no convincing evidence that they can be influenced by maternal dietary factors. However, Hartmann and Prosser (1982) noted that lactose concentration in human milk decreased from 78 to 60 g/liter both 5 to 6 days before and 6 to 7 days after ovulation. Other carbohydrates and their complexes are discussed below in the section "Nonlactose Carbohydrates in Human Milk".

Vitamins

A major factor influencing the vitamin content of human milk is the mother's vitamin status. In general, when maternal intakes of a vitamin are chronically low, the levels of that vitamin in human milk are also low. As maternal intakes of the vitamin increase, levels in milk also increase, but for many vitamins they plateau and do not respond further to supplementation through diet or pharmaceutical preparations. Although the milk concentrations of water-soluble vitamins are generally more responsive to maternal dietary intake than are concentrations of fat-soluble vitamins, there are important exceptions. These are discussed below for specific vitamins.

Fat-Soluble Vitamins

Vitamin A. The vitamin A content of human milk comprises principally retinyl esters (96%). The concentration of this vitamin in human milk decreases over the course of lactation from approximately 2,000 to 600 μg/liter (Chappell et al., 1986; Cumming and Briggs, 1983). Concentrations of carotene, a precursor of vitamin A, are reported to differ from 0 to 320 μg/liter (Butte and Calloway, 1981; Chappell et al., 1986; Department of Health and Social Security, 1977). This wide range may reflect mainly analytic difficulties and sampling errors (Jensen, 1989). β-Carotene is stored in the mammary gland during pregnancy and is rapidly secreted into milk during the first few days of lactation (Patton et al., 1990). Several reports indicate that the amount of vitamin A in human milk decreases with maternal deficiency of the vitamin and increases with excessive intake (Ajans et al., 1965; Butte and Calloway, 1981; Hrubetz et al., 1945).

Results of supplementation trials are equivocal. In vitamin A-depleted mothers, supplementation was found to increase the concentration of vitamin A in milk in some studies (e.g., Venkatachalam et al., 1962) but to have no effect in others (Belavady and Gopalan, 1960; Villard and Bates, 1987). Chappell et al. (1985b) noted no association between reported maternal intake of vitamin A and carotene with corresponding values in the milk of well-nourished Canadian women. In contrast, Gebre-Mehdin and coworkers (1976) reported that the concentration of retinyl esters was low in milk from disadvantaged Ethiopian women compared with that in milk from Ethiopian women of higher socioeconomic status and from Swedish women.

Vitamin D. Human milk normally contains 0.5 to 1.5 μg (20 to 60 IU) of vitamin D per liter (Greer et al., 1984a). Several studies indicate that the vitamin D activity of human milk is directly related to maternal vitamin D status. Hollis et al. (1983) reported that the vitamin D concentrations in human milk drop to undetectable levels during maternal deficiency and increase following supplementation and exposure to ultraviolet light. Potentially toxic amounts (175 μg, or >7,000 IU, per liter) of vitamin D could occur in human milk following daily administration of pharmacologic doses (2,500 μg, or 100,000 IU) of vitamin D_2 (ergocalciferol) to the mother (Greer et al., 1984b). The vitamin D activity of human milk is accounted for principally by vitamin D metabolites but also by vitamin D_2 and vitamin D_3 (cholecalciferol).

Vitamin K. The vitamin K content of mature human milk is typically 2 μg/liter (Haroon et al., 1982), and that of colostrum is approximately twice as high (von Kries et al., 1987, 1988). When mothers with low vitamin K intakes are given 20-mg supplements of vitamin K in the form of phylloquinone, milk levels of the vitamin are increased by twofold for at least 48 hours (Haroon et al., 1982; von Kries et al., 1987). However, even when the mother's vitamin K intake from food has been high or she has routinely taken supplements containing vitamin K, the amount of this vitamin obtained by the breastfed neonate in the first few days after birth may be insufficient to meet the infant's needs (see Chapter 7).

Vitamin E. Approximately 83% of the total vitamin E content of human milk is α-tocopherol. Small quantities of β-, γ, and δ-tocopherols are present as well (Kobayashi et al., 1975). Concentrations of tocopherols are high in colostrum (8 mg/liter) and decline and stabilize to 2 to 3 mg/liter in mature human milk. A single case report indicates that high maternal intakes (approximately 27 mg of vitamin E per day) resulted in an elevated plasma concentration of α-tocopherol equivalents (3.8 mg/dl compared with a normal concentration of 0.5 to 2.0 mg/dl) and a high milk content of 11 mg/liter on day 38 of lactation (Anderson and Pittard, 1985).

Water-Soluble Vitamins

Vitamin C. Bates and colleagues (1983) report that the vitamin C content of mature human milk levels off at 50 to 60 mg/liter if daily maternal intakes are equal to or exceed 100 mg (approximately the mother's Recommended Dietary Allowance [RDA] for this vitamin). When maternal vitamin C intake is relatively low, increases in intake are associated with an increased human milk content of this vitamin. These investigators also reported that the level of vitamin C in milk is 8 to 10 times that in maternal plasma.

Thiamin. There are large variations in the thiamin content of human milk between individuals and over the course of lactation. Thiamin concentrations are low in colostrum (10 μg/liter) and increase 7- to 10-fold in mature milk. Milk from mothers with beriberi contains less thiamin that that of healthy women in the same country. Infants nursed by mothers with beriberi develop the disease by 3 or 4 weeks of age (Hytten and Thomson, 1961). Pratt et al. (1951) have shown that the thiamin content of human milk can be sharply increased up to a certain limit, estimated to be 200 μg/liter.

Riboflavin and Niacin. Riboflavin content is high early in lactation and declines thereafter. The milk of well-nourished women contains riboflavin concentrations of approximately 350 μg/liter (Committee on Nutrition, 1985;

NRC, 1989). Lower concentrations found in riboflavin-deficient populations can be increased by supplementation (Bates et al., 1981). The average niacin concentration in human milk increases from 0.75 mg/liter in colostrum to approximately 1 mg/liter in mature human milk. Actual niacin levels are largely dependent on maternal intake; an observational study reported levels as high as 6 mg/liter among women who were successfully lactating (Pratt et al., 1951).

Vitamin B_6. The vitamin B_6 content is low in colostrum and varies between 50 and 250 μg/liter in mature milk. In the United States, levels in mature milk have been reported to be approximately 93 ± 8 (standard deviation [SD]) μg/liter, a value 10 times higher than levels in maternal serum. The vitamin B_6 content of milk is directly related (R = .8) to maternal intake (Styslinger and Kirksey, 1985). Roepke and Kirksey (1979) reported drastically reduced vitamin B_6 levels in milk from mothers with a long history (4 to 12 years) of oral contraceptive use before conception. Supplements of 20 mg/day were required to increase milk concentrations in those mothers and to reverse neurologic symptoms of deficiency in their infants (Kirksey and Roepke, 1981). However, the contraceptives taken by these women contained higher levels of estrogen than those that are now used in contraceptive formulations; current interrelationships among contraceptive use, vitamin B_6 intake, and vitamin B_6 concentrations in human milk are unknown. Further discussion of vitamin B_6 in human milk is included in Chapter 9.

Folate and Vitamin B_{12}. Folate and vitamin B_{12} in human milk are bound to whey proteins; therefore, maternal factors regulating protein secretion are more likely to affect milk levels of these vitamins over the short term than are fluctuations in maternal vitamin intake.

Improved methods of analysis have permitted detection of much higher folate levels in human milk than previously reported. Milk folate is quantitatively bound to folate-binding protein; folylpolyglutamates account for a considerable portion of total folate. In the United States, folate concentrations in human milk average 85 ± 37 (SD) μg/liter during the first 3 months of lactation (Brown et al., 1986a); in Japan, they average 141 ± 43 (SD) μg/liter during the first 6 months of lactation (Tamura, 1980). In apparently well-nourished women in industrialized countries, no correlation was found between maternal serum and milk folate levels (before or after maternal supplementation) (Salmenperä et al., 1986b; Smith et al., 1983; Tamura et al., 1980). However, milk folate levels were found to increase from 5 to 60 μg/liter after 4 days of oral folate supplementation of two lactating women with megaloblastic anemia resulting from dietary folate insufficiency (Metz et al., 1968). Folate levels in human milk typically increase with the progression of lactation, even as levels in maternal serum and red blood cells decrease (Smith et al., 1983). There is evidence that folate is preferentially partitioned to mammary tissue and secreted in milk during maternal deficiency (Metz et al., 1968). As a result, the folate content of milk is maintained at the expense of the mother's folate status.

The reported vitamin B_{12} concentration of mature human milk from U.S. women ranges from 0.3 to 3.2 μg/liter (average, 0.97 μg/liter) (Sandberg et al., 1981). These investigators reported that the vitamin B_{12} concentrations were not related to maternal dietary intake and did not respond to supplementation. However, the vitamin B_{12} content of milk produced by complete vegetarians, generally malnourished women, or mothers who have latent pernicious anemia secondary to hypothyroidism is very low—between 0.05 and 0.075 μg/liter (Johnson and Roloff, 1982).

Biotin. The biotin content in human milk is exceedingly variable: values were reported to range from 0 to 27 μg/liter when maternal plasma concentrations varied from 142 to 1,090 ng/liter (Salmenperä et al., 1985). The biotin content of human milk increases with the progression of lactation, is directly related to maternal plasma biotin concentration ($R = .21$ to $.44$ from 2 to 6 months of lactation), and markedly increases from approximately 13 to 485 μg/liter when a daily dose of 3 mg of biotin is added to the diet (Hood and Johnson, 1980). The biotin content of human milk is hundreds of times greater than the content in maternal plasma, suggesting that biotin is actively transported from the plasma through the alveolar cell into the milk.

Pantothenic Acid. The pantothenic acid content of human milk averages about 2.6 μg/liter and is significantly correlated ($R = .51$) with maternal dietary intake (Song et al., 1984). These investigators found that four women receiving pantothenic acid in supplements (>1.0 mg/day) had significantly higher milk pantothenic acid values (4.8 μg/liter) than those of nonsupplemented women (2.6 μg/liter).

Major Minerals

The concentrations of calcium, phosphorus, and magnesium in maternal serum are tightly regulated. Thus, there is little reason to expect that maternal intake of these nutrients will strongly influence their levels in human milk. Two-thirds of the calcium is bound to casein; the rest forms a soluble citrate complex. Phosphorus and magnesium are also largely bound to casein. Mean concentrations of calcium, phosphorus, and magnesium in mature human milk are approximately 280, 140, and 35 mg/liter, respectively (see Table 6-1).

Electrolytes

The concentrations of electrolytes (sodium, potassium, and chloride) in milk are determined by an electrical potential gradient in the secretory cell rather than by maternal nutritional status. The average concentrations of sodium, potassium, and chloride in mature human milk (7, 15, and 12 meq/liter, respectively) account for approximately 2, 3 and 4% of total osmoles, respectively, and are lower than their respective levels in colostrum by approximately 66, 31, and 36%, respectively (Macy, 1949). Similar values were found in more recent investigations (Picciano et al., 1981).

Although some investigators have reported that 5- to 40-fold increases in sodium and occasionally chloride levels in human milk are associated with emotional stress, mastitis, and diminished milk production in the mother (Anand et al., 1980; Arboit and Gildengers, 1980; Seale et al., 1982; Whitelaw and Butterfield, 1977), a common cause of high electrolyte levels of the milk and associated dehydration and malnutrition of infants appears to be lack of suckling or inadequate suckling (Naylor, 1981). Inadequate stimulation from suckling leads to involution of the mammary glands, which is characterized by reduction in lactose synthesis and elevated electrolyte concentrations in milk (Hartmann and Kulski, 1978). In the early stages, reinitiation of adequate suckling can reverse this process (Alpert and Cormier, 1983).

Trace Minerals

The concentrations of various trace elements in human milk may be influenced to widely varying degrees by maternal nutrition.

Iron, Copper, and Zinc

The concentrations of iron, copper, and zinc in human milk are highest immediately following parturition (Cavell and Widdowson, 1964). Reported mean values for the concentration of iron in mature human milk range from 0.2 to 0.9 mg/liter (Picciano and Guthrie, 1976; Siimes et al., 1979, respectively). Siimes and colleagues (1979) pointed out that some women have very high concentrations; therefore, the median of 0.3 mg/liter is lower than the mean. The iron concentration in milk is not influenced by the mother's iron status (Dallman, 1986; Murray et al., 1978; Siimes et al., 1984).

Over the first 4 months of lactation, the concentration of copper in human milk gradually declines and then remains stable up to month 12 (Casey et al., 1989; Salmenperä et al., 1986a; Vuori, 1979). In mature milk, copper concentrations range from 0.1 to 0.6 mg/liter, but most are at the lower end of the range (Dewey et al., 1984; Picciano and Guthrie, 1976; Salmenperä et al., 1986a). There is no relationship between maternal copper status and concentrations in human milk (Lönnerdal et al., 1981). Copper secretion into milk apparently is controlled, since milk copper concentrations are three to four times lower than serum concentrations (Lönnerdal et al., 1981).

Zinc concentrations in human milk decrease over the course of lactation. In colostrum, the zinc content is quite high (>10 mg/liter) (Casey et al., 1986). The concentration declines steeply during the first month and then declines gradually (Casey et al., 1989). Reported concentration ranges for months 1, 3, and 12 of lactation are 3 to 4, 1 to 1.5, and 0.5 mg/liter, respectively (Casey et al., 1989; Picciano and Guthrie, 1976; Vuori, 1979). Most of the evidence indicates that maternal dietary zinc intake does not influence concentrations in milk (Feeley et al., 1983; Kirksey et al., 1979; Moser and Reynolds, 1983; Vaughan et al., 1979; Vuori et al., 1980). Two reports suggest that zinc supplementation has a slight influence on milk zinc concentration in late lactation: after 6 months of supplementation with 13 mg of zinc per day (Krebs et al., 1985) and after 34 days of supplementation with 50 mg/day (Karra et al., 1989). However, the number of women in the comparison groups decreased markedly during the course of this intervention trial, making cross-sectional comparison somewhat questionable.

In summary, milk concentrations of iron, copper, or zinc appear to be maintained over different levels of maternal intake (Lönnerdal, 1986a). However, since the adequacy of maternal intake of these micronutrients has been questioned (see Chapter 4), this may place the mother at risk.

Manganese

The concentration of manganese in mature milk from women in industrialized nations declines from approximately 6 μg/liter during the first month of lactation to 3 μg/liter by the third month (Stastny et al., 1984; Vuori et al., 1980). Vuori and colleagues (1980) reported that the manganese concentration in milk may be influenced by maternal diet.

Selenium

Selenium concentrations in milk are high at the initiation of lactation (41 μg/liter) and decrease as lactation progresses (Smith et al., 1982). Mean values in mature milk (10 to 30 μg/liter) differ geographically both within countries and internationally (Kumpulainen, 1989). Mannan and Picciano (1987) report that the concentration of selenium in mature human milk is seven times higher than that in maternal plasma. These investigators also noted that the selenium concentration in human milk is directly related to maternal plasma concentration when plasma concentrations are less than 100 μg/liter. Worldwide, there are major differences in the selenium content of the soil and therefore in the local food supply. A study of rural African women living in an area where the selenium content of the diet varies with food availability indicates that milk selenium concentrations are low when maternal intake is low and also decrease with increasing parity (Funk et al., 1990). Debski et al. (1989) reported that the milk of vegetarians in California contained high concentrations of this trace element.

The enzyme glutathione peroxidase contains selenium. Its activity in milk correlates positively with the activity of this enzyme in maternal plasma and with both the linoleic acid and selenium contents of the milk. The enzyme's presence in milk may protect milk lipids from oxidative damage (Ellis et al., 1990). This suggests that the types of fatty acids consumed by the mother and the adequacy of her energy intake may influence the form and quantity of selenium secreted.

Fluoride

Several investigators have reported mean fluoride levels of 7 to 11 μg/liter in human milk (Ekstrand et al., 1984a; Esala et al., 1982; Spak et al., 1983); the American Academy of Pediatrics (Committee on Nutrition, 1985) suggests that 16 μg/liter be used as a normative value. Reports indicate that there is relatively little effect of maternal fluoride intake on the fluoride concentration of milk. Ekstrand and coworkers (1984b) observed that when a large fluoride dose (11.25 mg) was administered to a mother, only 0.2% of the dose was transferred through her milk to the infant. Spak et al. (1983) reported no significant difference in fluoride concentration of human milk when the fluoride content of the mother's drinking water was increased fivefold (from 0.2 ppm to 1.0 ppm). Although Esala et al. (1982) reported 50% higher levels in the milk of mothers whose drinking water contained 1.7 ppm of fluoride compared with mothers in areas with drinking water containing 0.2 ppm fluoride, the total amount of fluoride delivered through the milk of mothers in both groups was small. Singer and Armstrong (1960) suggested that plasma fluoride concentrations (and thus milk fluoride concentrations) do not increase unless water fluoride content exceeds 1.4 ppm.

Iodine

Iodine is unique among the trace elements because the mammary gland avidly accumulates it. Its level in human milk correlates directly with maternal intake; major sources of iodine in the United States are bread, dairy products, iodized salt, and seafood (NRC, 1989). The mean iodine value for the milk of U.S. women in the 1980s was 178 μg/liter. In one study, iodine values in human milk were reported to be as high as 731 μg/liter (Gushurst et al., 1984). Such milk would provide more than 500 μg of iodine to the nursing infant per day. This level of intake is approximately 10 times greater than the RDA for infants (NRC, 1989). In contrast, the concentration of iodine in human milk is 20 μg/liter in northwestern Zaire, where the iodine supply to the lactating woman is low and iodine deficiency is evident in approximately 75% of the population (Delange, 1985).

CONSTITUENTS OF HUMAN MILK WITH OTHER BIOLOGIC FUNCTIONS

Very few studies have been conducted to investigate the effects of maternal nutrition on the composition of nonnutritive substances in human milk. Research in this area is warranted, however, because of the important biologic functions of many of these substances. Briefly, these constituents have the following functions.

- nutrient synthesis, assembly, and utilization;
- direct protection against microbial pathogens;
- modulation of inflammatory processes;
- promotion of growth and maturation of selected systems by supplying inducers, such as growth factors and hormones;
- enhancement of neural transmission;
- catalysis (increasing the rate) of some metabolic reactions (Hamosh and Hamosh, 1988; Koldovský, 1989).

The many complex functions of milk constituents can be illustrated by describing the role of the milk protein α-lactalbumin, which constitutes approximately 25 to 30% of the total protein in human milk and thus is a major supplier of amino acids to the developing infant. It also is one of the two protein components of the system that synthesizes lactose within the mammary gland. In addition, α-lactalbumin is a metalloenzyme with calcium- and zinc-binding sites and is structurally similar to lysozyme (an antibacterial enzyme discussed below) (Hall and Campbell, 1986). Other examples of nonnutritive functions of milk proteins are given below and in Table 6-3.

TABLE 6-3 Examples of the Multiple Functions of Proteins in Human Milk[a]

	Proteins				
Function	α-Lactalbumin	Lactoferrin	Secretory IgA	BSS Lipase	EGF
Synthesis of a nutrient	x	o	o	x	o
Carrying metals	x	x	o	o	o
Preventing infection	?	x	x	o	o
Preventing inflammation	?	x	x	o	x
Promoting growth	o	x	o	o	x
Catalyzing reactions	o	o	o	x	x

[a]Abbreviations: IgA = immunoglobulin A; BSS = bile salt stimulated; EGF = epidermal growth factor. x indicates that the protein exhibits this function; o indicates that it does not.

TABLE 6-4   Spectra of Antimicrobial Effects of Five Major Types of Soluble Defense Factors in Human Milk[a]

Types of Pathogenic Microorganisms	Antimicrobial Effects of Defense Factors				
	Lipids	Oligosaccharides and Glycoconjugates	Lysozyme	Lactoferrin	Secretory IgA[b]
Enveloped viruses	x	o	o	o	x
Rotaviruses	o	o	o	o	x
Polioviruses	o	o	o	o	x
Respiratory syncytial virus	o	o	o	o	x
Enteric bacteria	o	x	x	x	x
Respiratory bacteria	o	x	x	x	x
Intestinal parasites	x	o	o	o	x

[a]From Goldman and Goldblum (1989b) with permission. x indicates a positive effect; o indicates no known effect.
[b]IgA = Immunoglobulin A.

Antiinfectious Agents

In human milk, there is a complex system of antimicrobial factors (Goldman and Goldblum, 1989b, 1990) (Table 6-4) with the following main characteristics:

- The factors are biochemically heterogeneous.
- Most of the factors are produced throughout lactation.
- The factors are relatively resistant to the digestive processes of the infant's gastrointestinal tract.
- Many of the factors interact in inhibiting or killing microbial pathogens.
- The immunologic factors protect by noninflammatory mechanisms.
- The factors of the system are common to mucosal sites and appear to protect principally the digestive tract and the respiratory system of the infant.

Nonlactose Carbohydrates in Human Milk

There is an array of moderate-chain-length carbohydrates (oligosaccharides and glucoconjugates) in human milk (Cleary et al., 1983; György et al., 1974; Holmgren et al., 1981; Kobata, 1972; Otnæss and Svennerholm, 1982; Otnæss et al., 1983; Svanborg-Edén et al., 1983). Some of these appear to be protective even though they are present in low concentrations. Nitrogen-containing sugars promote the growth of lactobacilli (György et al., 1974), the dominant bacteria in the lower intestinal tract of breastfed infants (Gyllenberg and Roine, 1957; Smith and Crabb, 1961). These lactobacilli appear to protect against the colonization of bacterial pathogens by secreting inhibitory organic compounds such as acetic acid. Specialized oligosaccharides, including monosialogangliosides and glucoconjugates, inhibit the binding of selected bacterial pathogens or their toxins to epithelial cells by acting as receptor analogs (Holmgren et al., 1981; Otnæss and Svennerholm, 1982; Otnæss et al., 1983).

Lipids

The hydrolysis of fats in human milk appears to generate fatty acids and monoglycerides with antiviral properties (Isaacs et al., 1986; Welsh and May, 1979; Welsh et al., 1979). This process may be catalyzed by the infant's own lipases as well as by the action of bile salt-stimulated lipase from human milk in the digestive tract of the recipient infant. The action of the antiviral lipids may be limited to a few enteric pathogens such as *Giardia lamblia* (Gillin et al., 1983, 1985) or encapsulated coronaviruses (Resta et al., 1985).

Proteins

Many of the whey proteins in human milk have direct protective effects against infection. Lactoferrin, one of the dominant whey proteins in human milk throughout lactation (Table 6-5) (Butte et al., 1984a; Goldman et al., 1982, 1983a,b), inhibits the multiplication of siderophilic (iron-absorbing) bacteria by competing with these microorganisims for ferric iron (Bullen et al., 1978; Stephens et al., 1980). The features of lactoferrin in human milk that are responsible for its antimicrobial effect are as follows:

• Approximately 80% is in the apo- (unconjugated) form (Fransson and Lönnerdal, 1980).
• The protein is relatively resistant to proteolysis (Brines and Brock, 1983; Samson et al., 1980).
• Lactoferrin appears to interact with several other host resistance factors in the inhibition or killing of bacterial pathogens.
• Certain forms of lactoferrin that do not bind to iron may inhibit the replication of some viruses (Furmanski et al., 1989).

Antibodies are abundant in human milk throughout lactation; they are

TABLE 6-5 Concentrations of Immunologic Factors in Human Milk During Several Phases of Lactation[a]

Factors	Mean Concentration, mg/ml ± SD,[b] by Stage of Lactation				
	2–3 days	1 month	6 months	1 year	2 years
Lactoferrin	5.3 ± 12.9	1.9 ± 0.3	1.4 ± 0.4	1.0 ± 0.2	1.2 ± 0.1
Secretory IgA[c]	2 ± 2.5	1 ± 0.3	0.5 ± 0.1	1 ± 0.3	1.1 ± 0.2
Lysozyme	0.09 ± 0.03	0.02 ± 0.03	0.25 ± 0.12	0.2 ± 0.1	0.19 ± 0.03

[a]From Goldman and Goldblum (1989b) with permission.
[b]SD = Standard deviation.
[c]IgA = Immunoglobulin A.

Secretory IgA Antibodies Commonly Found in Human Milk

Enteric Pathogens	Respiratory Pathogens
Bacteria, Toxins, Virulence Factors	Bacteria
Clostridium difficile	*Haemophilus influenzae*
Escherichia coli	*Streptococcus pneumoniae*
Klebsiella pneumoniae	Viruses
Salmonella spp.	Influenza viruses
Shigella spp.	Respiratory syncytial virus
Vibrio cholerae	Fungi
Parasites	*Candida albicans*
Giardia lamblia	Food proteins
Viruses	Cow's milk
Polioviruses	Soy
Rotaviruses	

From Goldman and Goldblum (1989b) with permission.

directed against pathogens encountered in the environment that are common to both the mother and infant (see box above) (Goldman and Goldblum, 1989b). These maternal antibodies are of particular importance because the secretory immune system of the infant does not mature for several months after birth (Burgio et al., 1980; Hanson et al., 1983).

The main antibody in human milk is secretory IgA (dimeric IgA coupled to secretory component) (Butte et al., 1984a; Goldman and Goldblum, 1989b; Goldman et al., 1982, 1983a,b). IgM and IgG are also found in human milk but in much lower concentrations (Goldman and Goldblum, 1989a). The IgA-producing cells in the mammary gland tissues originate from B cells from either the small intestine or the respiratory tract and enter the systemic circulation. Then, lactogenic hormones stimulate the B cells to travel to the mammary gland (Weisz-Carrington et al., 1978), where they are transformed to plasma cells that produce dimeric IgA. Because these B cells originate at maternal sites where exposure to environmental pathogens is high, the IgA is protective against pathogens to which the infant might be exposed.

Secretory IgA has at least three other important features: it is particularly suited to act at mucosal surfaces, since it is relatively resistant to proteolysis (Lindh, 1975); it protects by noninflammatory mechanisms (Goldman et al., 1986, 1990); and it acts in synergy with several other host resistance agents in human milk to achieve antimicrobial effects.

Lysozyme is a protein in human milk that affords protection in two different ways: it breaks down susceptible bacteria by cleaving peptidoglycans from their cell walls (Chipman and Sharon, 1969), and it acts in concert with other components in human milk to kill microbial pathogens. High concentrations of this protein are found in human milk throughout lactation (Butte et al., 1984b; Goldman et al., 1982, 1983a,b), whereas concentrations in cow's milk are very much lower. Like many other host resistance factors in human milk, lysozyme is relatively resistant to proteolysis and to denaturation resulting from the high acidity within the stomach.

Fibronectin, a protein that enhances phagocytosis, has recently been found in human milk (Friss et al., 1988). Serum levels of this protein are higher in breastfed than in nonbreastfed infants, but that finding cannot be explained solely by the amount of fibronectin in human milk.

Very low levels of the components of the classical and alternative pathways of the complement system have been found in human milk (Ballow et al., 1974; Nakajima et al., 1977). With the exception of the third component of complement (C3), these levels are unlikely to generate inflammation.

Few studies have addressed whether the nutritional status of women affects the immunologic composition of their milk. In a study of the milk from economically privileged and underprivileged women from Guatemala ($N = 86$) and Ethiopia ($N = 12$) and privileged women from Sweden ($N = 64$), Cruz and associates (1982) compared the concentrations and daily output of secretory IgA and secretory IgA antibodies to somatic antigens to serotypes of *E. coli.* Although it was implied that the underprivileged women were more poorly nourished, indices of nutritional status were not reported. Somewhat similar studies were conducted in India by Reddy et al. (1977) and Reddy and Srikantia (1978). They found no differences in the levels of IgA, IgM, IgG, lactoferrin, or lysozyme in the colostrum from well nourished and poorly nourished women. In that study, poor nutritional status was defined by low body weight and by low weight-to-height ratios. In a study conducted in India, Narula and colleagues (1982) found lower levels of IgG but similar levels of IgA in colostrum from well nourished and poorly nourished women.

A study that more completely defined maternal nutritional status was conducted with 23 Columbian women during the first 2 months of lactation (Miranda et al., 1983). Malnutrition was characterized by lower weight-to-height ratios and by lower creatinine-height indices and serum concentrations of total proteins, albumin, IgG, and IgA. The levels of albumin and IgG in the milk were much lower in malnourished women than in well nourished women. There were also significant but less striking decreases in IgA and C4 levels in milk from malnourished women, whereas no differences were found in C3 and lysozyme levels or in specific antibodies to respiratory syncytial virus.

More recently, Robertson and coworkers (1988) investigated the effects of maternal nutrition upon the avidity of secretory IgA antibodies to *E. coli* polysaccharides and diphtheria toxin in human milk. Decreased avidity was found in antibodies from the malnourished group.

In summary, the effects of maternal nutritional status upon the immunologic system in human milk remain controversial. Although some studies suggest that malnutrition may decrease the production or secretion of some of the components of the immunologic system in human milk, further investigations are needed to characterize more precisely the nutritional status of the mothers and the daily secretion of the immunologic factors.

Leukocytes

In addition to the soluble immunologic agents mentioned above, human milk contains living white blood cells (leukocytes) (Crago et al., 1979; Smith and Goldman, 1968). Neutrophils and macrophages account for approximately 90% of the white blood cells in human milk; the remaining white blood cells are lymphocytes. The neutrophils have phagocytic activity and intracellular killing power similar to those of neutrophils in human blood (Ho and Lawton, 1978; Robinson et al., 1978; Smith and Goldman, 1968; Tsuda et al., 1984) and the bactericidal power of these cells appears to be spared in malnourished women (Bhaskaram and Reddy, 1981). However, the neutrophils in milk are less motile than their counterparts in blood. Moreover, unlike blood neutrophils, they do not appear to increase many of their functions in response to bacteria- or serum-derived chemotactic agents (Thorpe et al., 1986).

The morphology of human milk macrophages suggests that they are activated; indeed, that is born out by the fact that they are more motile than their precursors in blood are (Özkaragöz et al., 1988). The macrophages in human milk are involved in antigen processing and presentation to T lymphocytes and thus may serve in the recognition of foreign materials. Furthermore, these macrophages display class II major histocompatibility antigens (Leyva-Cobián and Clemente, 1984), which suggests that they may participate in the process of immunogenesis in the infant.

Thymic-dependent lymphocytes (T cells) account for the majority of lymphocytes in milk; the relative proportions of the major subpopulations of these cells may be similar to those in blood (Keller et al., 1986). Although their cytotoxic capacities are poor, they can generate certain lymphokines when stimulated in vitro (Keller et al., 1981; Kohl et al., 1980; Lawton et al., 1979). The fate of these cells in the body is not known.

In the study of Narula et al. (1982) in poorly nourished Indian women whose malnutrition was defined by a body weight/height index, the total cell counts in milk collected on the second day of lactation were significantly lower than those found in well nourished Indian women. Cell counts obtained thereafter for as long as 180 days of lactation were similar in the well nourished and poorly nourished populations. Since appropriate cytochemical studies were not performed, it was difficult to determine whether any major alterations in cell populations in milk occurred as a result of changes in maternal nutritional status. More precise studies will be required to examine this question.

Antiinflammatory Agents

Human milk lacks inflammatory mediators or their initiating systems (Goldman et al., 1986), but it contains a host of antiinflammatory agents including agents that double as direct protective agents, antioxidants, enzymes that degrade inflammatory mediators, antienzymes, cytoprotective agents, and modulators of leukocyte activation (Goldman et al., 1986, 1990). Some of these agents are also components of the antimicrobial system in human milk, whereas others that have antioxidant activity, such as α-tocopherol and β-carotene, are also nutrients.

Enzymes

Human milk contains numerous proteins with enzyme activity (Hamosh, 1989; Hamosh et al., 1985a; Jenness, 1979; Shahani et al., 1980) (see Table 6-6 for examples of enzymes and enzyme functions). Little is known about the effects of maternal nutritional status on the amounts or activity levels of enzymes in milk. However, it is known that the regulation of enzyme activity in the lactating mammary gland differs from that of identical enzymes in other organs. Thus, in the lactating mammary gland the activity of lipoprotein lipase, which is markedly reduced in adipose tissue by fasting, is unaffected by fasting (Hamosh and Hamosh, 1983). The major fat-digesting enzyme in human milk (bile salt-stimulated lipase) is not affected by feeding pattern or diurnal variation (Hamosh et al., 1985b) or by nutritional status of the mother (Hernell et al., 1977).

Hormones, Growth Factors, and Inducers

Human milk contains many hormones, growth factors, and inducers of certain biologic processes (see reviews by Koldovský [1989] and Koldovský et al. [1987]). The hormones include cortisol (Koldovský [1989]), somatostatin (Werner et al., 1985), insulin (Cevreska et al., 1975), thyroid hormones, and the lactogenic hormones oxytocin (Leake et al., 1981) and prolactin (Healy et al., 1980). There is agreement among investigators concerning the measurement of most of these agents, but there is considerable disagreement regarding measurement of thyroid hormones and some others (see review by Koldovský et al. [1987]). The growth factors include epidermal growth factor (Carpenter, 1980), insulin (Cevreska et al., 1975), lactoferrin (Nichols et al., 1987), and factors that are specifically derived from the mammary gland epithelium (Kidwell et al., 1987). There is laboratory evidence for the presence of activators of monocytes such as tumor necrosis factor-α (Mushtaha et al., 1989a,b). Bendich and coworkers (1984) and Tengerdy et al. (1981) presented evidence that the vitamin α-tocopherol in human milk may stimulate the immune system in the

TABLE 6-6 Enzyme Functions in Human Milk[a]

Function	Enzyme	Process
Biosynthesis of milk components in the mammary gland	Phosphoglucomutase	Synthesis of lactose
	Lactose synthetase	
	Fatty acid synthetase	Synthesis of medium-chain fatty acids
	Thioesterase	
Digestive function in the infant	Lipoprotein lipase	Uptake of circulating triglyceride fatty acids
	Amylase	Hydrolysis of polysaccharides
	Lipase (bile salt dependent)	Hydrolysis of triglycerides
	Proteases	Proteolysis (not verified)
Transport	Xanthine oxidase	Carrier of iron, molybdenum
	Glutathione peroxidase	Carrier of selenium
	Alkaline phosphatase	Carrier of zinc, magnesium
Preservation of milk components	Antiprotease	Protection of bioactive proteins, i.e., enzymes and immunoglobulins
	Sulfhydryl oxidase	Maintenance of structure and function of proteins containing disulfide bonds
Antiinfective agents	Lysozyme	Bactericidal
	Peroxidase	
	Lipases (lipoprotein lipase, bile salt-dependent lipase)	Release of free fatty acids that have antibacterial, antiviral, and antiprotozoan actions

[a]From Hamosh (1989) with permission.

infant. Zimecki and coworkers (1987) reported that certain protein fractions in human milk may aid in generating helper cell responses and in performing other immunoregulatory functions. Finally, the presence of antiidiotypic antibodies in milk may act as immunizing agents; these antibodies mimic other antibodies in the infant that in turn are directed against the original stimulating microbial antigens in the mother; thus, they may be natural, safe immunizing agents (Okamoto and Ogra, 1989).

SUMMARY

A wealth of evidence indicates that human milk possesses many unique characteristics related to its content of nutrients, protective substances, and other components. Some evidence suggests that maternal and environmental influences are stronger than previously recognized and appreciated. If maternal intake of one or more nutrients is chronically low, certain nutrients and nonnutrient constituents of milk may decrease, with the potential for a negative impact on the nursing infant. There is mounting evidence that the concentrations of some constituents are preserved in milk at the expense of maternal reserves.

CONCLUSIONS

- There is abundant evidence that women are able to produce milk with adequate content of protein, fat, carbohydrate, and most minerals even when their supply of nutrients is limited. The nutrients in human milk most likely to be present in lower than normal concentrations in response to chronically low maternal intakes are the vitamins, especially vitamins B_6, B_{12}, A, and D. Those maintained at the expense of maternal stores or tissues include the macronutrients, most minerals, and folate.
- The kinds of fatty acids present in human milk are strongly influenced by maternal diet: the type and amount of fat in the diet and the adequacy of energy intake. However, maternal total fat and cholesterol intake have no apparent influence on the total fat and cholesterol contents of human milk.

RECOMMENDATIONS FOR CLINICAL PRACTICE

- Encourage breastfeeding mothers to consume good sources of all essential nutrients for their own health as well as to maintain adequate concentrations of nutrients in milk. Nutrients of special concern from the standpoint of milk composition are vitamin B_6 and, for complete vegetarians, vitamins B_{12} and D.
- Since many nutrients are secreted in human milk at the expense of maternal reserves, give breastfeeding women dietary guidance to maintain their own health as well as that of their infants (see Chapter 9).

• Advise lactating women to avoid excessive intake of vitamin D or iodine from pharmaceutical preparations because potentially toxic amounts of these nutrients can be secreted into human milk. There is no advantage to taking these nutrients in amounts exceeding the RDAs.

• Reassure lactating women that occasional days with low nutrient intake by the mother are unlikely to harm the baby. The nutrient content of milk decreases relatively slowly, or not at all, with short-term decreases in dietary intake.

REFERENCES

Ajans, Z.A., A. Sarrif, and M. Husbands. 1965. Influence of vitamin A on human colostrum and early milk. Am. J. Clin. Nutr. 17:139-142.

Alpert, S.E., and A.D. Cormier. 1983. Normal electrolyte and protein content in milk from mothers with cystic fibrosis: an explanation for the initial report of elevated milk sodium concentration. J. Pediatr 102:77-80.

Anand, S.K., C. Sandborg, R.G. Robinson, and E. Liberman. 1980. Neonatal hyper-natremia associated with elevated sodium concentration of breast milk. J. Pediatr. 96:66-68.

Anderson, D.M., and W.B. Pittard III. 1985. Vitamin E and C concentrations in human milk with maternal megadosing: a case report. J. Am. Diet. Assoc. 85:715-717.

Anderson, G.H., S.A. Atkinson, and M.H. Bryan. 1981. Energy and macronutrient content of human milk during early lactation from mothers giving birth prematurely and at term. Am. J. Clin. Nutr. 34:258-265.

Arboit, J.M., and E. Gildengers (letter). 1980. Breast-feeding and hypernatremia. J. Pediatr. 97:335-336.

Ballow, M., F. Fang, R.A. Good, N.K. Day. 1974. Developmental aspects of complement components in the newborn. The presence of complement components and C3 proactivator (properdin factor B) in human colostrum. Clin. Exp. Immunol. 18:257-266.

Bates, C.J., A.M. Prentice, A.A. Paul, B.A. Sutcliffe, M. Watkinson, and R.G. White-head. 1981. Riboflavin status in Gambian pregnant and lactating women and its implications for Recommended Dietary Allowances. Am. J. Clin. Nutr. 34:928-935.

Bates, C.J., A.M. Prentice, A. Prentice, W.H. Lamb, and R.G. Whitehead. 1983. The effect of vitamin C supplementation on lactating women in Keneba, a West African rural community. Int. J. Vitam. Nutr. Res. 53:68-76.

Belavady, B., and C. Gopalan. 1960. Effect of dietary supplementation on the composition of breast milk. Indian J. Med. Res. 48:518-523.

Bendich, A., P. D'Apolito, E. Gabriel, and L.J. Machlin. 1984. Interaction of dietary vitamin C and vitamin E on guinea pig immune responses to mitogens. J. Nutr. 114:1588-1593.

Berkow, S.W., L.M. Freed, M. Hamosh, J. Bitman, D.L. Wood, B. Happ, and P. Hamosh. 1984. Lipases and lipids in human milk: effect of freeze-thawing and storage. Pediatr. Res. 18:1257-1262.

Bhaskaram, P., and V. Reddy. 1981. Bacterial activity of human milk leukocytes. Acta Paediatr. Scand. 70:87-90.

Bitman, J., D.L. Wood, N.R. Mehta, P. Hamosh, and M. Hamosh. 1983. Lipolysis of triglycerides in human milk at low temperatures: a note of caution. J. Pediatr. Gastroenterol. Nutr. 2:521-524.

Blanc, B. 1981. Biochemical aspects of human milk—comparison with bovine milk. World Rev. Nutr. Diet. 36:1-89.

Brines, R.D., and J.H. Brock. 1983. The effect of trypsin and chymotrypsin on the in vitro antimicrobial and iron-binding properties of lactoferrin in human milk and bovine colostrum. Biochim. Biophys. Acta 759:229-235.

Brown, C.M., A.M. Smith, and M.F. Picciano. 1986a. Forms of human milk folacin and variation patterns. J. Pediatr. Gastroenterol. Nutr. 5:278-282.

Brown, K.H., N.A. Akhtar, A.D. Robertson, and M.G. Ahmed. 1986b. Lactational capacity of marginally nourished mothers: relationships between maternal nutritional status and quantity and proximate composition of milk. Pediatrics 78:909-919.

Bullen, J.J., H.J. Rogers, and E. Griffiths. 1978. Role of iron in bacterial infection. Curr. Top. Microbiol. Immunol. 80:1-35.

Burgio, G.R., A. Lanzavecchia, A. Plebani, S. Jayakar, and A.G. Ugazio. 1980. Ontogeny of secretory immunity: levels of secretory IgA and natural antibodies in saliva. Pediatr. Res. 14:1111-1114.

Butte, N.F., and D.H. Calloway. 1981. Evaluation of lactational performance of Navajo women. Am. J. Clin. Nutr. 34:2210-2215.

Butte, N.F., R.M. Goldblum, L.M. Fehl, K. Loftin, E.O. Smith, C. Garza, and A.S. Goldman. 1984a. Daily ingestion of immunologic components in human milk during the first four months of life. Acta Paediatr. Scand. 73:296-301.

Butte, N.F., C. Garza, J.E. Stuff, E.O. Smith, and B.L. Nichols. 1984b. Effect of maternal diet and body composition on lactational performance. Am. J. Clin. Nutr. 39:296-306.

Carlson, S.E. 1985. Human milk nonprotein nitrogen: occurrence and possible functions. Adv. Pediatr. 32:43-70.

Carpenter, G. 1980. Epidermal growth factor is a major growth-promoting agent in human milk. Science 210:198-199.

Casey, C.E., M.R. Neifert, J.M. Seacat, and M.C. Neville. 1986. Nutrient intake by breast-fed infants during the first five days after birth. Am. J. Dis. Child. 140:933-936.

Casey, C.E., M.C. Neville, and K.M. Hambidge. 1989. Studies in human lactation: secretion of zinc, copper, and manganese in human milk. Am. J. Clin. Nutr. 49:773-785.

Cavell, P.A., and E.M. Widdowson. 1964. Intakes and excretions of iron, copper, and zinc in the neonatal period. Arch. Dis. Child. 39:496-501.

Cevreska, S., V.P. Kovacev, M. Stankovski, and E. Kamamaras. 1975. The presence of immunologically reactive insulin in milk of women during the first week of lactation and its relation to changes in plasma insulin concentrations. God. Zb. Med. Fak. Skopje. 21:35-41.

Chappell, J.E., M.T. Clandinin, and C. Kearney-Volpe. 1985a. *Trans* fatty acids in human milk lipids: influence of maternal diet and weight loss. Am. J. Clin. Nutr. 42:49-56.

Chappell, J.E., T. Francis, and M.T. Clandinin. 1985b. Vitamin A and E content of human milk at early stages of lactation. Early Hum. Dev. 11:157-167.

Chappell, J.E., T. Francis, and M.T. Clandinin. 1986. Simultaneous high performance chromatography analysis of retinol esters and tocopherol isomers in human milk. Nutr. Res. 6:849-852.

Chipman, D.M., and N. Sharon. 1969. Mechanism of lysozyme action. Science 165:454-465.

Cleary, T.G., J.P. Chambers, and L.K. Pickering. 1983. Protection of suckling mice from the heat-stable enterotoxin of *Escherichia coli* by human milk. J. Infect. Dis. 148:1114-1119.

Committee on Nutrition. 1985. Composition of human milk: normative data. Pp. 363-368 in Pediatric Nutrition Handbook, 2nd ed. American Academy of Pediatrics, Elk Grove Village, Ill.

Crago, S.S., S.J. Prince, T.G. Pretlow, J.R. McGhee, and J. Mestecky. 1979. Human colostral cells. I. Separation and characterization. Clin. Exp. Immunol. 38:585-597.

Cruz, J.R., B. Carlsson, and B. García. 1982. Studies in human milk. III. Secretory IgA quantity and antibody levels against Escherichiae coli in colostrum and milk from underprivileged and privileged mothers. Pediatr. Res. 16:272-276.

Cumming, F.J., and M.H. Briggs. 1983. Changes in plasma vitamin A in lactating and non-lactating oral contraceptive users. Br. J. Obstet. Gynaecol. 90:73-77.

Dallman, P.R. 1986. Iron deficiency in the weanling: a nutritional problem on the way to resolution. Acta Paediatr. Scand. Suppl. 323:59-67.

Deb, A.K., and H.R. Cama. 1962. Studies on human lactation. Dietary nitrogen utilization during lactation, and distribution of nitrogen in mother's milk. Br. J. Nutr. 16:65-73.

Debski, B., D.A. Finley, M.F. Picciano, B. Lönnerdal, and J.A. Milner. 1989. Selenium content and glutathione peroxidase activity of milk from vegetarian and nonvegetarian women. J. Nutr. 119:215-220.

Delange, F. 1985. Physiopathology of iodine nutrition. Pp. 291-299 in R.K. Chandra, ed. Trace Elements in Nutrition of Children. Nestle Nutrition Workshop Series, Vol. 8. Raven Press, New York.

Department of Health and Social Security. 1977. Composition of Mature Human Milk. Report on Health and Social Security. 12. Her Majesty's Stationery Office, London.

Dewey, K.G., D.A. Finley, and B. Lönnerdal. 1984. Breast milk volume and composition during late lactation (7-20 months). J. Pediatr. Gastroenterol. Nutr. 3:713-720.

Ekstrand, J., C.J. Spak, J. Falch, J. Afseth, and H. Ulvestad. 1984a. Distribution of fluoride to human breast milk: following intake of high doses of fluoride. Caries Res. 18:93-95.

Ekstrand, J., L.I. Hardell, and C.J. Spak. 1984b. Fluoride balance studies on infants in a 1-ppm-water-fluoride area. Caries Res. 18:87-92.

Ellis, L., M.F. Picciano, A.M. Smith, M. Hamosh, and N.R. Mehta. 1990. The impact of gestational length on human milk selenium concentration and glutathione peroxidase activity. Pediatr. Res. 27:32-50.

Esala, S., E. Vuori, and A. Helle. 1982. Effect of maternal fluorine intake on breast milk fluorine content. Br. J. Nutr. 48:201-204.

Feeley, R.M., R.R. Eitenmiller, J.B. Jones, Jr., and H. Barnhart. 1983. Copper, iron, and zinc contents of human milk at early stages of lactation. Am. J. Clin. Nutr. 37:443-448.

Finley, D.A., B. Lönnerdal, K.G. Dewey, and L.E. Grivetti. 1985. Breast milk composition: fat content and fatty acid composition in vegetarians and non-vegetarians. Am. J. Clin. Nutr. 41:787-800.

Forsum, E., and B. Lönnerdal. 1980. Effect of protein intake on protein and nitrogen composition of breast milk. Am. J. Clin. Nutr. 33:1809-1813.

Fransson, G.B., and B. Lönnerdal. 1980. Iron in human milk. J. Pediatr. 96:380-384.

144   NUTRITION DURING LACTATION

Friss, H.E., L.G. Rubin, S. Carsons, J. Baranowski, and P.J. Lipsitz. 1988. Plasma fibronectin concentrations in breast fed and formula fed neonates. Arch. Dis. Child. 63:528-532.

Funk, M.A., L. Hamlin, M.F. Picciano, A. Prentice, and J.A. Milner. 1990. Milk selenium of rural African women: influence of maternal nutrition, parity, and length of lactation. Am. J. Clin. Nutr. 51:220-224.

Furmanski, P., L. Zhen-Pu, M.B. Fortuna, C.V.B. Swamy, and M. Ramachandra Das. 1989. Multiple molecular forms of human lactoferrin: identification of a class of lactoferrins that possess ribonuclease activity and lack iron-binding capacity. J. Exp. Med. 170:415-429.

Gaull, G.E., R.G. Jensen, D.K. Rassin, and M.H. Malloy. 1982. Human milk as food. Adv. Perinat. Med. 2:47-120.

Gebre-Medhin, M., A. Vahlquist, Y. Hofvander, L. Uppsäll, and B. Vahlquist. 1976. Breast milk composition in Ethiopian and Swedish mothers. I. Vitamin A and β-carotene. Am. J. Clin. Nutr. 29:441-451.

Gillin, F.D., D.S. Reiner, and C.S. Wang. 1983. Human milk kills parasitic intestinal protozoa. Science 221:1290-1292.

Gillin, F.D., D.S. Reiner, and M.J. Gault. 1985. Cholate-dependent killing of Giardia lamblia by human milk. Infect. Immun. 47:619-622.

Goldman, A.S., and R.M. Goldblum. 1989a. Immunoglobulins in human milk. Pp. 43-51 in S.A. Atkinson and B. Lönnerdal, eds. Protein and Non-Protein Nitrogen in Human Milk. CRC Press, Boca Raton, Fla.

Goldman, A.S., and R.M. Goldblum. 1989b. Immunologic system in human milk: characteristics and effects. Pp. 135-142 in E. Lebenthal, ed. Textbook of Gastroenterology and Nutrition in Early Infancy, 2nd ed. Raven Press, New York.

Goldman, A.S., and R.M. Goldblum. 1990. Human milk: immunologic-nutritional relationships. Ann. N.Y. Acad. Sci. 587:236-245.

Goldman, A.S., C. Garza, B.L. Nichols, and R.M. Goldblum. 1982. Immunologic factors in human milk during the first year of lactation. J. Pediatr. 100:563-567.

Goldman, A.S., R.M. Goldblum, and C. Garza. 1983a. Immunologic components in human milk during the second year of lactation. Acta Paediatr. Scand. 72:461-462.

Goldman, A.S., R.M. Goldblum, C. Garza, B.L. Nichols, and E.O. Smith. 1983b. Immunologic components in human milk during weaning. Acta Paediatr. Scand. 72:133-134.

Goldman, A.S., L.W. Thorpe, R.M. Goldblum, and L.A. Hanson. 1986. Anti-inflammatory properties of human milk. Acta Paediatr. Scand. 75:689-695.

Goldman, A.S., S.A. Atkinson, and L.A. Hanson. 1987. Human Lactation 3: The Effects of Human Milk on the Recipient Infant. Plenum Press, New York. 400 pp.

Goldman, A.S., R.M. Goldblum, and L.A. Hanson. 1990. Anti-inflammatory systems in human milk. Adv. Exp. Med. Biol. 262:69-76.

Greenberg, R., and M.L. Graves. 1984. Plasmin cleaves human beta-casein. Biochem. Biophys. Res. Commun. 125:463-468.

Greer, F.R., B.W. Hollis, D.J. Cripps, and R.C. Tsang. 1984a. Effects of maternal ultraviolet B irradiation on vitamin D content of human milk. J. Pediatr. 105:431-433.

Greer, F.R., B.W. Hollis, and J.L. Napoli. 1984b. High concentrations of vitamin D_2 in human milk associated with pharmacologic doses of vitamin D_2. J. Pediatr. 105:61-64.

Guerrini, P., G. Bosi, R. Chierici, and A. Fabbri. 1981. Human milk: relationship of fat content with gestational age. Early Hum. Dev. 5:187-194.

Gushurst, C.A., J.A. Mueller, J.A. Green, and F. Sedor. 1984. Breast milk iodide: reassessment in the 1980s. Pediatrics 73:354-357.

Gyllenberg, H., and P. Roine. 1957. The value of colony counts in evaluating the abundance of "Lactobacillus" bifidus in infant faeces. Acta Pathol. Microbiol. Scand. 41:144.

György, P., R.W. Jeanloz, H. von Nicolai, and F. Zilliken. 1974. Undialyzable growth factors for Lactobacillus Bifidus Var. Pennsylvanicus: protective effect of sialic acid bound to glycoproteins and oligosaccharides against bacterial degradation. Eur. J. Biochem. 43:29-33.

Hachey, D.L., M.R. Thomas, E.A. Emken, C. Garza, L. Brown-Booth, R.O. Adlof, and P.D. Klein. 1987. Human lactation: maternal transfer of dietary triglycerides labeled with stable isotopes. J. Lipid Res. 28:1185-1192.

Hachey, D.L., G.H. Silber, W.W. Wong, and C. Garza. 1989. Human lactation II: endogenous fatty acid synthesis by the mammary gland. Pediatr. Res. 25:63-68.

Hall, L., and P.N. Campbell. 1986. α-Lactalbumin and related proteins: a versatile gene family with an interesting parentage. Essays Biochem. 22:1-26.

Hamosh, M. 1989. Enzymes in human milk: their role in nutrient digestion, gastrointestinal function, and nutrient delivery to the newborn infant. Pp. 121-134 in E. Lebenthal, ed. Textbook of Gastroenterology and Nutrition in Infancy, 2nd ed. Raven Press, New York.

Hamosh, M., and A.S. Goldman, eds. 1986. Human Lactation 2: Maternal and Environmental Factors. Plenum Press, New York. 657 pp.

Hamosh, M., and P. Hamosh. 1983. Lipoprotein lipase: its physiological and clinical significance. Mol. Aspects Med. 6:199-289.

Hamosh, P., and M. Hamosh. 1987. Differences in composition of preterm, term and weaning milk. Pp. 129-141 in Xanthou, M., ed. New Aspects of Nutrition in Pregnancy, Infancy and Prematurity. Elsevier Science Publishers. B.V. (Biomedical Division).

Hamosh, M., and P. Hamosh. 1988. Mother to infant biochemical and immunological transfer through breast milk. Pp. 155-160 in G.H. Wiknjosastro, W.H. Prakoso, and K. Maeda, eds. Perinatology. Excerpta Medica, Amsterdam.

Hamosh, M., T.R. Clary, S.S. Chernick, and R.O. Scow. 1970. Lipoprotein lipase activity of adipose and mammary tissue and plasma triglyceride in pregnant and lactating rats. Biochim. Biophys. Acta 210:473-482.

Hamosh, M., L.M. Freed, J.B. Jones, S.E. Berkow, J. Bitman, N.R. Mehta, B. Happ, and P. Hamosh. 1985a. Enzymes in human milk. Pp. 251-266 in R.G. Jensen and M.C. Neville, eds. Human Lactation: Milk Components and Methodologies. Plenum Press, New York.

Hamosh, M., J. Bitman, C.S. Fink, L.M. Freed, C.M. York, D.L. Wood, N.R. Mehta, and P. Hamosh. 1985b. Lipid composition of preterm human milk and its digestion by the infant. Pp. 153-164 in J. Schaub, ed. Composition and Physiological Properties of Human Milk. Elsevier, Amsterdam.

Hanson, L.A., T. Söderström, C. Brinton, B. Carlsson, P. Larsson, L. Mellander, and C.S. Eden. 1983. Neonatal colonization with *Escherichia coli* and the ontogeny of the antibody response. Prog. Allergy 33:40-52.

Haroon, Y., M.J. Shearer, S. Rahim, W.G. Gunn, G. McEnery, and P. Barkhan. 1982. The content of phylloquinone (vitamin K_1) in human milk, cows' milk and infant formula foods determined by high-performance liquid chromatography. J. Nutr. 112:1105-1117.

Hartmann, P.E., and J.K. Kulski. 1978. Changes in the composition of the mammary secretion of women after abrupt termination of breastfeeding. J. Physiol. (Lond) 275:1-11.

Hartmann, P.E., and C.G. Prosser. 1982. Acute changes in the composition of milk during the ovulatory menstrual cycle in lactating women. J. Physiol. (Lond) 324:21-30.

Healy, D.L., S. Rattigan, P.E. Hartmann, A.C. Herington, and H.G. Burger. 1980. Prolactin in human milk: correlation with lactose, total protein, and α-lactalbumin levels. Am. J. Physiol. 238:E83-E86.

Hernell, O., M. Gebre-Medhin, and T. Olivecrona. 1977. Breast milk composition in Ethiopian and Swedish mothers. IV. Milk lipases. Am. J. Clin. Nutr. 30:508-511.

Ho, P.C., and J.W.M. Lawton. 1978. Human colostral cells: phagocytosis and killing of E. coli, and C. albicans. J. Pediatr. 93:910-915.

Hollis, B.W., B.A. Roos, and P.W. Lambert. 1982. Vitamin D compounds in human and bovine milk. Advances Nutr. Res. 4:49-75.

Hollis, B.W., P.W. Lambert, and R.L. Horst. 1983. Factors affecting the antirachitic sterol content of native milk. Pp. 157-182 in M.F. Holick, T.K. Gray, and C.S. Anast, eds. Perinatal Calcium and Phosphorous Metabolism. Elsevier, Amsterdam.

Holmgren, J., A.M. Svennerholm, and C. Ahren. 1981. Nonimmunoglobulin fraction of human milk inhibits bacterial adhesion (hemagglutination) and enterotoxin binding of Escherichiae coli and Vibrio cholerae. Infect. Immun. 33:136-141.

Hood, R.L., and A.R. Johnson. 1980. Supplementation of infant formulations with biotin. Nutr. Reports Internat. 21:727-731.

Hrubetz, M.C., H.J. Deuel, Jr., and B.J. Hanley. 1945. Studies on carotenoid metabolism. V. The effect of a high vitamin A intake on the composition of human milk. J. Nutr. 29:245-254.

Hustead, V.A., J.L. Greger, and G.R. Gutcher. 1988. Zinc supplementation and plasma concentration of vitamin A in preterm infants. Am. J. Clin. Nutr. 47:1017-1021.

Hytten, F.E. 1954a. Clinical and chemical studies in human lactation. I. Collection of milk samples. Br. Med. J. 1:175-176.

Hytten, F.E. 1954b. Clinical and chemical studies in human lactation. IV. Trends in milk composition during course of lactation. Br. Med. J.:249-253.

Hytten, F.E. 1954c. Clinical and chemical studies in human lactation. V. Individual differences in composition of milk. Br. Med. J. 1:253-255.

Hytten, F.E., and A.M. Thomson. 1961. Nutrition of the lactating woman. Pp. 3-46 in Kon, S.K. and A.T. Cowie, eds. Milk: the Mammary Gland and Its Secretion. Academic Press, New York.

Insull, W., Jr., J. Hirsch, T. James, and E.H. Ahrens, Jr. 1959. The fatty acids of human milk. II. Alterations produced by manipulation of caloric balance and exchange of dietary fats. J. Clin. Invest. 38:443-450.

Isaacs, C.E., H. Thormar, and T. Pessolano. 1986. Membrane-disruptive effect of human milk: inactivation of enveloped viruses. J. Infect. Dis. 154:966-971.

Janas, L.M., and M.F. Picciano. 1982. The nucleotide profile of human milk. Pediatr. Res. 16:659-662.

Jelliffe, D.B. 1966. The Assessment of the Nutritional Status of the Community. Monograph Series No. 53. World Health Organization, Geneva. 271 pp.

Jenness, R. 1979. The composition of human milk. Semin. Perinatol. 3:225-239.

Jensen, R.G. 1989. The Lipids of Human Milk. CRC Press, Boca Raton, Fla. 213 pp.

Jensen, R.G., and M.C. Neville, eds. 1985. Human Lactation: Milk Components and Methodologies. Plenum Press, New York. 307 pp.

Johnson, P.R., Jr., and J.S. Roloff. 1982. Vitamin B_{12} deficiency in an infant strictly breast-fed by a mother with latent pernicious anemia. J. Pediatr. 100:917-919.

Karra, M.V., A. Kirksey, O. Galal, N.S. Bassily, G.G. Harrison, and N.W. Jerome. 1989. Effect of short-term oral zinc supplementation on the concentration of zinc in milk from American and Egyptian women. Nutr. Res. 9:471-478.

Keller. M.A., R.M. Kidd, Y.J. Bryson, J.L. Turner, and J. Carter. 1981. Lymphokine production by human milk lymphocytes. Infect. Immun. 32:632-636.

Keller, M.A., J. Faust, L.J. Rolewic, and D.D. Stewart. 1986. T cell subsets in human colostrum. J. Pediatr. Gastroenterol. Nutr. 5:439-443.

Kidwell, W.R., D.S. Salomon, S. Mohanam, and G.I. Bell. 1987. Production of growth factors by normal human mammary cells in culture. Pp. 227-239 in A.S. Goldman, S.A. Atkinson, and L.A. Hanson, eds. Human Lactation 3: The Effects of Human Milk on the Recipient Infant. Plenum Press, New York.

Kirksey, A., and J.L.B. Roepke. 1981. Vitamin B_6 nutriture of mothers of three breast-fed neonates with central nervous system disorders. Fed. Proc., Fed. Am. Soc. Exp. Biol. 40:864.

Kirksey, A., J.A. Ernst, J.L. Roepke, and T.L. Tsai. 1979. Influence of mineral intake and use of oral contraceptives before pregnancy on the content of human colostrum and of more mature milk. Am. J. Clin. Nutr. 32:30-39.

Kobata, A. 1972. Isolation of oligosaccharides from human milk. Pp. 262-271 in V. Ginsburg, ed. Methods in Enzymology, Vol. 28: Complex Carbohydrates, Part B. Academic Press, New York.

Kobayashi, H., C. Kanno, K. Yamauchi, and T. Tsugo. 1975. Identification of α-,β-, γ-, and δ-tocopherols and their contents in human milk. Biochim. Biophys. Acta 380:282-290.

Kohl, S., L.K. Pickering, T.G. Cleary, K.D. Steinmetz, and L.S. Loo. 1980. Human colostral cytotoxicity. II. Relative defects in colostral leukocyte cytotoxicity and inhibition of peripheral blood leukocyte cytotoxicity by colostrum. J. Infect. Dis. 142:884-891.

Koldovsky, O. 1989. Hormones in milk: their possible physiological significance for the neonate. Pp. 97-119 in E. Lebenthal, ed. Textbook of Gastroenterology and Nutrition in Infancy, 2nd ed. Raven Press, New York.

Koldovsky, O., A. Bedrick, P. Pollack, R.K. Rao, and W. Thornburg. 1987. Hormones in milk: their presence and possible physiological significance. Pp. 183-196 in A.S. Goldman, S.A. Atkinson, and L.A. Hanson, eds. Human Lactation 3: The Effects of Human Milk on the Recipient Infant. Plenum Press, New York.

Krebs, N.F., K.M. Hambidge, M.A. Jacobs, and J.O. Rasbach. 1985. The effects of dietary zinc supplement during lactation on longitudinal changes in maternal zinc status and milk zinc concentrations. Am. J. Clin. Nutr. 41:560-570.

Kulski, J.K., and P.E. Hartmann. 1981. Changes in body composition during the initiation of lactation. Aust. J. Exp. Bio. Med. Sci. 59:101-114.

Kumpulainen, J. 1989. Selenium: requirement and supplementation. Acta Paediatr. Scand. Suppl. 351:114-117.

Lawton, J.W.M., K.F. Shortridge, R.L.C. Wong, and M.H. Ng. 1979. Interferon synthesis by human colostral leucocytes. Arch. Dis. Child. 54:127-130.

Leake, R.D., R.E. Weitzman, and D.A. Fisher. 1981. Oxytocin concentrations during the neonatal period. Biol. Neonate 39:127-131.

Leyva-Cobián, F., and J. Clemente. 1984. Phenotypic characterization and functional activity of human milk macrophages. Immunol. Lett. 8:249-256.

Lindblad, B.S., and R.J. Rahimtoola. 1974. A pilot study of the quality of human milk in a lower socio-economic group in Karachi, Pakistan. Acta Paediatr. Scand. 63:125-128.

Lindh, E. 1975. Increased resistance of immunoglobulin A dimers to proteolytic degradation after binding of secretory component. J. Immunol. 114:284-286.

Lönnerdal, B. 1985a. Biochemistry and physiological function of human milk proteins. Am. J. Clin. Nutr. 42:1299-1317.

Lönnerdal, B. 1985b. Methods for studying the total protein content of human milk. Pp. 25-31 in R.G. Jensen and M.C. Neville, eds. Human Lactation: Milk Components and Methodologies. Plenum Press, New York.

Lönnerdal, B. 1986a. Effects of maternal dietary intake on human milk composition. J. Nutr. 116:499-513.

Lönnerdal, B. 1986b. Effects of maternal nutrition on human lactation. Pp. 301-323 in M. Hamosh and A.S. Goldman, eds. Human Lactation 2: Maternal and Environmental Factors. Plenum Press, New York.

Lönnerdal, B., E. Forsum, M. Gebre-Medhin, and L. Hambraeus. 1976a. Breast milk composition in Ethiopian and Swedish mothers. II. Lactose, nitrogen and protein contents. Am. J. Clin. Nutr. 29:1134-1141.

Lönnerdal, B., E. Forsum, and L. Hambraeus. 1976b. A longitudinal study of the protein, nitrogen, and lactose contents of human milk from Swedish well-nourished mothers. Am. J. Clin. Nutr. 29:1127-1133.

Lönnerdal, B., E. Forsum, and L. Hambraeus. 1976c. The protein content of human milk. I. A transversal study of Swedish normal material. Nutr. Rep. Int. 13:125-134.

Lönnerdal, B., C.L. Keen, and L.S. Hurley. 1981. Iron, copper, zinc, and manganese in milk. Annu. Rev. Nutr. 1:149-174.

Lönnerdal, B., L.R. Woodhouse, and C. Glazier. 1987. Compartmentalization and quantitation of human milk protein. J. Nutr. 117:1385-1395.

Macy, I.G. 1949. Composition of human colostrum and milk. Am. J. Dis. Child. 78:589-603.

Macy, I.G., H.H. Williams, J.P. Pratt, and B.M. Hamil. 1945. Human milk studies. XIX. Implications of breast feeding and their investigation. Am. J. Dis. Child. 70:135-141.

Mannan, S., and M.F. Picciano. 1987. Influence of maternal selenium status on human milk selenium concentration and glutathione peroxidase activity. Am. J. Clin. Nutr. 46:95-100.

Metz, J., R. Zalusky, and V. Herbert. 1968. Folic acid binding by serum and milk. Am. J. Clin. Nutr. 21:289-297.

Miranda, R., N.G. Saravia, R. Ackerman, N. Murphy, S. Berman, and D.N. McMurray. 1983. Effect of maternal nutritional status on immunological substances in human colostrum and milk. Am. J. Clin. Nutr. 37:632-640.

Moser, P.B., and R.D. Reynolds. 1983. Dietary zinc intake and zinc concentrations of plasma, erythrocytes, and breast milk in antepartum and postpartum lactating and nonlactating women: a longitudinal study. Am. J. Clin. Nutr. 38:101-108.

Murray, M.J., A.B. Murray, N.J. Murray, and M.B. Murray. 1978. The effect of iron status of Nigerien mothers on that of their infants at birth and 6 months, and on the concentration of Fe in breast milk. Br. J. Nutr. 39:627-630.

Mushtaha, A.A., F.C. Schmalstieg, T.K. Hughes, Jr., S. Rajaraman, H.E. Rudloff, and A.S. Goldman. 1989a. Chemokinetic agents for monocytes in human milk: possible role of tumor necrosis factor-α. Pediatr. Res. 25:629-633.

Mushtaha, A.A., F.C. Schmalstieg, T.K. Hughes, Jr., H.E. Rudloff, and A.S. Goldman. 1989b. Chemokinetic effects of exogenous and endogenous tumor necrosis factor-α on human blood monocytes. Int. Arch. Allergy Appl. Immunol. 90:11-15.

Nakajima, S., A.S. Baba, and N. Tamura. 1977. Complement system in human colostrum: presence of nine complement components and factors of alternative pathway in human colostrum. Int. Arch. Allergy Appl. Immunol. 54:428-433.

Narula, P., S.K. Mittal, S. Gupta, and K. Saha. 1982. Cellular and humoral factors of human milk in relation to nutritional status in lactating mothers. Indian J. Med Res. 76:415-423.

Naylor, A.J. 1981. Elevated sodium concentration in human milk: its clinical significance. Refrig. Sci. Technol. 1981-2:79-84.

Nichols, B.L., K.S. McKee, J.F. Henry, and M. Putman. 1987. Human lactoferrin stimulates thymidine incorporation into DNA of rat crypt cells. Pediatr. Res. 21:563-567.

Nommsen, L.A., C.A. Lovelady, M.J. Heinig, B. Lönnerdal, and K.G. Dewey. In press. Determinants of energy, protein, lipid and lactose concentrations in human milk during the first 12 months of lactation: the DARLING Study. J. Clin. Nutr.

NRC (National Research Council). 1989. Recommended Dietary Allowances, 10th ed. Report of the Subcommittee on the Tenth Edition of the RDAs, Food and Nutrition Board, Commission on Life Sciences. National Academy Press, Washington, D.C. 284 pp.

O'Connor, D.L., M.F. Picciano, T. Tamura, and B. Shane. 1990a. Impaired milk folate secretion is not corrected by supplemental folate during iron deficiency in rats. J. Nutr 120:499-506.

O'Connor, D.L., T. Tamura, and M.F. Picciano. 1990b. Presence of folylpolyglutamates in human milk. FASEB J. 4:A915 (abstract).

Okamoto, Y., and P.L. Ogra. 1989. Antiviral factors in human milk: implications in respiratory syncytial virus infection. Acta Paediatr. Scand., Suppl. 351:137-143.

Otnæss, A.B., and A.M. Svennerholm. 1982. Non-immunoglobulin fraction of human milk protects rabbits against enterotoxin-induced intestinal fluid secretion. Infect. Immun. 35:738-740.

Otnæss, A.B.K., A. Laegreid, and K. Ertresvåg. 1983. Inhibition of enterotoxin from Escherichia coli and Vibrio cholerae by gangliosides from human milk. Infect. Immun. 40:563-569.

Özkaragöz, F., H.B. Rudloff, S. Rajaraman, A.K. Mushtaha, F.C. Schmalstieg, and A.S. Goldman. 1988. The motility of human milk macrophages in collagen gels. Pediatr. Res. 23:449-452.

Patton, S., L.M. Canfield, G.E. Huston, A.M. Ferris, and R.G. Jensen. 1990. Carotenoids of human colostrum. Lipids 25:159-165.

Picciano, M.F. 1984a. The composition of human milk. Pp. 111-122 in P.L. White and N. Selvey, eds. Malnutrition: Determinants and Consequences. Alan R. Liss, New York.

Picciano, M.F. 1984b. What constitutes a representative human milk sample? J. Pediatr. Gastroenterol. Nutr. 3:280-283.

Picciano, M.F. 1985. Trace elements in human milk and infant formulas. Pp. 157-174 in R.K. Chandra (ed.). Trace Elements in Nutrition of Children. Nestle Nutrition Workshop Series, Vol. 8. Raven Press, N.Y.

Picciano, M.F., and H.A. Guthrie. 1976. Copper, iron, and zinc contents of mature human milk. Am. J. Clin. Nutr. 29:242-254.

Picciano, M.F., E.J. Calkins, J.R. Garrick, and R.H. Deering. 1981. Milk and mineral intakes of breastfed infants. Acta Paediatr. Scand. 70:189-194.

Pratt, J.P., B.M. Hamil, E.Z. Moyer, M. Kaucher, C. Roderuck, M.N. Coryell, S. Miller, H.H. Williams, and I.G. Macy. 1951. Metabolism of women during the reproductive cycle. XVIII. The effect of multi-vitamin supplements on the secretion of B vitamins in human milk. J. Nutr. 44:141-157.

Prentice, A., A.M. Prentice, and R.G. Whitehead. 1981. Breast-milk fat concentrations of rural African women. 2. Long-term variations within a community. Br. J. Nutr. 45:495-503.

Prentice, A., L.M. Jarjou, P.J. Drury, O. Dewit, and M.A. Crawford. 1989. Breast-milk fatty acids of rural Gambian mothers: effects of diet and maternal parity. J. Pediatr. Gastroenterol. Nutr. 8:486-490.

Rana, S.K., and T.A.B. Sanders. 1986. Taurine concentrations in the diet, plasma, urine and breast milk of vegans compared with omnivores. Br. J. Nutr. 56:17-27.

Rassin, D.K., J.A. Sturman, and G.E. Gaull. 1978. Taurine and other free amino acids in milk of man and other mammals. Early Hum. Dev. 2:1-13.

Reddy, V., and S.G. Srikantia. 1978. Interaction of nutrition and the immune response. Indian J. Med. Res. 66:48-57.

Reddy, V., C. Bhaskaram, N. Raghuramuhi, and V. Jagadeesan. 1977. Antimicrobial factors in human milk. Acta Paediatr. Scand. 66:229-232.

Resta, S., J.P. Luby, C.R. Rosenfeld, and J.D. Siegel. 1985. Isolation and propagation of a human enteric coronavirus. Science 229:978-981.

Robertson, D.M., B. Carlsson, K. Coffman, M. Han-Zoric, F. Salil, C. Jones, and L.A. Hanson. 1988. Avidity of IgA antibody to Escherichia coli polysaccharide and diphtheria toxin in breast milk from Swedish and Pakistani mothers. Scand. J. Immunol. 28:783-789.

Robinson, J.E., B.A.M. Harvey, and J.F. Soothill. 1978. Phagocytosis and killing of bacteria and yeast by human milk cells after opsonisation in aqueous phase of milk. Br. Med. J. 1:1443-1445.

Roepke, J.L.B., and A. Kirksey. 1979. Vitamin B_6 nutriture during pregnancy and lactation. I. Vitamin B_6 intake, levels of the vitamin in biological fluids, and condition of the infant at birth. Am. J. Clin. Nutr. 32:2249-2256.

Ruegg, M., and B. Blanc. 1982. Structure and properties of the particulate constituents of human milk. A review. Food Microstruct. 1:25-48.

Salmenperä, L., J. Perheentupa, J.P. Pispa, and M.A. Siimes. 1985. Biotin concentrations in maternal plasma and milk during prolonged lactation. Int. J. Vitam. Nutr. Res. 55:281-285.

Salmenperä, L., J. Perheentupa, P. Pakarinen, and M.A. Siimes. 1986a. Cu nutrition in infants during prolonged exclusive breast-feeding: low intake but rising serum concentrations of Cu and ceruloplasmin. Am. J. Clin. Nutr. 43:251-257.

Salmenperä, L., J. Perheentupa, and M.A. Siimes. 1986b. Folate nutrition is optimal in exclusively breast-fed infants but inadequate in some of their mothers and in formula-fed infants. J. Pediatr. Gastroenterol. Nutr. 5:283-289.

Samson, R.R., C. Mirtle, and D.B.L. McClelland. 1980. The effect of digestive enzymes on the binding and bacteriostatic properties of lactoferrin and vitamin B_{12} binder in human milk. Acta Paediatr. Scand. 69:517-523.

Sandberg, D.P., J.A. Begley, and C.A. Hall. 1981. The content, binding, and forms of vitamin B_{12} in milk. Am. J. Clin. Nutr. 34:1717-1724.

Sanders, T.H.B., T.R. Ellis, and J.W.T. Dickerson. 1978. Studies of vegans: the fatty acid composition of plasma choline-phosphoglycerides, erythrocytes, adipose tissue, breastmilk and some indicators of susceptibility to ischemic heart disease in vegans and omnivore controls. Am. J. Clin. Nutr. 31:805.

Sann, L., F. Bienvenu, C. Lahet, J. Bienvenu, and M. Bethenod. 1981. Comparison of the composition of breast milk from mothers of term and preterm infants. Acta Paediatr. Scand. 70:115-116.

Seale, T.W., O.M. Rennert, M.L. Shiftman, and P.T. Swender. 1982. Toxic breast milk: neonatal hypernatremia associated with elevated sodium in breast milk. Pediatr. Res. 16:176a.

Shahani, K.M., A.J. Kwan, and B.A. Friend. 1980. Role and significance of enzymes in human milk. Am. J. Clin. Nutr. 33:1861-1868.

Siimes, M.A., E. Vuori, and P. Kuitunen. 1979. Breast milk iron—a declining concentration during the course of lactation. Acta Paediatr. Scand. 68:29-31.

Siimes, M.A., L. Salmenperä, and J. Perheentupa. 1984. Exclusive breast-feeding for 9 months: risk of iron deficiency. J. Pediatr. 104:196-199.

Singer, L., and W.D. Armstrong. 1960. Regulation of human plasma fluoride concentration. J. Appl. Physiol. 15:508-510.

Smith, H.W., and W.E. Crabb. 1961. The faecal bacterial flora of animals and man: its development in the young. J. Pathol. Bacteriol. 82:53-66.

Smith, C.W., and A.S. Goldman. 1968. The cells of human colostrum. I. In vitro studies of morphology and functions. Pediatr. Res. 2:103-109.

Smith, A.M., M.F. Picciano, and J.A. Milner. 1982. Selenium intakes and status of human milk and formula fed infants. Am. J. Clin. Nutr. 35:521-526.

Smith, A.M., M.F. Picciano, and R.H. Deering. 1983. Folate supplementation during lactation: maternal folate status, human milk folate content, and their relationship to infant folate status. J. Pediatr. Gastroenterol. Nutr. 2:622-628.

Song, W.O., G.M. Chan, B.W. Wyse, and R.G. Hansen. 1984. Effect of pantothenic acid status on the content of the vitamin in human milk. Am. J. Clin. Nutr. 40:317-324.

Spak, C.J., L.I. Hardell, and P. de Chateau. 1983. Fluoride in human milk. Acta Paediatr. Scand. 72:699-701.

Stastny, D., R.S. Vogel, and M.F. Picciano. 1984. Manganese intake and serum manganese concentration of human milk-fed and formula-fed infants. Am. J. Clin. Nutr. 39:872-878.

Stephens, S., J.M. Dolby, J. Montreuil, and G. Spik. 1980. Differences in inhibition of the growth of commensal and enteropathogenic strains of *Escherichia coli* by lactotransferrin and secretory immunoglobulin A isolated from human milk. Immunology 41:597-603.

Styslinger, L., and A. Kirksey. 1985. Effects of different levels of vitamin B_6 supplementation on vitamin B_6 concentrations in human milk and vitamin B_6 intakes of breastfed infants. Am. J. Clin. Nutr. 41:21-31.

Svanberg, U., M. Gebre-Medhin, B. Ljunqvist, and M. Olsson. 1977. Breast milk composition in Ethiopian and Swedish mothers. III. Amino acids and other nitrogenous substances. Am. J. Clin. Nutr. 30:499-507.

Svanborg-Edén, C., B. Andersson, L. Hagberg, L.A. Hanson, H. Leffler, G. Magnusson, G. Noori, J. Dahmen, and T. Söderström. 1983. Receptor analogues and anti-pili antibodies as inhibitors of bacterial attachment in vivo and in vitro. Ann. N.Y. Acad. Sci. 409:580-592.

Tamura, T., Y. Yoshimura, and T. Arakawa. 1980. Human milk folate and folate status in lactating mothers and their infants. Am. J. Clin. Nutr. 33:193-197.

Tengerdy, R.P., M.M. Mathias, and C.F. Nockels. 1981. Vitamin E, immunity and disease resistance. Adv. Exp. Med. Biol. 135:27-42.

Thorpe, L.W., H.E. Rudloff, L.C. Powell, and A.S. Goldman. 1986. Decreased response of human milk leukocytes to chemoattractant peptides. Pediatr. Res. 20:373-377.

Tsuda, H., K. Takeshige, Y. Shibata, and S. Minakami. 1984. Oxygen metabolism of human colostral macrophages: comparison with monocytes and polymorphonuclear leukocytes. J. Biochem. 95:1237-1245.

Vaughan, L.A., C.W. Weber, and S.R. Kemberling. 1979. Longitudinal changes in the mineral content of human milk. Am. J. Clin. Nutr. 32:2301-2306.

Venkatachalam, P.S., B. Belavady, and C. Gopalan. 1962. Studies on vitamin A nutritional status of mothers and infants in poor communities of India. J. Pediatr. 61:262-268.

Villard, L., and C.J. Bates. 1987. Effect of vitamin A supplementation on plasma and breast milk vitamin A levels in poorly nourished Gambian women. Hum. Nutr.: Clin. Nutr. 41C:47-58.

von Kries, R., M. Shearer, P.T. McCarthy, M. Haug, G. Harzer, and U. Göbel. 1987. Vitamin K$_1$ content of maternal milk: influence of the stage of lactation, lipid composition, and vitamin K$_1$ supplements given to the mother. Pediatr. Res. 22:513-517.

von Kries, R., M.J. Shearer, and U. Göbel. 1988. Vitamin K in infancy. Eur. J. Pediatr. 147:106-112.

Vuori, E. 1979. Intake of copper, iron, manganese and zinc by healthy, exclusively-breast-fed infants during the first 3 months of life. Br. J. Nutr. 42:407-411.

Vuori, E., S.M. Mäkinen, R. Kara, and P. Kuitunen. 1980. The effects of the dietary intakes of copper, iron, manganese, and zinc on the trace element content of human milk. Am. J. Clin. Nutr. 33:227-231.

Weisz-Carrington, P., M.E. Roux, M. McWilliams, J.M. Phillips-Quagliata, and M.E. Lamm. 1978. Hormonal induction of the secretory immune system in the mammary gland. Proc. Natl. Acad. Sci. U.S.A. 75:2928-2932.

Welsh, J.K., and J.T. May. 1979. Anti-infective properties of breast milk. J. Pediatr. 94:1-9.

Welsh, J.K., M. Arsenakis, R.J. Coelen, and J.T. May. 1979. Effect of antiviral lipids, heat, and freezing on the activity of viruses in human milk. J. Infect. Dis. 140:322-328.

Werner, H., T. Amarant, R.P. Millar, M. Fridkin, and Y. Koch. 1985. Immunoreactive and biologically active somatostatin in human and sheep milk. Eur. J. Biochem. 148:353-357.

Whitelaw, A., and A. Butterfield. 1977. High breast-milk sodium in cystic fibrosis. Lancet 2:1288.

WHO (World Health Organization). 1985. The Quantity and Quality of Breast Milk. Report on the WHO Collaborative Study on Breast-Feeding. World Health Organization, Geneva. 148 pp.

Wurtman, J.J., and J.D. Fernstrom. 1979. Free amino acid, protein, and fat contents of breast milk from Guatemalan mothers consuming a corn-based diet. Early Hum. Dev. 3:67-77.

Zimecki, M., A. Pierce-Cretel, G. Spik, and Z. Wieczorek. 1987. Immunoregulatory properties of the proteins present in human milk. Arch. Immunol. Ther. Exp. 35:351-360.

Zinder, O., M. Hamosh, T.R.C. Fleck, and R.O. Scow. 1974. Effect of prolactin on lipoprotein lipase in mammary gland and adipose tissue of rats. Am. J. Physiol. 226:744-748.

7

Infant Outcomes

Because the exclusively breastfed infant is entirely dependent upon the mother for nutrition, the subcommittee examined the evidence relating maternal nutrition to infant health. In addition to nutrients in human milk, it considered constituents that have important nonnutritive functions (see Chapter 6).

As discussed in Chapters 5 and 6, the adequacy of the maternal diet may affect the formation, composition, or secretion of milk. As nutritional demands of the infant increase, milk production becomes correspondingly greater (see Chapter 5). Thus, there is a complex interrelationship between maternal nutrition, volume and composition of the milk, and the vigor of the infant.

Since infant nutrition, growth, development, and health are interrelated, the effects of breastfeeding and maternal nutrition on each of these outcomes were reviewed. The health-related outcomes include resistance to infectious diseases, allergic disorders, and chronic diseases with an immunologic basis that develop later in childhood; the passage of infectious or toxic agents in milk to the recipient; and infant mortality. Because of the specific tasks assigned to the subcommittee, this review was limited to effects on full-term infants.

In reviewing the relevant literature, the subcommittee had to contend with several confounding factors that potentially alter the interpretation of the results. For example, sick infants may be unable to breastfeed because they are separated from their mothers or because they are unable to suckle adequately. In such circumstances, if the mother does not continue lactation by pumping, breastfeeding is difficult to resume if or when the child recovers. Thus, illness may cause the cessation of breastfeeding, rather than the absence of breastfeeding causing illness. In many cultures, there is a strong relationship between the type of infant feeding and the social status and functioning of the family. In the United States, breastfeeding rates increase with an increase in socioeconomic status. The favorable environment of these women and their infants is associated with a lower risk of many illnesses. In addition, since surveys indicate that the breastfeeding mother is less likely to smoke, her infant is at lower risk of respiratory problems from exposure to passive cigarette smoke. Further, the young infant in day care—often because the mother is working (and therefore less likely to breastfeed)—may be exposed to communicable diseases more often than the infant cared for exclusively at home. Thus, the lower risks of morbidity reported for breastfed infants may be in part due to factors other than breastfeeding. Other potential sources of bias are reviewed by Kramer (1987).

INFANT NUTRITION: VITAMINS AND MINERALS

Human milk serves as the nutritional standard for infants. Certain nutrients (vitamins A, D, K, B_{12}, riboflavin, and folate; iron; copper; zinc; and fluoride) are reviewed in this section to illustrate the uniqueness of human milk and relationships, if any, of the infant's nutritional status to maternal nutrient stores and maternal diet. Other essential nutrients are of no less importance to the infant; information about them is presented in Chapter 6.

Three major factors contribute to the nutritional status of the exclusively breastfed infant: nutrient stores, especially those accumulated in utero; the amount and bioavailability of nutrients supplied by human milk; and environmental and genetic factors that influence the efficiency of nutrient utilization. Nutrient stores at birth are determined by the rate of placental nutrient transfer and by the duration of gestation. The stores of many nutrients increase substantially during the last trimester of pregnancy and tend to be higher in infants with higher birth weight or greater gestational age. The infant's total nutrient intake is determined by nutrient concentrations in human milk and by the volume of milk consumed. The amount of nutrient absorbed by the infant is further influenced by the bioavailability of that nutrient in human milk.

Providing the breastfed infant with supplemental foods has a complex effect on the total amount of nutrient absorbed. For example, infants consuming such foods as formula or infant cereal generally decrease their intake of human milk (see Chapter 5) and, thus, the nutrients and other specialized components it supplies. Thus, the intake of supplementary foods may add nutrients in a less bioavailable form, decrease the bioavailability of nutrients in human milk, and decrease the intake of other important factors in human milk.

Growth, infections, and differences in the efficiency of nutrient utilization affect the infant's rate of nutrient utilization, which in turn can influence the infant's nutritional status. Birth weight is inversely associated with the rate of nutrient utilization. For example, infants who are small at birth usually experience catch-up growth during infancy. Disease or injury may adversely affect nutrient utilization either directly by increasing rates of catabolism or urinary and fecal losses or indirectly by sequestrating a nutrient in tissue compartments.

Finally, other environmental influences, such as the degree of exposure to ultraviolet light (ordinarily from sunshine) in the case of the synthesis of vitamin D, may be important determinants of the nutritional status of the infant.

Fat-Soluble Vitamins

Vitamin D

Plasma levels of 25-hydroxycholecalciferol (a vitamin D metabolite used as a measure of vitamin D status) in the mother are positively correlated with those in the neonate, providing evidence that maternal vitamin D status affects the infant's vitamin D stores (Hillman and Haddad, 1974; Hoogenboezem et al., 1989; Markestad, 1983; Markestad et al., 1983). Several investigators have found that plasma concentrations of 25-hydroxycholecalciferol in the neonate are within the normal range for adults (10 to 40 ng/ml) (Markestad, 1983; Roberts et al., 1981), whereas Ala-Houhala (1985) reported that 25-hydroxycholecalciferol plasma levels in Finnish neonates were abnormally low in winter (mean, <10 ng/ml) compared with the range of values found in summer (12 to 18 ng/ml, $p < .001$). These studies suggest that infants born to mothers with inadequate vitamin D status are highly dependent on a regular supply of vitamin D through diet, supplements, or exposure to ultraviolet light.

Plasma 25-hydroxycholecalciferol levels in unsupplemented breastfed infants have been compared with those of formula-fed infants or breastfed infants receiving approximately 10 μg of supplemental vitamin D per day. In six reports, plasma 25-hydroxycholecalciferol levels were substantially lower in unsupplemented breastfed infants (Ala-Houhala, 1985; Chan et al., 1982; Greer et al., 1982; Lichtenstein et al., 1986; Markestad, 1983; Roberts et al., 1981). Four studies (Ala-Houhala, 1985; Greer et al., 1982; Hoogenboezem et al., 1989; Markestad, 1983) have shown plasma levels of this compound at or below the lower limits of normal ($\leq$10 ng/ml) (Nutrition Foundation, 1984) in the unsupplemented groups. Ala-Houhala (1985) reported that in the winter months, 10 of 18 unsupplemented breastfed infants had plasma levels of less than 5 ng/ml, which may lead to rickets (Nutrition Foundation, 1984). Despite reports of rickets in breastfed infants (Arnaud et al., 1976; O'Connor, 1977; Ozsoylu, 1977) and the low vitamin D content of human milk, breastfeeding has long been considered to be protective against rickets (Belton, 1986; Lakdawala and Widdowson, 1977).

Breastfed infants require approximately 30 minutes of exposure to sunlight per week if wearing only a diaper, or 2 hours per week if fully clothed without a hat, to maintain normal serum 25-hydroxycholecalciferol levels (Specker et al., 1985). Darkly pigmented infants require a greater exposure to sunshine to initiate the synthesis of vitamin D in the skin (Clemens et al., 1982).

In a study by Greer and colleagues (1982), which included randomization of breastfed infants to a placebo or to a daily supplement of 10 μg of vitamin D, the bone mineral content of the placebo group was significantly lower in the first few months after birth but slightly higher than that of the supplemented group by the end of the first year.

In summary, exclusive breastfeeding results in normal infant bone mineral content when maternal vitamin D status is adequate and the infant is regularly exposed to sunlight. If the infant or mother is not exposed regularly to sunlight, or if the mother's intake of vitamin D is low, supplements for the infant may be indicated (5 to 7.5 μg/day).

Vitamin A

Although vitamin A concentrations in human milk are dependent on the mother's vitamin A status, vitamin A deficiency is rare among breastfed infants, even in parts of the world with endemic vitamin A deficiency (Sommer, 1982). Even after breastfeeding is discontinued, it appears to confer a protective effect (Sommer, 1982; West et al., 1986), presumably because some of the vitamin A provided by human milk is stored in the liver. Infants who consume human milk that provides 100 to 151 μg of retinol equivalents per day grow well and do not show signs of vitamin A deficiency. In the United States, human milk provides approximately twice this amount (FAO, 1988; NRC, 1989). These U.S. concentrations are used as the international standard for adequate vitamin A intakes in infancy (FAO, 1988; NRC, 1989). In the United States, there is no indication to routinely supplement either the infant or the mother with vitamin A.

Vitamin K

Vitamin K is essential for the formation of several proteins required for blood clotting. This vitamin has two major forms: vitamin K_1 (phylloquinone), synthesized by plants, and vitamin K_2 (menaquinone), synthesized by bacteria. Most of the vitamin K in human milk is phylloquinone; the extent to which infants absorb menaquinone produced by gut microflora is not known. Vitamin K stores at birth are extremely low. Therefore, newborns are immediately dependent on an external source of the vitamin, but the amount provided by human milk is low—approximately 2 μg/liter (Committee on Nutrition, 1985; NRC, 1989). Bacteria that colonize the intestinal tracts of breastfed infants produce less menaquinone than do those in formula-fed infants.

A deficiency of the vitamin produces a syndrome in infants called hemorrhagic disease of the newborn. This vitamin K-dependent disease has two different clinical forms. The classic early-onset form occurs at age 2 to 10 days in 1 of 200 to 400 unsupplemented newborns. The late-onset form occurs around 1 month of age in 1 of 1,000 to 2,000 unsupplemented newborns. Late-onset hemorrhagic disease of the newborn is a devastating, often fatal disease (Gleason and Kerr, 1989). Both forms occur more often in unsupplemented breastfed than formula-fed infants.

Although maternal supplementation with vitamin K in the last weeks of pregnancy (Owen et al., 1967) or unusually high milk intakes (>500 ml) during the first 3 days of postnatal life (Motohara et al., 1989) may reduce the risk of hemorrhagic disease of the newborn, the most dependable method of preventing this serious disorder is to inject the infant with 0.5 to 1.0 mg of vitamin K at birth or to give an oral 1.0- to 2.0-mg dose, as recommended by the American Academy of Pediatrics (Committee on Nutrition, 1985) and required by many states.

Water-Soluble Vitamins

Vitamin B_{12}

Full-term infants of adequately nourished women are born with a total body vitamin B_{12} content of 30 to 40 μg (FAO, 1988). Assuming that 0.10 μg/day is required during infancy (FAO, 1988), these stores would supply an infant's needs for approximately 8 months. The 0.4 μg of vitamin B_{12} per day usually provided by human milk to the exclusively breastfed infant provides for ample accumulation of stores (FAO, 1988; NRC, 1989). Vitamin B_{12} concentrations in milk, and thus the infant's intake of this vitamin, are dependent on the mother's B_{12} intake and stores.

Breastfed infants born to women who eat little or no animal foods are at risk for developing vitamin B_{12} deficiency. In a study of six vitamin B_{12}-deficient, exclusively breastfed infants in India, vitamin B_{12} concentrations in their mother's milk ranged from 0.03 to 0.07 μg/liter (Jadhav et al., 1962). Vitamin B_{12} deficiency has also been found in breastfed infants of complete vegetarian mothers in industrialized countries (Close, 1983; Davis et al., 1981; Gambon et al., 1986; Higgenbottom et al., 1978; Rendle-Short et al., 1979; Sklar, 1986). Urinary methylmalonic acid (UMMA) concentrations of the breastfed infants of omnivorous mothers were significantly lower ($p = .05$) than those of infants of complete vegetarians; maternal serum B_{12} concentrations were negatively associated with maternal UMMA ($p = .003$) and infant UMMA ($p < .001$) levels (Specker et al., 1988). In general, the deficiency syndrome is usually not clinically apparent until the latter half of infancy. An important finding is that breastfed infants may develop clinical signs of vitamin B_{12} deficiency before their mothers do (Lampkin and Saunders, 1969; McPhee et al., 1988).

For infants of mothers eating a mixed diet that includes animal foods, human milk is a generous source of vitamin B_{12}; it provides for the infant's needs throughout the first year of life. For mothers who are complete vegetarians, it is desirable to find an acceptable food source or supplement of vitamin B_{12} that will meet their needs and those of the nursing infant.

Folate

The full-term infant is born with adequate folate stores, even when maternal folate is suboptimal (Salmenperä et al., 1986b). The bioavailability of folate in human milk is high: to maintain equivalent folate status in formula-fed infants, approximately 50% more folate is required from formula than from human milk (Ek and Magnus, 1982). Serum and red cell folate levels are adequate in breastfed infants; indeed, they are several-fold greater than adult reference levels (Ek and Magnus, 1979; Salmenperä et al., 1986b; Smith et al., 1985). This is reported for infants exclusively breastfed for up to 1 year (Salmenperä et al., 1986b).

Maternal folate levels in serum and milk do not appear to be correlated; however, there are strong associations between maternal and infant serum folate levels at 6 weeks and at 3 months after birth (Smith et al., 1983) and at 4 and 9 months after birth (Salmenperä et al., 1986b). Those associations suggest that folate stores accumulated in utero are more important determinants of folate status during infancy than are levels of folate in milk.

Riboflavin

Biochemical data concerning the riboflavin status of infants are difficult to interpret. Hovi and colleagues (1979) reported a transient increase in the activation coefficient of erythrocyte glutathione reductase (EGR) in full-term healthy breastfed newborns—a finding that suggests riboflavin deficiency. The increase became even greater when the infants had received phototherapy for treatment of hyperbilirubinemia (Gromisch et al., 1977; Hovi et al., 1979; Tan et al., 1978); however, this was not accompanied by clinical signs of riboflavin deficiency. The increase in the activation coefficient did not occur with daily maternal riboflavin supplements of 0.5 mg/kg of body weight, but neither was this increase evident after 2 weeks in the infants of unsupplemented women (Nail et al., 1980). The riboflavin concentration in human milk is dependent on maternal riboflavin status (Bates et al., 1982).

High EGR activation coefficients have been reported for breastfed infants who receive only 0.13 to 0.21 mg of riboflavin per day from human milk (Bates et al., 1982). The average intake of riboflavin in exclusively breastfed infants in the United States is estimated to be 0.26 mg/day. Using several criteria, including riboflavin levels in urine and blood, Snyderman and coworkers (1949) found that riboflavin intakes of 0.3 to 0.4 mg/day provide adequate riboflavin status. Among infants undergoing phototherapy, comparable intakes of riboflavin maintain normal EGR activation coefficients (Tan et al., 1978). No longitudinal studies of representative populations have been conducted in developed countries to determine the adequacy of riboflavin status among breastfed infants. No reports of riboflavin deficiency among exclusively breastfed infants in the United States were encountered in the review of the literature by the subcommittee.

Minerals

Iron

Iron deficiency and iron deficiency anemia remain important problems in the United States and the rest of the world. The estimated worldwide prevalence of anemia in children from birth to age 4 years is 43%. There are remarkable differences in the prevalence rates of iron deficiency anemia in economically developed regions (~12%) and developing areas (~51%) of the world (FAO, 1988). In the United States, children aged 1 to 2 years have a higher prevalence of iron deficiency (9.3%) than do people in other age groups (DHHS, 1988). Although inadequate iron intakes are not the sole cause of anemia in infants and children, diets low in iron play a major etiologic role.

A heavy demand is placed on the iron reserves of breastfed infants: the estimated daily physiologic requirement is 0.7 mg for growth and 0.2 mg to replace basal losses (Dallman, 1986). Human milk provides from 0.15 to 0.68 mg of iron per day. Approximately 50% of iron is absorbed from human milk compared with 7% from iron-fortified formula and 4% from infant cereals (Dallman, 1986). The iron concentration in milk is not influenced by the mother's iron status (Dallman, 1986; Murray et al., 1978; Siimes et al., 1984). Body stores of iron and ferritin levels increase during the first 3 months of postnatal life and then drop during the fourth to sixth months (Duncan et al., 1985; Garry et al., 1981; Saarinen et al., 1977). Despite those changes, iron deficiency is uncommon in breastfed infants during their first 6 months (Duncan et al., 1985; Garry et al., 1981; Owen et al., 1981; Picciano and Deering, 1980; Saarinen and Siimes, 1979a; Saarinen et al., 1977).

Woodruff and colleagues (1977) suggest that partially breastfed infants younger than 6 months are at risk of iron deficiency: they found a hemoglobin level lower than 11.0 g/dl in 1 of 12 breastfed infants and a transferrin saturation of less than 16% in 4 of them. Mothers in that study were instructed to feed supplementary foods to the infants at age 3 months; foods high in iron content were offered in limited amounts. Supplementary foods lead to decreased intake of human milk and possibly impair the absorption of iron from human milk (Oski and Landaw, 1980).

Two studies of a total of 43 infants indicated that there is a risk of iron deficiency by age 9 months if human milk is the infant's only food (Pastel et al., 1981; Siimes et al., 1984). Therefore, foods with bioavailable iron,

iron-fortified foods, or an iron supplement should be given beginning at age 6 months (or earlier, if supplementary foods are introduced before that time).

Copper

Full-term infants have relatively large copper stores at birth (Brückmann and Zondek, 1939; Widdowson et al., 1972). The relationship between maternal copper status and concentration in human milk is weak (Munch-Peterson, 1950; Salmenperä et al., 1986a; Vuori et al., 1980). Serum copper levels were higher among the older infants in a cross-sectional study of breastfed infants ranging from newborns through age 12 months (Ohtake, 1977). Salmenperä and coworkers (1986a) found that ceruloplasmin as well as serum copper consistently rose during 12 months of exclusive breastfeeding, despite the low copper intakes characteristic of breastfed infants. The daily intakes from months 4 to 9 ranged from 0.03 to 0.26 mg/day—less than the Food and Nutrition Board's estimated safe and adequate daily dietary intake of 0.4 to 0.6 mg/day for infants aged 0 to 6 months (NRC, 1989). Neither the subcommittee nor Mason (1979) could find case reports of copper deficiency of exclusively breastfed infants. Thus, the evidence suggests that the bioavailability of copper in human milk is high and that the copper status of breastfed infants is adequate during the first year of life.

Zinc

Human milk has been regarded as a good source of zinc (Lönnerdal et al., 1984); this form of zinc is highly bioavailable (Sandström et al., 1983). The zinc concentration in human milk does not appear to be influenced by the mother's diet (Lönnerdal et al., 1981), but the evidence is not consistent (see Chapter 6).

Plasma zinc levels in breastfed infants are similar to those of adults and of infants fed zinc-fortified formula (Hambidge et al., 1979), and they are substantially greater than those of infants fed formula not fortified with zinc (Hambidge et al., 1979; Vigi et al., 1984). Erythrocyte and hair zinc levels also are similar in breastfed infants and infants fed formula fortified with zinc (Hatano et al., 1985; MacDonald et al., 1982). The full-term breastfed infant who is born with usual liver zinc stores is at very low risk of zinc deficiency.

Fluoride

Although fluoride is not considered to be an essential nutrient, it is beneficial to humans in the prevention of dental caries (NRC, 1989). Fluoride supplementation during infancy helps prevent caries in deciduous teeth; however, caries is a multifactorial disease, and breastfeeding may affect the prevalence of caries in ways other than by the provision of fluoride. The subcommittee found no studies that directly assessed the relationship between the mode of feeding in infancy and the incidence of caries.

From the fluoride concentrations in human milk estimated by the Committee on Nutrition (1985), one could project that an exclusively breastfed infant would consume only 0.012 mg of fluoride per day. Fluoride levels are not easily increased by maternal dietary or supplementary fluoride (see Chapter 6). The only other likely source of fluoride in the infant's diet is water. The subcommittee supports the recommendations of the American Academy of Pediatrics that infants receive 0.25-mg fluoride supplements daily if their water supply contains less than 0.3 ppm of fluoride (Committee on Nutrition, 1986).

GROWTH AND DEVELOPMENT

Historically, growth has been used as the basis to judge the adequacy of nutrient intake by the infant. A major question before the subcommittee was whether nutrition of the lactating woman influences infant growth. Because slow infant growth is sometimes used as a reason for supplementing infants with formula or solid foods or for discontinuing breastfeeding, it was essential to include a brief review of the assessment of infant growth. Interrelationships among infant growth, other indices of development, and maternal nutritional status were found to be difficult to ascertain, since few sound studies had been conducted to address them.

Pattern of Growth

Although the most commonly used indicators of infant growth have been body weight and weight gain, it is desirable to consider simultaneously length in order to assess linear growth and adiposity (the relationship of weight to length, also indicated by skinfold thickness).

Healthy, full-term infants lose an average of approximately 5 to 8% of their body weight during the first week after birth; the percentage lost is somewhat higher among breastfed infants (7.4%) than formula-fed infants (4.9%) (Podratz et al., 1986) but is unlikely to be of clinical importance. After the first week, the pattern of weight gain in infancy depends on the initial size of the infant, whether the infant is breastfed or formula fed, and other environmental and physiologic factors. In industrialized countries, the rate of weight gain of breastfed infants is similar to that of formula-fed infants and to National Center for Health Statistics (NCHS) reference data for infants up to age 2 to 3 months; however, it is less rapid over the subsequent 9 months (Chandra, 1982; Czajka-Narins and Jung, 1986; Dewey et al., 1990a; Duncan et al., 1984; Forsum and Sadurskis, 1986; Garza et al., 1987; Hitchcock et al., 1985; Saarinen and Siimes, 1979b; Salmenperä et al., 1985; Whitehead and Paul, 1984). In developing countries, breastfed infants tend to grow more rapidly than their formula-fed counterparts throughout the first 6 months of postnatal life (Mahmood and Feachem, 1987; Seward and Serdula, 1984; Unni and Richard, 1988). This difference may reflect a greater risk of infection and malnutrition among formula-fed infants in low-income populations living in areas with poor sanitation (Brown et al., 1989).

Although most studies have linked differences in the rate of weight gain with the mode of feeding, differences in linear growth between breastfed and formula-fed infants are small if differences in size at birth are controlled (Czajka-Narins and Jung, 1986; Dewey et al., 1989; Hitchcock and Coy, 1989; Nelson et al., 1989). Weight for length tends to be somewhat lower for breastfed infants than for formula-fed infants after age 6 months (Czajka-Narins and Jung, 1986; Dewey et al., 1989; Hitchcock and Coy, 1989). Thus, it is likely that the differences in weight gain patterns represent primarily differences in adiposity.

In affluent populations, the difference in rate of growth associated with mode of feeding during infancy is consistent with energy intakes of breastfed and formula-fed infants. At 3 to 4 months of age, reported average energy intakes of breastfed infants are lower than those of formula-fed infants—74 to 91 kcal/kg of body weight compared with 92 to 104 kcal/kg, respectively (Axelsson et al., 1987; Butte et al., 1984; Dewey and Lönnerdal, 1983; Dewey et al., in press; Shepherd et al., 1988). The subcommittee found only one study of infants older than 5 months that compared intakes by feeding method. Dewey et al. (in press) reported that average gross energy intakes of breastfed infants are consistently lower than those of formula-fed infants—84 and 98 kcal/kg, respectively, at 6 months; 87 and 97 kcal/kg, respectively, at 9 months; and 92 and 95 kcal/kg respectively, at 12 months—even though both groups received solid foods beginning at 4 to 6 months. As discussed in Chapter 5, these lower intakes by breastfed infants are governed primarily by infant demand, not by insufficient milk volume.

Assessment of Growth of Breastfed Infants

Growth charts used to assess infant growth are based on data derived primarily from formula-fed infants (Hamill et al., 1977). The commonly used NCHS infant growth charts are based on information collected by the Fels Research Institute from 867 infants born between 1929 and 1975. In that study, the mode of feeding was known for 75% of the infants. Of those, only 17% were exclusively breastfed and few were breastfed for more than 3 months. Furthermore, the infant formulas used at that time were less similar to human milk (for example, they were higher in total proteins, total fats, and saturated fatty acids) and the infants were more likely to be given solid foods before age 4 months than they are today (Fomon, 1987). Therefore, a number of investigators suggest that NCHS growth charts are inappropriate for breastfed infants (Dewey et al., 1990; Duncan et al., 1984; Hitchcock et al., 1985; Whitehead and Paul, 1984).

Similarly, it has been noted (Dewey et al., 1989) that it can be misleading to assess growth of breastfed infants by using current reference data for the increment in weight or length during specified age intervals, such as data presented by Roche and colleagues (1989) based on the Fels Research Institute population. The 5th percentile of these reference data was suggested by Roche et al. as a cutoff to indicate infants at risk of malnutrition. Caution is needed in applying this cutoff because the data are based on predicted values obtained from measurements at 3- rather than 1-month intervals, which obscures some of the short-term variation in infant growth. Thus, more than 5% of all infants, regardless of feeding mode, would be expected to be below the Fels 5th percentile in any given month.

Furthermore, Dewey and coworkers (1989) found that the percentage of breastfed infants who fell below the 5th percentile for weight gain was much larger than would be expected, averaging 31% over the six 1-month intervals up to age 6 months and 52% over the six 1-month intervals between ages 6 and 12 months. On average, infants grew less rapidly than the 5th percentile during 4.4 months out of the first 12 months. Although these percentages seem alarming, these were healthy infants who fed on demand and received solid foods beginning at 4 to 6 months. Furthermore, with regard to morbidity, activity levels, or time sleeping during the first year of life, the breastfed infants with growth rates below the 5th percentile were not different from the breastfed infants with faster growth rates (Dewey et al., in press). Therefore, it is highly likely that their growth rates were normal and not a sign of malnutrition.

Recently, data have been published on weight and length gain of 419 breastfed and 720 formula-fed infants enrolled in growth studies in Iowa between 1965 and 1987 (Nelson et al., 1989). These infants were measured up to 112 days of age. One shortcoming of the study was that the breastfed infants were allowed up to 240 ml of formula per day, and before 1979, all infants were allowed solid foods beginning at 1 month of age. Therefore, additional data are necessary to construct appropriate growth charts for infants exclusively breastfed for the first 4 to 6 months and extensively breastfed throughout the remainder of the first year.

Long-Term Growth Status

Few investigators have examined whether the differences in growth rates between breastfed and formula-fed infants during the first year of life are maintained later on in childhood. Birkbeck et al. (1985) measured children at 7 years of age who were either breastfed for at least 12 weeks ($N = 283$) or formula fed from birth ($N = 383$). Children who had been breastfed were taller, but the difference was not statistically significant when controlled for birth weight, parental stature, and socioeconomic status. Similarly, Pomerance (1987) found no differences in growth rate from 3 to 12 years of age between formula-fed children and those who had been breastfed for at least 2 months. These studies indicate no long-term difference in growth status attributable to breastfeeding. However, more data are needed on children breastfed for 4 months or longer.

Maternal Nutrition and Infant Growth

It is often assumed that maternal nutrition during lactation will affect milk volume and composition and, therefore, infant growth. However, Chapters 5 and 6 provide evidence that some of these assumptions are not necessarily valid. For example, the influence of maternal nutrition on milk volume is difficult to demonstrate, even in populations at substantial risk of malnutrition. The links among maternal nutrition, the composition of human milk, and growth rates of breastfed infants are problematic for several reasons. First, infant growth is not a very good indicator of milk or energy intake because the amount of energy required for growth is a relatively small fraction of total energy needs. In the first 2 months of postnatal life, growth accounts for approximately 30% of energy requirements, but this decreases to 5 to 10% at 4 to 6 months and to about 3% at 10 to 12 months (Butte, 1988). Second, several factors, such as intestinal malabsorption following digestive tract infections, may affect growth independently of energy intake. Finally, the energy content of fat tissue is much higher than that of lean tissue, so some consideration of the changes in body composition is necessary in evaluating different infant growth patterns.

The results of studies in Taiwan (Adair and Pollitt, 1985), Colombia (Herrera et al., 1980), and Guatemala (Lechtig and Klein, 1980) indicate that maternal nutrition during lactation has little direct impact on infant growth. In these studies, mothers were provided food supplements during both pregnancy and lactation, and infant weight gain was a main outcome variable. In only two cases was maternal supplementation associated with increased infant growth: among a subgroup of thinner breastfeeding women in the Colombia study (Herrera et al., 1980) and in a subset of the women in the Guatemala study for whom complete information was available (Delgado et al., 1982).

Several factors limit the interpretation of results from these studies: the provision of supplements to infants as well as to the mothers (Herrera et al., 1980; Lechtig and Klein, 1980), higher mean birth weights of the infants born to the supplemented mothers (Herrera et al., 1980), lack of information of the impact of the supplement on total maternal energy intake, and self-selection bias among women consuming greater amounts of the supplement in the Guatemala study (Lechtig and Klein, 1980).

Growth of breastfed infants during the first 4 to 6 months is similar in industrialized and developing countries (Whitehead and Paul, 1984). The initial starting point—birth weight—may differ among populations, but the shape of the weight curve among exclusively breastfed infants from 0 to 6 months is remarkably consistent.

Development

As noted below, several developmental indices have been associated with the mode of infant feeding. However, no reports have been published concerning the influence of maternal nutrition on any of these indices within a group of breastfed infants.

Gastrointestinal and Metabolic Responses

Compared with formula-fed infants, breastfed infants have slower rates of gastric filling (Lucas et al., 1981a) and faster rates of gastric emptying (Cavell, 1979, 1981). These differences may contribute to some of the differences in hormonal responses, such as the decreased insulin and gastric inhibitory polypeptide responses and the higher blood ketone levels, in breastfed as compared with formula-fed infants (Lucas et al., 1981b). These responses may have long-term effects on the fat deposition of the infant (see the section "Obesity" below).

Studies in animals suggest that several components of human milk may contribute to gastrointestinal maturation (Koldovskỳ et al., 1988; Menard and Arsenault, 1988; Sheard and Walker, 1988). This is the subject of ongoing research but is beyond the scope of this report.

Other Physiologic Responses

Measurements of breastfed and formula-fed infants made during the first 3 postnatal days indicate a distinct physiologic state and a greater reactivity to stimuli among breastfed infants, in that their heart rates are slower and more variable and their vagal tone is elevated (DiPietro et al., 1987). Butte and coworkers (1990) reported that sleeping metabolic rate and body temperature are slightly lower in breastfed infants than in formula-fed infants at ages 1 and 4 months. Elias et al. (1986) and Wright and colleagues (1983) reported that breastfed infants are more likely to awaken at night than are formula-fed infants during the first 2 years, whereas Weissbluth et al. (1984) found no such difference among 4- to 8-month-old infants.

Cognitive Development

Several studies have compared the cognitive development of children aged 6 months to 15 years who were breastfed or formula fed (Fergusson et al., 1982; Menkes, 1977; Morley et al., 1988; Morrow-Tlucak et al., 1988;

Rodgers, 1978; Taylor and Wadsworth, 1984). Slight but statistically significant differences favoring children who had been breastfed were reported. In the most complete studies (Fergusson et al., 1982; Morrow-Tlucak et al., 1988; Taylor and Wadsworth, 1984), the influence of covariates such as maternal intelligence, educational level, socioeconomic status, child-rearing attitudes, and home environment were controlled for in the analysis. With these adjustments, the differences between groups, although smaller, remained statistically significant. The biologic importance of the findings is unclear. It is possible that the differences resulted from other confounding variables that were not identified or from enhanced maternal-infant interactions rather than from the specific biologic properties of human milk.

BREASTFEEDING AND MORBIDITY

Short-Term Effects

Infectious Diseases

Breastfeeding may protect the recipient infant against common infectious diseases in four different ways:

• Human milk inhibits the growth of many types of microbial pathogens. By avoiding foods other than human milk through exclusive breastfeeding, the infant's exposure to environmental pathogens is limited.

• Breastfeeding enhances the nutritional status of infants under conditions in which poor sanitary environments and the low quality of weaning foods reduce the nutritional well-being of infants.

• Through its contraceptive effects, breastfeeding may increase the interval between births (Habicht et al., 1985; Hobcraft, 1987; Thapa et al., 1988) and may thus both reduce the number of infectious contacts within households (Aaby et al., 1984; Hanson, 1986) and permit more human resources and other benefits to be directed to fewer children.

• Human milk contains an array of antimicrobial agents (Goldman and Goldblum, 1989), antiinflammatory agents (Goldman et al., 1986, 1990b), and immunologic stimulating agents (Goldman and Goldblum, 1989, 1990), most of which are absent from infant formula, or are present only in limited quantities, and are produced by the young infant only in limited amounts.

The frequency of gastrointestinal infections appears to be much lower in breastfed infants than in formula-fed infants in many industrialized countries (Cunningham, 1981; Cushing and Anderson, 1982; Palti et al., 1984) and developing countries (Clemens et al., 1986; Glass and Stoll, 1989; Mata et al., 1967, 1969; Plank and Milanesi, 1973; Ruiz-Palacios et al., 1986). The protection against gastrointestinal infections is more evident in populations in which sanitary standards are low and potable water is not readily available.

However, a lower incidence of gastrointestinal infections in breastfed infants in the United States (Myers et al., 1984) and lower perinatal mortality from infectious disease among breastfed, compared with formula-fed, infants in England (Carpenter et al., 1983) suggest that the protective effects of breastfeeding are important in industrialized as well as in developing countries. Moreover, since breastfed infants may remain asymptomatic even after exposure to enteropathogens (microorganisms that infect the intestinal tract) contaminating the nipples and areola of the nursing mother (Mata and Urrutia, 1971; Wyatt and Mata, 1969), the protection afforded by breastfeeding is attributable to factors in the milk in addition to an avoidance of pathogens.

For some infections, the duration is shorter and the intensity is less in breastfed infants than in formula-fed infants, but the attack rate (the incidence during a defined period of risk) is similar (Duffy et al., 1986; Glass et al., 1983; Mata et al., 1967, 1969). For example, in Bangladesh, protection against infections but not against colonization with *Vibrio cholerae* correlated with the amount of secretory immunoglobulin A (IgA) antibodies to that bacterium in the human milk (Glass and Stoll, 1989; Glass et al., 1983). In the United States, the protection afforded to infants against rotavirus appeared to result from factors in human milk other than specific antibodies (Duffy et al., 1986).

Protective effects of breastfeeding against certain respiratory infections have also been reported. For example, respiratory syncytial virus infections are less severe among breastfed infants than among formula-fed babies, although the attack rate is the same (Chiba et al., 1987; Downham et al., 1976; Pullan et al., 1980). In addition, serum interferon-α levels are higher in breastfed infants following respiratory syncytial virus infection (Chiba et al., 1987), even though the concentration of this antiviral agent is negligible in human milk. This suggests that the breastfed infant's immune system may be primed by human milk to respond to certain respiratory viral pathogens more rapidly and to a greater degree than is the case for formula-fed infants.

The incidence of otitis media is lower in breastfed than in formula-fed infants (Saarinen, 1982; Schaefer, 1971), but it is unclear whether this is a result of components of human milk or of other factors associated with the feeding method, such as higher enrollment of formula-fed infants in day-care centers, differences in the sucking mechanisms, or the adverse effects of foreign proteins in formula-fed infants.

The relationship between the nutritional status of the lactating woman and the susceptibility of the breastfed infant to infections requires further study.

Allergies

The effects of various infant-feeding practices on the age of onset and severity of allergies have been extensively investigated. Breastfeeding appears to be protective against food allergies (see the review by Kramer [1988]).

Evidence concerning such protective effects against other types of allergies is conflicting. When suspected food allergens were excluded from the diets of pregnant and lactating women whose families were at high risk for atopic dermatitis (Chandra, 1987; Chandra et al., 1985), the incidence of this condition was lowered among breastfed infants compared with its incidence in a group of controls. Recently, Hattevig and colleagues (1990) also found that maternal dietary restrictions for 3 months during lactation resulted in a lower rate of atopic dermatitis among the mothers' infants for 6 months. Several case reports suggest that components of foods ingested by the mother pass into the milk and then cause allergic reactions in the infant, and that these problems can be prevented by excluding the allergens from the maternal diet (Cant et al., 1985; Harmatz et al., 1987; Jakobsson and Lindberg, 1978, 1983; Kilshaw and Cant, 1984; Shannon, 1921). Nonetheless, the benefit of prophylactic use of allergen-restricted diets for the general population of pregnant and lactating women is not well established (Hattevig et al., 1990).

Early observations that atopic eczema in infants is associated with abnormal serum lipids (Hansen, 1937; Hansen et al., 1947) have recently been confirmed and extended (Bordoni et al., 1988; Manku et al., 1982; Rocklin, 1986; Wright, 1989). The findings suggest that in affected infants, the conversion of dietary linoleic acid to long-chain polyunsaturated metabolites is defective (Wright, 1985). The administration of γ-linolenic acid, a normal constituent of human milk, helps alleviate the eczema (Biagi et al., 1988; Meigel et al., 1987; Morse et al., 1989). In keeping with that finding, human milk consumed by infants with atopic dermatitis had lower concentrations of dihomo-γ-linolenic acid (a metabolite of linolenic acid) than did milk from control subjects (Morse et al., 1989).

Although the lay literature implies that maternal diet may contribute to colic (crying greatly in excess of 1 hour/day [Brazelton, 1962; Carey, 1984; Hunziker and Barr, 1986]) among breastfed infants, the subcommittee found only one study concerning this relationship. Results from that small study in Denmark (Jakobsson and Lindberg, 1978) suggest that the passage of food allergens, especially from cow's milk, through human milk accounts for 30% of the cases of colic in breastfed infants. It is difficult to generalize from that report, however, since the subjects may not have been representative of the overall population of infants with colic.

Chronic Diseases with an Immunologic Basis

Because human milk contains a host of direct-acting antimicrobial factors, antiinflammatory agents, and substances that may hasten the maturation of the infant's immune system, there is reason to believe that development of chronic diseases having an infectious or immunologic basis may be influenced by the method of infant feeding. Recent investigations suggest that breastfeeding exerts long-term protective effects against three such diseases: type I diabetes mellitus (Borch-Johnsen et al., 1984; Mayer et al., 1988), lymphoma (Davis et al., 1988), and Crohn's disease (Koletzko et al., 1989). Potential risk factors were identified for 114 cases of Crohn's disease and 180 controls (unaffected siblings) within 107 families. The children with this disease were less likely to have been breastfed (relative risk of 3.6 for formula-fed infants). Even though each of these studies was retrospective and depended on long-term recall, the finding that breastfeeding may reduce the risks of developing serious disorders in later life warrants further investigation.

Effects of Infectious Agents

A discussion of infectious agents in human milk requires consideration of both exposure to the pathogen and development of overt disease. Collected human milk contains many common epidermal bacteria that are not harmful to the recipient infant. With appropriate management, it is uncommon for the infant to become infected from women with mastitis or breast abscesses (Rench and Baker, 1989; Thomsen et al., 1984). Enteropathogens such as *Shigella* and *Salmonella* species may contaminate human milk through the areola and nipples of the breast, especially if those bacteria are prevalent in the environment (Mata et al., 1967, 1969; Wyatt and Mata, 1969). However, symptomatic infections with those enteropathogens are unusual in the recipient infant, seemingly because of the activity of the host defense system in human milk.

Of more concern are the reports that human milk contains viral pathogens including cytomegalovirus, hepatitis B virus, rubella virus, human T lympho-cytotropic virus type 1 (HTLV-1), and human immunodeficiency virus type 1 (HIV-1). Cytomegalovirus is common in milk produced by seropositive women (Ahlfors and Ivarsson, 1985; Dworsky et al., 1983; Stagno et al., 1980). As many as 70% of seropositive lactating women have the virus in their milk at some time (Ahlfors and Ivarsson, 1985). Although the infants become infected by ingesting the virus, the colonization does not progress to disease (Dworsky et al., 1983; Stagno et al., 1980), possibly because of specific IgG antibodies transferred via the placenta during pregnancy and immune substances provided in the mother's milk.

Both the wild and vaccine strains of rubella virus have been recovered from human milk (Buimovici-Klein et al., 1977; Klein et al., 1980; Losonsky et al., 1982). As a consequence of this transmission, mild clinical rubella has been reported, but severe disease has not.

Women who live in regions endemic for hepatitis B commonly have the surface antigens in their milk, but there is no evidence that breastfeeding is a route through which hepatitis B virus is transmitted and infection results (Boxall et al., 1974; Linnemann and Goldberg, 1974).

In parts of the West Indies, Africa, and the southwestern area of Japan, HTLV-1 (the retrovirus that causes adult T-cell leukemia) is endemic (Wong-Staal and Gallo, 1985). This virus is commonly found in milk from carrier women. Recently, epidemiologic evidence of the transmission of this virus via breastfeeding was found in an endemic population in the Nagasaki Prefecture in Japan (Hino, 1989). Since the annual incidence of adult T-cell leukemia in that population is estimated to be 0.1 to 0.2%, the demonstration of HTLV-1 in human milk is of great concern there. In a small sample investigated in Hino's study, 30% of breastfed, 10% of mixed-fed, and none of the totally formula-fed infants became positive carriers for the virus. Although it is not known whether the seropositive infants will develop the disease in later life, Hino has recommended that breastfeeding cease in that region of Japan to interrupt the spread of the disease. Follow-up studies are needed to validate or refute that recommendation. Although HTLV-1 is not a major disease in the United States, it is possible that a public health problem may develop if infected individuals immigrate to this country from endemic areas.

Of more immediate concern is the growing epidemic of HIV-1 infections in the United States and other countries and the possibility that HIV-1 may be transmitted to the infant via breastfeeding. Transplacental transmission of HIV-1 infections to the fetus occurs in about 30 to 40% of cases when women are seropositive during pregnancy. In contrast, the risk of transmitting HIV-1 via breastfeeding is not well established. Human milk contains $CD4^+$ T cells and macrophages that are prime targets for the virus. There are two reports of the detection of HIV-1 in human milk (Thiry et al., 1985; Vogt et al., 1986). Moreover, there are several reports of the postnatal acquisition by the mother of HIV-1 by transfusion of contaminated blood and the subsequent transmission of the infection to the infant, ostensibly by breastfeeding (see the review by Davis [1989]). The risk of transmitting the infection under more natural conditions remains uncertain.

More recent studies suggest that there is little likelihood that HIV-1 is a frequent contaminant of human milk or that breastfeeding is an important route of transmission of the virus. In a preliminary report (Yolken et al., 1990), the HIV-1 virion, RNA, messenger RNA, or integrated complementary DNA could not be demonstrated in the milk of HIV-1-infected women by the polymerase chain reaction. In addition, specific antibodies to HIV-1 (Yolken et al., 1990) and other factors that inhibit the binding of HIV-1 envelope proteins (gp120) to $CD4^+$ T cells (Newburg and Yolken, 1990) have been found in human milk.

Finally, a preliminary report of a European collaborative study on perinatal HIV-1 infections suggests that the risk of transmitting HIV-1 infections by breastfeeding women who were found to be seropositive during pregnancy is low (M.L. Newell, Institute of Child Health, London, United Kingdom, personal communication, 1990). However, the results of that study are inconclusive since only small numbers of infants were investigated; a more extensive follow-up of the infants will be required to ascertain whether there is a discernible risk of HIV-1 attributable to breastfeeding. In addition, studies are needed to determine whether breastfeeding provides health benefits to the infant who is infected with HIV-1 during intrauterine life.

Until more definitive information is available, the reader should consult two public health pronouncements on this subject: in the United States, the Centers for Disease Control (CDC, 1985) advised mothers who are seropositive for HIV-1 not to breastfeed; the World Health Organization (WHO, 1987) took the view that the risk of transmitting the virus in human milk is uncertain and that breastfeeding should be encouraged, especially in developing countries, because of the known health benefits of human milk.

Obesity

The effects of early feeding practices—both type of feeding (formula or human milk) and timing of introduction of solid foods—on immediate and subsequent weight have been extensively studied (see reviews by Hamosh [1988], Hamosh and Hamosh [1987], Himes [1979], and Kovar et al. [1984]). However, there are limitations in many of those studies. For example, the duration and degree of breastfeeding were seldom reported, and data on infant feeding practices were often based on parental recall rather than recorded information (see reviews by Hamosh and Hamosh (1987) and Kramer [1981, 1987]).

Nevertheless, no association between breastfeeding and obesity in the adult has been established. In general, early studies indicated that breastfed infants were much leaner than formula-fed ones (Taitz, 1977; Weil, 1977), whereas later studies show a weaker association (Dubois et al., 1979; Ferris et al., 1980; Hofvander et al., 1982; Saarinen and Siimes, 1979b; Shukla et al., 1972; Sveger et al., 1975; Vobecky et al., 1983). This difference may be attributable to the introduction of new formulas in the 1980s (the later formulations are more similar to human milk) and to changes in parental attitudes that have led to less overfeeding of formula-fed infants (reviewed by Hamosh [1988], Hamosh and Hamosh [1987], and Whitehead et al. [1986]). Furthermore, Birkbeck and colleagues (1985) controlled for familial differences in socioeconomic status and stature, but their results failed to show that breastfeeding prevents obesity in children.

The genesis of obesity appears to involve many factors (Hamosh and Hamosh, in press), including critical periods of pre- or postnatal adipose tissue development, genetics (Bouchard et al., 1990; Mueller, 1983; Ravussin et al., 1988; Stunkard et al., 1986, 1990), eating style (Agras et al., 1987), energy expenditure (Berkowitz et al., 1985; Bogardus et al., 1986; Bray, 1987; Elliot et al., 1989; Ravussin et al., 1988; Roberts et al., 1988), and social factors (Agras et al., 1987; Berkowitz et al., 1985; Roberts et al., 1988). Thus, the precise role of breastfeeding in this process remains undetermined.

Atherosclerosis

For years there has been interest in whether the cholesterol content of human milk, which is higher than that of commercial infant formulas, has a beneficial or adverse effect on later development of atherosclerosis. Studies in animals, including rats, guinea pigs, and baboons, have failed to provide clear-cut evidence that the mode of feeding affects blood cholesterol levels (see the review by Hamosh [1988]), but they suggest that feeding cholesterol may affect the mechanism of handling cholesterol in the body (Mott et al., 1990). Human studies (Fomon et al., 1984; Friedman and Goldberg, 1975; Hodgson et al., 1976; Huttunen et al., 1983; Marmot et al., 1980) show only small and inconsistent differences in serum cholesterol levels between formula-fed and breastfed children and young adults. Confounding genetic factors and dietary intake after weaning may not have been adequately considered in the interpretation of study results (Wissler and McGill, 1983). Furthermore, the extent and duration of breastfeeding have not been considered with sufficient rigor in most studies. Thus, the specific effects of the types of infant feeding on the development of atherosclerosis cannot be assessed at present.

BREASTFEEDING AND MORTALITY

Research Through 1950 in Developed Countries

Since the latter part of the last century, a great deal of attention has been given to the relationship of the mode of infant feeding with the infant's subsequent survival (see Appendix A).

Differences in postneonatal mortality rates between breastfed and bottle-fed infants in the developed countries from 1850 to 1950 are vividly summarized in Figure 7-1. The trends are striking and straightforward: there were markedly lower mortality rates among breastfed than among bottle-fed infants throughout. Although mortality rates, and thus absolute differences in mortality rates between the two groups, fell dramatically during the period, the relative advantage of breastfed infants persisted throughout, such that the postneonatal death rates of breastfed infants continued to remain at least half those of bottle-fed infants. While infant mortality rates among both breastfed and bottle-fed groups are now very low, there is no current information on whether breastfeeding confers any advantages for infant survival in the developed countries.

Research in Developing Countries

Some generalizations that can be made from the studies abstracted in Appendix B may also be relevant to policy in developed societies. First, there is a consistently increased risk of mortality among formula-fed infants under

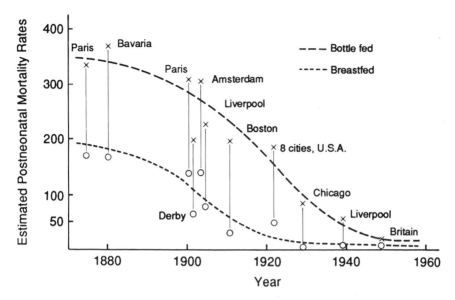

FIGURE 7-1 Estimated postneonatal mortality rates among breastfed and bottle-fed infants, various locations, 1870-1950. From Wray (1990) with permission.

1 year of age than among breastfed infants. Second, most studies suggest that infants receiving both human milk and formula have lower death rates than those of infants given only formula, but that exclusive breastfeeding is associated with the lowest mortality rates.

There are fewer data on the incidence of infectious disease than on the severity of the infection (that is, case fatality). During the neonatal period, the incidence of infectious disease appears to be lower among exclusively breastfed infants. After the neonatal period, incidence appears to be relatively less affected by mode of feeding, but severity appears to be much lessened among infants who have been breastfed. However, there are several exceptions to these generalizations: for example, Plank and Milanesi (1973) found little protection from breastfeeding among infants who were simultaneously receiving supplemental food.

The association between breastfeeding and mortality after 1 year of age has been inconsistent. For example, while Cantrelle and Leridon (1971) found no protection during the second and third years of life, Briend et al. (1988), in a careful prospective study in rural Bangladesh, observed that breastfeeding provided persistent and strong protection against mortality throughout the age span studied (up to the infants' third birthday). It does appear that even in primitive conditions excess mortality is not inevitable among those weaned after the first birthday, but the situations in which protection is not conferred by breastfeeding are not understood.

In general, the relationship of breastfeeding to child mortality in developing countries has been found to be less strong with increased educational and social status of the mother. See, for example, the results of Palloni and Tienda (1986) from studies conducted in Peru.

Recently there has been renewed focus on the effect of child spacing among breastfed infants (see Chapter 8) on child survival (Hobcraft, 1987; Thapa et al., 1988). In countries with high infant and child mortality rates, Hobcraft (1987) estimated that a closely spaced preceding birth (a birth interval of less than 2 years) is associated with a 50% increase in the risk of mortality before age 5 for the new (index) infant. At a birth interval of less than 12 months, the risk is even higher. If another infant is born before the index child's second birthday, the index child's risk of dying before age 5 was estimated to increase by 55%. Controlling for birth weight did not influence these estimated effects, suggesting that they were in addition to the shortened interpregnancy intervals resulting from preterm delivery. In developed countries, the overall impact of child spacing on survival is probably minimal (Fedrick and Adelstein, 1973), but further research is needed to assess whether there is an impact among disadvantaged families.

Research in Developed Countries Since 1950

The subcommittee found only six published studies relating mode of infant feeding with mortality based on data collected since 1950 in the developed world (see Appendix A); three of these were concerned with sudden infant death syndrome (SIDS) (one of them focused on botulism). Naeye and colleagues (1976) found an odds ratio of 1.3 (not significant) for increased risk of SIDS among infants who were not breastfed. An odds ratio of 3.06 for formula-fed versus either breastfed or mixed-fed infants was calculated by the subcommittee from the data of Biering-Sorensen et al. (1978). Arnon and colleagues (1982) found significantly higher rates of breastfeeding among infants hospitalized with botulism than among controls but a decreased likelihood of sudden death from botulism among those who were ever breastfed.

In a study in Sheffield, England, covering the years between 1970 and 1979, Carpenter et al. (1983) attributed a decrease of 0.8 postperinatal infant deaths per 1,000 births to increased rates of breastfeeding, but no direct comparison of the rates of breastfed and bottle-fed infants was presented. A study from Canada (Department of National Health and Welfare Canada, 1963) was concerned exclusively with Canadian Indians, a relatively deprived and therefore atypical population.

Differences, even of large magnitude, may be difficult to detect in the developed countries, with their generally low infant and child death rates.

Larger and more sophisticated studies are needed to determine whether or not breastfeeding leads to lowered infant mortality in developed countries, especially among poor mothers and children.

There are many other unanswered questions about breastfeeding and infant mortality: (1) What are the relative impacts on infant mortality of improvements in nutritional status, immunologic competence, or protection from a contaminated food supply? (2) Up to what age is breastfeeding protective? (3) What are the relative merits of exclusive breastfeeding compared with partial breastfeeding supplemented by other foods? (4) What is the relative impact of breastfeeding on the incidence of infection as opposed to the severity of infection?

For further information, see the reviews by Cunningham (1981), Jason et al. (1984), Kovar et al. (1984), Kramer (1987), Winikoff (1981), and Wray (1978, 1990). Those of Cunningham (1981) and Wray (1978, 1990) are particularly informative. Since there are many sources of confounding possible when comparing death rates between breastfed and other infants, the reader is referred to the information on sources of bias at the beginning in this chapter and to the review by Kramer (1987).

MEDICATIONS, LEGAL AND ILLEGAL DRUGS, AND ENVIRONMENTAL AGENTS

The subcommittee's understanding of nutrition during lactation would be incomplete without consideration of foreign, potentially toxic substances passed from mother to infant via human milk. Such substances are discussed briefly below.

Certain drugs and environmental chemicals that enter a mother's body may appear in her milk. The hazard, if any, posed by extraneous substances in milk is dependent upon a number of factors:

• the pharmacokinetics of the foreign substance, including its molecular size, solubility, ionization, protein binding, acidity, metabolism, storage, and excretion (Wilson, 1981);

• the mode of entry of the agent, as well as its absorption, efficiency of metabolism, and excretion by the mother (Lawrence, 1989; Rivera-Calimlim, 1987);

• the physiologic maturity of the infant, which influences whether or not the compound can be absorbed by the neonatal gut, detoxified, or excreted, or whether the infant is otherwise unusually susceptible to the effects of the foreign substance.

Medications

Maternal medication is usually not a reason to discourage breastfeeding.

If the mother requires a drug that poses a risk for her infant for only a short time, she can pump her breasts to maintain lactation and discard the milk. This applies to diagnostic radiopharmaceuticals, antiprotozoal compounds, and a few antibiotics that cannot be safely given to an infant (such as chloramphenicol). Compounds such as sulfadiazine may be contraindicated for the breastfeeding mother in the early postpartum period but are well tolerated when the infant is at least 1 month of age. Certain other drugs are contraindicated during breast-feeding. They include antineoplastic drugs, therapeutic radiopharmaceuticals, lithium, lactation-suppressing drugs, certain antithyroid drugs, and synthetic anticoagulants (for specific information, see Briggs et al. [1986], Committee on Drugs [1989], and Lawrence [1989]).

Caffeine or Coffee

The use of caffeine to treat immature infants with apnea has provided an opportunity to study the absorption, distribution, metabolism, and excretion of this drug in neonates. The milk-to-plasma ratio ranges between 0.5 and 0.8—an amount less than 1% of the maternal dose. However, when an infant receives frequent doses, caffeine can accumulate, causing wakefulness or irritability. Maternal consumption of one or two caffeine-containing beverages per day is not associated with unacceptable levels of caffeine in human milk (Committee on Drugs, 1989; Wilson, 1981; Wilson et al., 1985).

There is evidence from a study in Costa Rica that maternal consumption of three or more cups of coffee per day during pregnancy and lactation can affect iron concentrations in milk and infant iron status at 1 month of age (Muñoz et al., 1988). Studies in rats suggest that this effect is not due to caffeine but to some other component(s) in coffee (Muñoz et al., 1986). There is a need for further investigations in other populations and in pregnant and lactating women consuming fewer than three cups of coffee per day.

Alcohol

Small amounts of alcohol have been recommended in many cultures as a means of stimulating milk secretion. On the other hand, excessive alcohol intake has been associated with failure to initiate the let-down reflex (see Chapter 5), high alcohol levels in the milk, and lethargic nurslings (Cobo, 1973), as well as with adverse health consequences for the mother. Wilson and colleagues (1980) comment: "The observation that acetaldehyde, the major metabolite of ethanol, is not excreted in the milk is significant since some have postulated that acetaldehyde contributes to the toxicity of alcohol" (p. 34). In a study of 1-year-old infants, Little and colleagues (1989) found a strong positive association between psychomotor development scores obtained with the Bayley Scales of Infant Development (Bayley, 1969) and a proxy measure for exposure to alcohol through breastfeeding. Actual differences in these scores were minor for groups at the extremes of alcohol exposure. The scores of infants of breastfeeding mothers who occasionally drank (e.g., one or two drinks per week) did not differ from those of infants who were not exposed to any alcohol through breastfeeding. The amount of alcohol in the milk, the impact of confounding socioeconomic factors, and deficits in maternal interactions with the infant were not reported in this study. Therefore, it remains unclear whether alcohol in human milk presents a problem to the infant.

Cigarette Smoking

Cigarette smoking may adversely affect milk volume (see Chapter 5). Neither Luck and Nau (1985) nor the subcommittee found reports of associations between nicotine levels present in the milk of heavy smokers and symptoms in their nursing infants.

Studies to compare nicotine and cotinine levels of breastfed and formula-fed infants are most appropriate if conducted after the infants are 8 days old to eliminate the effect of transplacental exposure. The blood levels of nicotine and cotinine in infants of smokers vary widely, regardless of feeding method. It appears that absorption of nicotine in the respiratory tract, which is rapid and complete, is greater than absorption of nicotine from human milk. The infant's exposures from inspired air and from milk amount to less than 5% of the average dose inhaled by an adult smoker. Ranges of measurable nicotine in the milk vary from 1.4 to 62 ng/ml and are usually higher than the corresponding serum level. The nicotine content tends to increase with increased depth of inhalation and with an increased number of puffs per cigarette (Luck and Nau, 1985).

Although no reports have been published associating nicotine from human milk with infant health problems, it is advisable to counsel mothers to avoid smoking for 2.5 hours before feeding (Luck and Nau, 1987) and to avoid smoking in the infant's presence.

Illegal Drugs

Marijuana appears in human milk as $\triangle$-9-tetrahydrocannabinol, which is poorly absorbed in this form but may be sufficient to cause lethargy and decreased feeding frequency and duration after prolonged exposure. Heroin and cocaine also appear in human milk and place the infant at significant risk of toxicity, despite the low bioavailability from milk (Chasnoff et al., 1987).

Environmental Contaminants

In high-exposure areas, the milk of some women contains insecticides.

Organochlorinated compounds were investigated worldwide after the first report in 1951 of the presence of dichlorodiphenyltrichloroethane (DDT) in the milk of healthy U.S. women (Laug et al., 1951). Polychlorinated biphenyls (PCBs), hexachlorobenzene, dieldrin, and heptachlor epoxide have also been identified in milk from women with known heavy exposures. In a study of hundreds of subjects at delivery in the Great Lakes region of New York State in 1978, PCB was not detectable in the cord blood of the infants or in the milk of the mothers, except when the women illegally ate contaminated lake fish at least once a week (Lawrence, 1989). In general, PCB levels in milk decline over the period of lactation and with the number of children nursed (Rogan et al., 1986) if there are no new exposures during this period.

The levels of DDT and other insecticides in human milk vary with the weight of the mother, the number of children, the duration of lactation, and the residence and occupation of the mother (Rogan and Gladen, 1985; Wilson et al., 1973). Insecticide levels in human milk tend to be higher than those in cow's milk, because humans are at the top of the food chain. Levels are higher at the end of a single nursing because the fat content of the milk is increased at that time.

In a study of 858 children from birth to 5 years of age whose mother's milk contained PCBs and dichlorodiphenyl ethane (DDE, a metabolite of DDT) after a heavy exposure, there was no evidence of change in growth rate or general health, nor were there adverse effects on weight gain or differences in the number of physician visits for illness. However, DDE in the human milk was associated with a shorter duration of breastfeeding (Gladen et al., 1988; Rogan et al., 1987). These children remain under surveillance.

Agent Orange (2,3,7,8-tetrachlorodibenzo-p-dioxin), the best known of the dioxins, has been found in human milk in pooled samples from women with known exposures to high levels in Vietnam. There is no evidence that the U.S. population at large is at risk (Schecter and Gasiewicz, 1987; Schecter et al., 1986, 1987).

Heavy metals—such as lead, mercury, arsenic, and cadmium—are found in higher concentrations in certain water supplies, cow's milk, and reconstituted formula than in human milk (Dabeka et al., 1986; Jensen, 1983). Thus, breastfed infants are exposed to lower amounts than their formula-fed counterparts are. Whenever there has been an exposure or a woman has been found to have elevated mercury or lead levels, the infant's serum and the milk levels should be checked (Perkins and Oski, 1976). In the case of lead poisoning, evidence suggests that maternal serum levels under 40 mg/dl are not associated with elevated lead values in the milk (Dillon et al., 1974). Lead levels in milk are lower than would be predicted from maternal serum levels (Wolff, 1983). Based on a single case study, Ryu and colleagues (1978) state that loss of lead from the body can be expected in breastfed infants exposed to lead in utero if their lead intake is less than 5 μg/kg of body weight per day.

Filer (1968) summarized the effects of radionuclides in several parts of North America upon infants and children. Staub and Murphy (1965) found less radiostrontium in human milk than in cow's milk specimens collected in Denver and Chicago during 1959 to 1961. The deposition of strontium-90 in deciduous teeth of infants in St. Louis was also much greater in formula-fed than in breastfed infants (Rosenthal et al., 1964). Filer (1968) recommended that one of the principal methods of limiting radionuclide intake by infants would be to increase the percentage of infants who are breastfed. For more current information concerning the problem of radionuclides in foods, the reader is referred to the report of Carter (1988) of the aftermath of the Chernobyl nuclear explosion.

If there is a possibility of heavy environmental contamination, the mother should discuss the concern with the physician and, when appropriate, testing can be arranged through a state-approved laboratory.

CONCLUSIONS

• For the biological reasons discussed in this chapter, breastfeeding is recommended for all infants in the United States under ordinary circumstances. Exclusive breastfeeding is the preferred method of feeding for normal full-term infants from birth to age 4 to 6 months. Breastfeeding complemented by the appropriate introduction of other foods is recommended for the remainder of the first year or longer, if desired. The subcommittee and advisory committee recognize that it is difficult for some women to follow the recommendations for social or occupational reasons, such as those discussed in Chapters 2 and 3.

• During the first 2 to 3 months of lactation, exclusively breastfed infants generally stay at approximately the same weight-for-age percentile or gain weight at a slightly faster rate, although they ingest less energy than do formula-fed infants. After the third month, exclusively breastfed infants tend to follow lower weight-for-age and length-for-age percentiles. In general, those patterns are not altered by the introduction of solid foods.

• The nutritional status of breastfed infants in the United States is generally excellent because of the uniqueness of the composition of human milk, including the high bioavailability of many of its constituents. In general, nutritional supplements are not needed for the breastfed infant. Nevertheless, certain nutritional interventions sometimes may be warranted, as described under the section "Recommendations for Clinical Practice" below.

• In general, breastfed infants have fewer gastrointestinal or respiratory infections than do formula-fed infants in both developed and developing countries, but the extent to which breastfeeding is protective may depend upon the type of microorganism and the degree to which the infant is exposed to that pathogen.

• Although some studies suggest that maternal nutrition may affect the immunologic components in human milk, no studies address the effect of such changes upon the susceptibility of the recipient infant to infectious diseases.

• Breastfeeding appears to protect against food allergy and eczema, but the protective mechanisms are not understood well. The subcommittee concluded that to reduce the chance of allergy or colic in their breastfed infants, mothers should not avoid important food sources of nutrients such as cow's milk in the absence of objective evidence provided by oral elimination-challenge trials (see later section "Maternal Diet"). Although there are some reports of untoward reactions in breastfed infants linked to extrinsic food allergens in human milk, the use of food allergen-restricted diets in pregnancy, lactation, or both should be limited to those cases for which the sensitization has been proven.

• Recent epidemiologic studies suggest that breastfeeding may lessen the risk of developing certain chronic diseases (such as lymphoma, Crohn's disease, and type I diabetes mellitus) later in life.

• Current evidence does not warrant the conclusion that breastfeeding will prevent obesity in the offspring.

• The effects of breastfeeding on infant and childhood mortality in the United States deserve study, especially among subgroups with higher than average mortality rates.

• In general, human milk has not been shown to transmit infections, but more research will be required to ascertain the risk to the recipient of HTLV-1 in human milk and whether HIV-1 is a major infectious agent in human milk.

RECOMMENDATIONS FOR CLINICAL PRACTICE

Infant Nutrition

The following steps should be taken to ensure adequate nutrition of breast-fed infants:

• All newborns should receive a 0.5- to 1.0-mg injection or a 1.0- to 2.0-mg oral dose of vitamin K immediately after birth, regardless of the type of feeding that will be offered the infant.

• The infant should be given a 5.0- to 7.5-μg supplement of vitamin D per day if his or her exposure to sunlight appears to be inadequate.

• Fluoride supplements should be provided only to breastfed infants who live in households in which the fluoride content of the water supply is low (<0.3 ppm).

• Human milk is a sufficient source of iron for the first 6 months of an infant's life, but foods with bioavailable iron, iron-fortified foods, or a low-dose iron supplement should be provided at 6 months, or earlier if supplementary foods are introduced before that time.

• The milk of complete vegetarians is likely to be deficient in vitamin B_{12}. In such cases, it is desirable to supplement the infant and either to find an acceptable food source of vitamin B_{12} for the mother or to provide her with a supplement of this vitamin (even if she is asymptomatic).

Infant Growth

• The subcommittee recommends that health care providers be informed about the differences in growth between healthy breastfed and formula-fed infants. On average, breastfed infants gain weight more slowly than do those fed formula. Slower weight gain, by itself, does not justify the use of supplemental formula. When in doubt, clinicians should evaluate adequacy of growth according to the guidelines described by Lawrence (1989).

Infant Health

Breastfeeding ordinarily confers health benefits to the infant, but in certain rare cases it may pose some health risks. The following recommendations address some aspects of infant health:

• Breastfeeding is recommended to reduce the incidence and severity of certain infectious gastrointestinal and respiratory diseases and other disorders in infancy.

• Mothers should be encouraged to continue breastfeeding, even if they develop mastitis, with certain rare exceptions, but they should be advised to seek early treatment (see Lawrence [1989] for specific recommendations).

• Neither cytomegalovirus nor hepatitis virus infections during lactation are contraindications to breastfeeding. In the case of hepatitis virus infections, immunizations are necessary regardless of the mode of feeding. Rubella immunization is warranted in seronegative women during the immediate postpartum period even if the woman chooses to breastfeed.

• For mothers requiring medication and desiring to breastfeed, the clinician should select the medication least likely to pass into the milk and to the infant.

• Medications rarely pose a problem during lactation; breastfeeding is contraindicated if certain drugs must be administered. Such drugs include antineoplastic agents, therapeutic radiopharmaceuticals, some but not all antithyroid agents, and antiprotozoan agents. Medications that can be given to infants can be taken by the lactating woman.

• In those rare cases when there is heavy exposure to pesticides, heavy metals, or other contaminants that may pass into the milk, breastfeeding is not recommended if maternal levels are high.

Maternal Diet

Objective evidence should be obtained from an oral elimination challenge trial before advising women to make long-term diet changes to reduce the problem of allergy or colic in their breastfed infants. In such studies, the suspected food allergen is first eliminated from the mother's diet to determine whether the breastfed infant will become asymptomatic. Oral challenges should then be conducted under careful medical supervision to ascertain whether the symptoms can be reproduced. Provoked reactions should be treated with appropriate medications as rapidly as possible. If a basic food must be eliminated from the diet for weeks to months, adequate nutrient intake should be promoted through special dietary planning.

REFERENCES

Aaby, P., J. Bukh, I.M. Lisse, and A.J. Smits. 1984. Overcrowding and intensive exposure as determinants of measles mortality. Am. J. Epidemiol. 120:49-63.

Adair, L.S., and E. Pollitt. 1985. Outcome of maternal nutritional supplementation: a comprehensive review of the Bacon Chow study. Am. J. Clin. Nutr. 41:948-978.

Agras, W.S., H.C. Kraemer, R.I. Berkowitz, A.F. Korner, and L.D. Hammer. 1987. Does a vigorous feeding style influence early development of adiposity? J. Pediatr. 110:799-804.

Ahlfors, K., and S.A. Ivarsson. 1985. Cytomegalovirus in breast milk of Swedish milk donors. Scand. J. Infect. Dis. 17:11-13.

Ala-Houhala, M. 1985. 25-Hydroxyvitamin D levels during breast-feeding with or without maternal or infantile supplementation of vitamin D. J. Pediatr. Gastroenterol. Nutr. 4:220-226.

Arnaud, S.B., G.B. Stickler, and J.C. Haworth. 1976. Serum 25-hydroxyvitamin D in infantile rickets. Pediatrics 57:221-225.

Arnon, S.S., K. Damus, B. Thompson, T.F. Midura, and J. Chin. 1982. Protective role of human milk against sudden death from infant botulism. J. Pediatr. 100:568-573.

Axelsson, I., S. Borulf, L. Righard, and N. Räihä. 1987. Protein and energy intake during weaning. I. Effects on growth. Acta Paediatr. Scand. 76:321-327.

Bates, C.J., A.M. Prentice, A.A. Paul, A. Prentice, B.A. Sutcliffe, and R.G. Whitehead. 1982. Riboflavin status in infants born in rural Gambia, and the effect of a weaning food supplement. Trans. R. Soc. Trop. Med. Hyg. 76:253-258.

Bayley, N. 1969. Manual for the Bayley Scales of Infant Development. Psychological Corp, New York. 178 pp.

Belton, N. 1986. Rickets—not only the "English Disease." Acta Paediatr. Scand. Suppl. 323:68-75.

Berkowitz, R.I., W.S. Agras, A.F. Korner, H.C. Kraemer, and C.H. Zeanah. 1985. Physical activity and adiposity: a longitudinal study from birth to childhood. J. Pediatr. 106:734-738.

Biagi, P.L., A. Bordoni, M. Masi, G. Ricci, C. Fanelli, A. Patrizi, E. Ceccolino. 1988. A long-term study of the use of evening primrose oil (Efamol) in atopic children. Drugs Exp. Clin. Res. 14:285-290.

Biering-Sørensen, F., T. Jørgensen, and J. Hilden. 1978. Sudden infant death in Copenhagen 1956-1971. I. Infant feeding. Acta Paediatr. Scand. 67:129-137.

Birkbeck, J.A., P.M. Buckfield, and P.A. Silva. 1985. Lack of long-term effect of the method of infant feeding on growth. Hum. Nutr.: Clin. Nutr. 39C:39-44.

Bogardus, C., S. Lillioja, E. Ravussin, W. Abbott, J.K. Zawadzki, A. Young, W.C. Knowler, R. Jacobowitz, and P.P. Moll. 1986. Familial dependence of the resting metabolic rate. N. Engl. J. Med. 315:96-100.

Borch-Johnsen, K., G. Joner, T. Mandrup-Poulsen, M. Christy, B. Zachau-Christiansen, K. Kastrup, and J. Nerup. 1984. Relationship between breast-feeding and incidence rates of insulin-dependent diabetes mellitus. A hypothesis. Lancet 2:1083-1086.

Bordoni, A., P.L. Biagi, M. Masi, G. Ricci, C. Fanelli, A. Patrizi, and E. Ceccolini. 1988. Evening primrose oil (Efamol) in the treatment of children with atopic eczema. Drugs Exp. Clin. Res. 14:291-297.

Bouchard, C., A. Tremblay, J.P. Despres, A. Nadeau, P.J. Lupien, G. Theriault, J. Dussault, S. Moorjani, S. Pinault, and G. Fournier. 1990. The response to long-term overfeeding in identical twins. N. Engl. J. Med. 322:1477-1482.

Boxall, E.H., T.H. Flewett, D.S. Dane, C.H. Cameron, F.O. MacCallum, and T.W. Lee. 1974. Hepatitis-B surface antigen in breast milk. Lancet 2:1007-1008.

Bray, G.A. 1987. Obesity—a disease of nutrient or energy imbalance? Nutr. Rev. 45:33-43.

Brazelton, T.B. 1962. Crying in infancy. Pediatrics 29:579-588.

Briend, A., B. Wojtyniak, and M.G. Rowland. 1988. Breast feeding, nutritional state, and child survival in rural Bangladesh. Br. Med. J. 296:879-882.

Briggs, G.G., R.K. Freeman, and S.J. Yaffe. 1986. Drugs in Pregnancy and Lactation. Williams & Wilkins, Baltimore. 495 pp.

Brown, K.H., R.E. Black, G. Lopez de Romaña, and H. Creed de Kanashiro. 1989. Infant-feeding practices and their relationship with diarrheal and other disease in Huascar (Lima), Peru. Pediatrics 83:31-40.

Brückmann, G., and S.G. Zondek. 1939. Iron, copper and manganese in human organs at various ages. Biochem. J. 33:1845-1857.

Buimovici-Klein, E., R.L. Hite, T. Byrne, and L.Z. Cooper. 1977. Isolation of rubella virus in milk after postpartum immunization. J. Pediatr. 91:939-941.

Butte, N.F. 1988. Energy requirements during infancy. Pp. 86-99 in R.C. Tsang and B.L. Nichols, eds. Nutrition During Infancy. Hanley & Belfus, Philadelphia.

Butte, N.F., C. Garza, E.O. Smith, and B.L. Nichols. 1984. Human milk intake and growth in exclusively breast-fed infants. J. Pediatr. 104:187-195.

Butte, N.F., W.W. Wong, C. Garza, and P.D. Klein. 1990. Adequacy of human milk for meeting energy requirements during early infancy. Pp. 103-116 in S.A. Atkinson, L.A. Hanson, and R. Chandra, eds. Human Lactation 4: Breastfeeding, Nutrition, Infection and Infant Growth in Developed and Emerging Countries. ARTS Biomedical Publishers and Distributors. St. John's, Newfoundland, Canada.

Cant, A., R.A. Marsden, and P.J. Kilshaw. 1985. Egg and cow's milk hypersensitivity in exclusively breast fed infants with eczema, and detection of egg protein in breast milk. Br. Med. J. 291:932-935.

Cantrelle, P., and H. Leridon. 1971. Breast feeding, mortality in childhood and fertility in a rural zone of Senegal. Popul. Stud. 25:505-533.

Carey, W.B. 1984. "Colic"—primary excessive crying as an infant-environmental interaction. Pediatr. Clin. North Am. 31:993-1005.

Carpenter, R.G., A. Gardner, M. Jepson, E.M. Taylor, A. Salvin, R. Sunderland, J.L. Emery, E. Pursall, and J. Roe. 1983. Prevention of unexpected infant death: evaluation of the first seven years of the Sheffield Intervention Programme. Lancet 1:723-727.

Carter, M.W. 1988. Radionuclides in the Food Chain. Springer-Verlag, New York, 518 pp.

Cavell, B. 1979. Gastric emptying in preterm infants. Acta Paediatr. Scand. 68:725-730.

Cavell, B. 1981. Gastric emptying in infants fed human milk or infant formula. Acta Paediatr. Scand. 70:639-641.

CDC (Centers for Disease Control). 1985. Recommendations for assisting in the prevention of perinatal transmission of human T-lymphotropic virus type III/lymphadenopathy-associated virus and acquired immunodeficiency syndrome. Morbid. Mortal. Wkly. Rep. 34:721-732.

Chan, G.M., C.C. Roberts, D. Folland, and R. Jackson. 1982. Growth and bone mineralization of normal breast-fed infants and the effects of lactation on maternal bone mineral status. Am. J. Clin. Nutr. 36:438-443.

Chandra, R.K. 1982. Physical growth of exclusively breast fed-infants. Nutr. Res. 2:275-276.

Chandra, R.K. 1987. Prevention of atopic disease: environmental engineering utilizing antenatal antigen avoidance and breast feeding. Pp. 269-274 in A.S. Goldman, S.A. Atkinson, and L.A. Hanson, eds. Human Lactation 3: The Effects of Human Milk on the Recipient Infant. Plenum Press, New York.

Chandra, R.K., S. Puri, and P.S. Cheema. 1985. Predictive value of cord blood IgE in the development of atopic disease and role of breast-feeding in its prevention. Clin. Allergy 15:517-522.

Chasnoff, I.J., D.E. Lewis, and L. Squires. 1987. Cocaine intoxication in a breast-fed infant. Pediatrics 80:836-838.

Chiba, Y., T. Minagawa, K. Mito, A. Nakane, K. Suga, T. Honjo, and T. Nakao. 1987. Effect of breast feeding on responses of systemic interferon and virus-specific lymphocyte transformation in infants with respiratory syncytial virus infection. J. Med. Virol. 21:7-14.

Clemens, J.B., B. Stanton, B. Stoll, N.S. Shahid, H. Banu, and A.K.M.A. Chowdhury. 1986. Breast-feeding as a determinant of severity in shigellosis: evidence for protection throughout the first three years of life in Bangladeshi children. Am. J. Epidemiol. 123:710-720.

Clemens, T.L., J.S. Adams, S.L. Henderson, and M.F. Holick. 1982. Increased skin pigment reduces capacity of skin to synthesize vitamin D_3. Lancet 1:74-76.

Close, G.Ć. 1983. Rastafarianism and the vegans syndrome. Br. Med. J. 286:473.

Cobo, E. 1973. Effect of different doses of ethanol on the milk-ejecting reflex in lactating women. Am. J. Obstet. Gynecol. 115:817-821.

Committee on Drugs. 1989. Transfer of drugs and other chemicals into human milk. Pediatrics 84:924-936.

Committee on Nutrition. 1985. Pediatric Nutrition Handbook, 2nd ed. American Academy of Pediatrics, Elk Grove Village, Ill. 421 pp.

Committee on Nutrition. 1986. Fluoride supplementation. Pediatrics 77:758-761.

Cunningham, A.S. 1981. Breast-feeding and morbidity in industrialized countries: an update. Pp. 128-168 in D.B. Jelliffe and E.F.P. Jelliffe, eds. Advances in International Maternal and Child Health, Vol. 1. Oxford University Press, Oxford.

Cushing, A.H., and L. Anderson. 1982. Diarrhea in breast-fed and non-breast-fed infants. Pediatrics 70:921-925.

Czajka-Narins, D.M., and E. Jung. 1986. Physical growth of breast-fed and formula-fed infants from birth to age two years. Nutr. Res. 6:753-762.

Dabeka, R.W., K.F. Karpinskl, A.D. McKenzie, and C.D. Bajdik. 1986. Survey of lead, cadmium and fluoride in human milk and correlation of levels with environmental and food factors. Food Chem. Toxicol. 24:913-921.

Dallman, P.R. 1986. Iron deficiency in the weanling: a nutritional problem on the way to resolution. Acta Paediatr. Scand. Suppl. 323:59-67.

Davis, J.R., Jr., J. Goldenring, and B.H. Lubin. 1981. Nutritional vitamin B_{12} deficiency in infants. Am. J. Dis. Child. 135:566-567.

Davis, M.K. 1989. The role of human milk in human immunodeficiency virus infection. Pp. 151-160 in S.A. Atkinson, L.A. Hanson, and R.K. Chandra, eds. Human Lactation 4: Breastfeeding, Nutrition, Infection and Infant Growth in Developed and Emerging Countries. ARTS Biomedical Publishers and Distributors, St. John's, Newfoundland, Canada.

Davis, M.K., D.A. Savitz, and B.I. Graubard. 1988. Infant feeding and childhood cancer. Lancet 2:365-368.

Delgado, H.L., V.E. Valverde, R. Martorell, and R.E. Klein. 1982. Relationship of maternal and infant nutrition to infant growth. Early Hum. Dev. 6:273-286.

Department of National Health and Welfare, Canada. 1963. Survey of Maternal and Child Health of Canadian Registered Indians 1962. Cited in Gerrard, J.W., and K.K.T. Tan. 1978. Hazards of formula feeding. Keeping Abreast. J. Hum. Nurturing. 3:20-25.

Dewey, K.G., and B. Lönnerdal. 1983. Milk and nutrient intake of breast-fed infants from 1 to 6 months: Relation to growth and fatness. J. Pediatr. Gastroenterol. Nutr. 2:497-506.

Dewey, K.G., M.J. Heinig, L.A. Nommsen, and B. Lönnerdal. 1989. Infant growth and breast-feeding. Am. J. Clin. Nutr. 50:1116-1117.

Dewey, K.G., M.J. Heinig, L.A. Nommsen, and B. Lönnerdal. 1990a. Growth patterns of breast-fed infants during the first year of life: the DARLING study. Pp. 269-282 in S.A. Atkinson, L.A. Hanson, and R. Chandra, eds. Human Lactation 4: Breastfeeding, Nutrition, Infection and Infant Growth in Developed and Emerging Countries. ARTS Biomedical Publishers and Distributors, St. John's, Newfoundland, Canada.

Dewey, K.G., M.J. Heinig, L.A. Nommsen, and B. Lönnerdal. 1990b. Low energy intakes and growth velocities of breast-fed infants: are there functional consequences? In B. Schürch and N.S. Scrimshaw, eds. Proceedings of an IDECG Workshop. IDECG - Nestle Foundation, Lausanne, Switzerland.

Dewey, K.G., M.J. Heinig, L.A. Nommsen, and B. Lönnerdal. In press. Maternal vs. infant factors related to breast milk intake and residual milk volume: the DARLING study. Pediatr.

DHHS (Department of Health and Human Services). 1988. The Surgeon General's Report on Nutrition and Health. DHHS (PHS) Publ. No. 88-50210. Public Health Service, U.S. Department of Health and Human Services. U.S. Government Printing Office, Washington, D.C. 727 pp.

Dillon, H.K., D.J. Wilson, and W. Schaffner. 1974. Lead concentrations in human milk. Am. J. Dis. Child. 128:491-492.

DiPietro, J., S.K. Larson, and S.W. Porges. 1987. Behavioral and heart rate pattern differences between breast-fed and bottle-fed neonates. Dev. Psychol. 23:467-474.

Downham, M.A.P.S., R. Scott, D.G. Sims, J.K.G. Webb, and P.S. Gardner. 1976. Breast-feeding protects against respiratory syncytial virus infections. Br. Med. J. 2:274-276.

Dubois, S., D.E. Hill, and G.H. Beaton. 1979. An examination of factors believed to be associated with infantile obesity. Am. J. Clin. Nutr. 31:1997-2007.

Duffy, L.C., M. Riepenhoff-Talty, T.E. Byers, L.J. La Scolea, M.A. Zielezny, D.M. Dryja, and P.L. Ogra. 1986. Modulation of rotavirus enteritis during breast-feeding. Am. J. Dis. Child. 140:1164-1168.

Duncan, B., C. Schaefer, B. Sibley, and N.M. Fonseca. 1984. Reduced growth velocity in exclusively breast-fed infants. Am. J. Dis. Child. 138:309-313.

Duncan, B., R.B. Schifman, J.J. Corrigan, Jr., and C. Schaefer. 1985. Iron and the exclusively breast-fed infant from birth to six months. J. Pediatr. Gastroenterol. Nutr. 4:421-425.

Dworsky, M., M. Yow, S. Stagno, R.F. Pass, and C. Alford. 1983. Cytomegalovirus infection of breast milk and transmission in infancy. Pediatrics 72:295-299.

Ek, J., and E.M. Magnus. 1979. Plasma and red blood cell folate in breastfed infants. Acta Paediatr. Scand. 68:239-243.

Ek, J., and E. Magnus. 1982. Plasma and red cell folate values and folate requirements in formula-fed term infants. J. Pediatr. 100:738-744.

Elias, M.F., N.A. Nicolson, C. Bora, and J. Johnston. 1986. Sleep/wake patterns of breast-fed infants in the first 2 years of life. Pediatrics 77:322-329.

Elliot, D.L., L. Goldberg, K.S. Kuehl, and C. Hanna. 1989. Metabolic evaluation of obese and nonobese siblings. J. Pediatr. 114:957-962.

FAO (Food and Agriculture Organization). 1988. Requirements of Vitamin A, Iron, Folate, and Vitamin B_{12}. Report of a Joint FAO/WHO Expert Consultation. FAO Food and Nutrition Series No. 23. Food and Agriculture Organization, Rome. 107 pp.

Fedrick, J., and P. Adelstein. 1973. Influence of pregnancy spacing on outcome of pregnancy. Br. Med. J. 4:753-756.

Fergusson, D.M., A.L. Beautrais, and P.A. Silva. 1982. Breast-feeding and cognitive development in the first seven years of life. Soc. Sci. Med. 16:1705-1708.

Ferris, A.G., M.J. Laus, D.W. Hosmer, and V.A. Beal. 1980. The effect of diet on weight gain in infancy. Am. J. Clin. Nutr. 33:2635-2642.

Filer, L.J., Jr. 1968. Evaluation and reduction of risks: Problems and applications of individual control measures. Pediatrics 41:308.

Fomon, S.J. 1987. Reflections on infant feeding in the 1970s and 1980s. Am. J. Clin. Nutr. Suppl. 46:171-182.

Fomon, S.J., R.R. Rogers, E.E. Ziegler, S.E. Nelson, and L.N. Thomas. 1984. Indices of fatness and serum cholesterol at age eight years in relation to feeding and growth during early infancy. Pediatr. Res. 18:1233-1238.

Forsum, E., and A. Sadurskis. 1986. Growth, body composition and breast milk intake of Swedish infants during early life. Early Hum. Dev. 14:121-129.

Friedman, G., and S.J. Goldberg. 1975. Concurrent and subsequent serum cholesterols of breast- and formula-fed infants. Am. J. Clin. Nutr. 28:42-45.

Gambon, R.C., M.J. Lentze, and E. Rossi. 1986. Megaloblastic anaemia in one of monozygous twins breast fed by their vegetarian mother. Eur. J. Pediatr. 145:570-571.

Garry, P.J., G.M. Owen, E.M. Hooper, and B.A. Gilbert. 1981. Iron absorption from human milk and formula with and without iron supplementation. Pediatr. Res. 15:822-828.

Garza, C., J. Stuff, and N. Butte. 1987. Growth of the breast-fed infant. Pp. 109-121 in A.S. Goldman, S.A. Atkinson, and L.A. Hanson, eds. Human Lactation 3: The Effects of Human Milk on the Recipient Infant. Plenum Press, New York.

Gladen, B.C., W.J. Rogan, P. Hardy, J. Thullen, J. Tingelstad, and M. Tully. 1988. Development after exposure to polychlorinated biphenyls and dichlorodiphenyl dichloroethene transplacentally and through human milk. J. Pediatr. 113:991-995.

Glass, R.I., and B.J. Stoll. 1989. The protective effect of human milk against diarrhea: a review of studies from Bangladesh. Acta Paediatr. Scand. Suppl. 351:131-136.

Glass, R.I., A.M. Svennerholm, B.J. Stoll, M.R. Khan, K.M.B. Hossain, M.I. Huq, and J. Holmgren. 1983. Protection against cholera in breast-fed children by antibodies in breast milk. N. Engl. J. Med. 308:1389-1392.

Gleason, W.A., Jr., and G.A. Kerr. 1989. Questions about quinones in infant nutrition. J. Pediatr. Gastroenterol. Nutr. 8:285-287.

Goldman, A.S., and R.M. Goldblum. 1989. Immunologic system in human milk: characteristics and effects. Pp. 135-142 in E. Lebenthal, ed. Textbook of Gastroenterology and Nutrition in Early Infancy, 2nd ed. Raven Press, New York.

Goldman, A.S., and R.M. Goldblum, 1990. Human milk: immunologic-nutritional relationships. Ann. N.Y. Acad. Sci. 587:236-245.

Goldman, A.S., L.W. Thorpe, R.M. Goldblum, and L.A. Hanson. 1986. Anti-inflammatory properties of human milk. Acta Paediatr. Scand. 75:689-695.

Goldman, A.S., R.M. Goldblum, and L.A. Hanson. 1990a. Anti-inflammatory systems in human milk. Adv. Exp. Med. Biol. 262:69-76.

Goldman, A.S., R.M. Goldblum, and L.A. Hanson. 1990b. Anti-inflammatory systems in human milk. Pp. 69-76 in A. Bendich, M. Phillips, and R.P. Tengerdy, eds. Antioxidant Nutrients and Immune Functions. Plenum Press, New York.

Greer, F.R., J.E. Searcy, R.S. Levin, J.J. Steichen, P.S. Steichen-Asche, and R.C. Tsang. 1982. Bone mineral content and serum 25-hydroxyvitamin D concentrations in breast-fed infants with and without supplemental vitamin D: one year follow-up. J. Pediatr. 100:919-922.

Gromisch, D.S., R. Lopez, H.S. Cole, and J.M. Cooperman. 1977. Light (phototherapy)-induced riboflavin deficiency in the neonate. J. Pediatr. 90:118-122.

Habicht, J.-P., J. DaVanzo, W.P. Butz, and L. Meyers. 1985. The contraceptive role of breastfeeding. Popul. Stud. 39:213-232.

Hambidge, K.M., P.A. Walravens, C.E. Casey, R.M. Brown, and C. Bender. 1979. Plasma zinc concentrations of breast-fed infants. J. Pediatr. 94:607-608.

Hamill, P.V.V., T.A. Drizd, C.L. Johnson, R.B. Reed, and A.F. Roche. 1977. NCHS Growth Curves for Children from Birth to 18 Years: United States. Vital and Health Statistics, Series 11, No. 165. DHHS Publ. No. (PHS) 78-1650. National Center for Health Statistics, Public Health Service, U.S. Department of Health, Education, and Welfare, Hyattsville, Md. 74 pp.

Hamosh, M. 1988. Does infant nutrition affect adiposity and cholesterol levels in the adult? J. Pediatr. Gastroenterol. Nutr. 7:10-16.

Hamosh, M., and P. Hamosh. 1987. Does nutrition in early life have long term metabolic effects? Can animal models be used to predict these effects in the human? Pp. 37-55 in A.S. Goldman, S.A. Atkinson, and L.A. Hanson, eds. Human Lactation 3: The Effects of Human Milk on the Recipient Infant. Plenum Press, New York.

Hamosh, M., and P. Hamosh. 1990. Obesity. Annales Nestlé 48:59-69.

Hansen, A.E. 1937. Serum lipids in eczema and in other pathologic conditions. Am. J. Dis. Child. 53:933-946.

Hansen, A.E., E.M. Knott, H.F. Wiese, E. Shaperman, and I. McQuarrie. 1947. Eczema and essential fatty acids. Am. J. Dis. Child. 73:1-18.

Hanson, L.A. 1986. The global responsibility towards child health. Aust. Paediatr. J. 22:157-159.

Harmatz, P.R., D.G. Hanson, M. Brown, R.E. Kleinman, W.A. Walker, and K.J. Bloch. 1987. Transfer of maternal food proteins in milk. Pp. 289-299 in A.S. Goldman, S.A. Atkinson, and L.A. Hanson, eds. Human Lactation 3: The Effects of Human Milk on the Recipient Infant. Plenum Press, New York.

Hatano, S., K. Aihara, Y. Nishi, and T. Usui. 1985. Trace elements (copper, zinc, manganese, and selenium) in plasma and erythrocytes in relation to dietary intake during infancy. J. Pediatr. Gastroenterol. Nutr. 4:87-92.

Hattevig, G., B. Kjellman, N. Sigurs, E. Grodzinsky, J. Hed, and B. Bjorksten. 1990. The effect of maternal avoidance of eggs, cow's milk, and fish during lactation on the development of IgE, IgG, and IgA antibodies in infants. J. Allergy Clin. Immunol. 85:108-115.

Herrera, M.G., J.O. Mora, B. de Paredes, and M. Wagner. 1980. Maternal weight/height and the effect of food supplementation during pregnancy and lactation. Pp. 252-263 in H. Aebi and R. Whitehead, eds. Maternal Nutrition During Pregnancy and Lactation. Hans Huber Publishers, Bern.

Higginbottom, M.C., L. Sweetman, and W.L. Nyhan. 1978. A syndrome of methylmalonic aciduria, homocystinuria, megaloblastic anemia and neurologic abnormalities in a vitamin B-12-deficient breast-fed infant of a strict vegetarian. N. Engl. J. Med. 299:317-323.

Hillman, L.S., and J.G. Haddad. 1974. Human perinatal vitamin D metabolism I: 25-hydroxyvitamin D in maternal and cord blood. J. Pediatr. 84:742-749.

Himes, J.H. 1979. Infant feeding practices and obesity. J. Am. Diet. Assoc. 75:122-125.

Hino, S. 1989. Milk-borne transmission of HTLV-I as a major route in the endemic cycle. Acta Paediatr. Jpn. 31:428-435.

Hitchcock, N.E., and J.F. Coy. 1989. The growth of healthy Australian infants in relation to infant feeding and social group. Med. J. Aust. 150:306-311.

Hitchcock, N.E., M. Gracey, and A.I. Gilmour. 1985. The growth of breast fed and artificially fed infants from birth to twelve months. Acta Paediatr. Scand. 74:240-245.

Hobcraft, J. 1987. Does family planning save children's lives? Technical background paper prepared for the International Conference on Better Health for Women and Children Through Family Planning, Nairobi, Kenya, October, 1987. Population Council, New York. 77 pp.

Hodgson, P.A., R.D. Ellefson, L.R. Elveback, L.E. Harris, R.A. Nelson, and W.H. Weidman. 1976. Comparison of serum cholesterol in children fed high, moderate, or low cholesterol milk diets during neonatal period. Metabolism 25:739-746.

Hofvander, Y., U. Hagman, C. Hillervik, and S. Sjolin. 1982. The amount of milk consumed by 1-3 months old breast- or bottle-fed infants. Acta Paediatr. Scand. 71:953-958.

Hoogenboezem, T., H.J. Degenhart, S.M.P.F. de Muinck Keizer-Schrama, R. Bouillon, W.F.A. Grose, W.H.L. Hackeng, and H.K.A. Visser. 1989. Vitamin D metabolism in breast-fed infants and their mothers. Pediatr. Res. 25:623-628.

Hovi, L., R. Hekali, and M.A. Siimes. 1979. Evidence of riboflavin depletion in breastfed newborns and its further acceleration during treatment of hyperbilirubinemia by phototherapy. Acta Paediatr. Scand. 68:567-570.

Hunziker, U.A., and R.G. Barr. 1986. Increased carrying reduces infant crying: a randomized controlled trial. Pediatrics 77:641-648.

Huttunen, J.K., U.M. Saarinen, E. Kostiainen, and M.A. Siimes. 1983. Fat composition of the infant diet does not influence subsequent serum lipid levels in man. Atherosclerosis 46:87-94.

Jadhav, M., J.K.G. Webb, S. Vaishnava, and S.J. Baker. 1962. Vitamin-B_{12} deficiency in Indian infants: a clinical syndrome. Lancet 2:903-907.

Jakobsson, I., and T. Lindberg. 1978. Cow's milk as a cause of infantile colic in breast-fed infants. Lancet 2:437-439.

Jakobsson, I., and T. Lindberg. 1983. Cow's milk proteins cause infantile colic in breast-fed infants: a double-blind crossover study. Pediatrics 71:268-271.

Jason, J.M., P. Nieburg, and J.S. Marks. 1984. Mortality and infectious disease associated with infant-feeding practices in developing countries. Pediatrics 74:702-727.

Jensen, A.A. 1983. Chemical contaminants in human milk. Residue Rev. 89:1-128.

Kilshaw, P.J., and A.J. Cant. 1984. The passage of maternal dietary proteins into human breast milk. Int. Arch. Allergy Appl. Immunol. 75:8-15.

Klein, E.B., T. Byrne, and L.Z. Cooper. 1980. Neonatal rubella in a breast-fed infant after postpartum maternal infection. J. Pediatr. 97:774-775.

Koldovský, O., A. Bedrick, P. Pollack, R.K. Rao, and W. Thornburg. 1988. Possible physiological role of hormones and hormone-related substances present in milk. Pp. 123-139 in L.A. Hanson, ed. Biology of Human Milk. Nestle Nutrition Workshop Series, Vol. 15. Raven Press, New York.

Koletzko, S., P. Sherman, M. Corey, A. Griffiths, and C. Smith. 1989. Role of infant feeding practices in development of Crohn's disease in childhood. Br. Med. J. 298:1617-1618.

Kovar, M.G., M.K. Serdula, J.S. Marks, and D.W. Fraser. 1984. Review of the epidemiologic evidence for an association between infant feeding and infant health. Pediatrics 74:615-638.

Kramer, M.S. 1981. Do breast-feeding and delayed introduction of solid foods protect against subsequent obesity? J. Pediatr. 98:883-887.

Kramer, M.S. 1987. Breast feeding and child health: methodologic issues in epidemiologic research. Pp. 339-360 in A.S. Goldman, S.A. Atkinson, and L.A. Hanson, eds. Human Lactation 3: The Effects of Human Milk on the Recipient Infant. Plenum Press, New York.

Kramer, M.S. 1988. Does breast feeding help protect against atopic disease? Biology, methodology, and a golden jubilee of controversy. J. Pediatr. 112:181-190.

Lakdawala, D.R., and E.M. Widdowson. 1977. Vitamin-D in human milk. Lancet 1:167-168.

Lampkin, B.C., and E.F. Saunders. 1969. Nutritional vitamin B_{12} deficiency in an infant. J. Pediatr. 75:1053-1055.

Laug, E.P., F.M. Kunze, and C.S. Prickett. 1951. Occurrence of DDT in human fat and milk. Arch. Ind. Hyg. 3:245-246.

Lawrence, R.A. 1989. Breastfeeding: A Guide for the Medical Profession, 3rd ed. C.V. Mosby, St. Louis. 652 pp.

Lechtig, A., and R.E. Klein. 1980. Maternal food supplementation and infant health: results of a study in rural areas of Guatemala. Pp. 285-313 in H. Aebi and R. Whitehead, eds. Maternal Nutrition During Pregnancy and Lactation. Hans Huber, Bern.

Lewis, D.S., H.A. Bertrand, E.J. Masoro, H.C. McGill, Jr., K.D. Carey, and C.A. McMahan. 1983. Preweaning nutrition and fat development in baboons. J. Nutr. 113:2253-2259.

Lichtenstein, P., B.L. Specker, R.C. Tsang, F. Mimouni, and C. Gormley. 1986. Calcium-regulating hormones and minerals from birth to 18 months of age: a cross-sectional study. I. Effects of sex, race, age, season, and diet on vitamin D status. Pediatrics 77:883-890.

Linnemann, C.C., Jr., and S. Goldberg. 1974. HBAg in breast milk. Lancet 2:155.

Little, R.E., K.W. Anderson, C.H. Ervin, B. Worthington-Roberts, and S.K. Clarren. 1989. Maternal alcohol use during breast-feeding and infant mental and motor development at one year. N. Engl. J. Med. 321:425-430.

Lönnerdal, B., C.L. Keen, and L.S. Hurley. 1981. Iron, copper, zinc, and manganese in milk. Annu. Rev. Nutr. 1:149-174.

Lönnerdal, B., C.L. Keen, and L.S. Hurley. 1984. Zinc binding ligands and complexes in zinc metabolism. Adv. Nutr. Res. 6:139-167.

Losonsky, G.A., J.M. Fishaut, J. Strussenberg, and P.L. Ogra. 1982. Effect of immunization against rubella on lactation products. II. Maternal-neonatal interactions. J. Infect. Dis. 145:661-666.

Lucas, A., P.J. Lucas, and J.D. Baum. 1981a. Differences in the pattern of milk intake between breast and bottle fed infants. Early Hum. Dev. 5:195-199.

Lucas, A., S. Boyes, S.R. Bloom, and A. Aynsley-Green. 1981b. Metabolic and endocrine responses to a milk feed in six-day-old term infants: differences between breast and cow's milk formula feeding. Acta Paediatr. Scand. 70:195-200.

Luck, W., and H. Nau. 1985. Nicotine and cotinine concentrations in serum and urine of infants exposed via passive smoking or milk from smoking mothers. J. Pediatr. 107:816-820.

Luck, W., and H. Nau. 1987. Nicotine and cotinine concentrations in the milk of smoking mothers: influence of cigarette consumption and diurnal variation. Eur. J. Pediatr. 146:21-26.

MacDonald, L.D., R.S. Gibson, and J.E. Miles. 1982. Changes in hair zinc and copper concentrations of breast fed and bottle fed infants during the first six months. Acta Paediatr. Scand. 71:785-789.

Mahmood, D.A., and R.G. Feachem. 1987. Feeding and nutritional status among infants in Basrah City, Iraq: a cross-sectional study. Hum. Nutr.: Clin. Nutr. 41C:373-381.

Manku, M.S., D.F. Horrobin, N. Morse, V. Kyte, K. Jenkins, S. Wright, and J.L. Burton. 1982. Reduced levels of prostaglandin precursors in the blood of atopic patients: defective delta-6-desaturase function as a biochemical basis for atopy. Prostaglandins, Leukot. Med. 9:615-628.

Markestad, T. 1983. Effect of season and vitamin D supplementation on plasma concentrations of 25-hydroxyvitamin D in Norwegian infants. Acta Paediatr. Scand. 72:817-821.

Markestad, T., L. Aksnes, P.H. Finne, and D. Aarskog. 1983. Vitamin D nutritional status of premature infants supplemented with 500 IU vitamin D_2 per day. Acta Paediatr. Scand. 72:517-520.

Marmot, M.G., C.M. Page, E. Atkins, and J.W.B. Douglas. 1980. Effect of breast-feeding on plasma cholesterol and weight in young adults. J. Epidemiol. Commun. Health 34:164-167.

Mason, K.E. 1979. A conspectus of research on copper metabolism and requirements of man. J. Nutr. 109:1979-2066.

Mata, L.J., and J.J. Urrutia. 1971. Intestinal colonization of breast-fed children in a rural area of low socioeconomic level. Ann. N.Y. Acad. Sci. 176:93-109.

Mata, L.J., J.J. Urrutia, and J.E. Gordon. 1967. Diarrhoeal disease in a cohort of Guatemalan village children observed from birth to age two years. Trop. Geogr. Med. 19:247-257.

Mata, L.J., J.J. Urrutia, B. García, R. Fernández, and M. Behar. 1969. Shigella infection in breast-fed Guatemalan Indian neonates. Am. J. Dis. Child. 117:142-146.

Mayer, E.J., R.F. Hamman, E.C. Gay, D.C. Lezotte, D.A. Savitz, and G.J. Klingensmith. 1988. Reduced risk of IDDM among breast-fed children: the Colorado IDDM Registry. Diabetes 37:1625-1632.

McPhee, A.J., G.P. Davidson, M. Leahy, and T. Beare. 1988. Vitamin B_{12} deficiency in a breast fed infant. Arch. Dis. Child. 63:921-923.

Meigel, W., T. Dettke, E.M. Meigel, and U. Lenze. 1987. Additional oral treatment of atopical dermatitis with unsaturated fatty acids. Z. Hautkr. 62 Suppl. 1:100-103.

Menard, D., and P. Arsenault. 1988. Epidermal and neural growth factors in milk: effects of epidermal growth factor on the development of the gastrointestinal tract. Pp. 105-122 in Biology of Human Milk. Nestle Nutrition Workshop Series, Vol. 15. Raven Press, New York.

Menkes, J.H. 1977. Early feeding history of children with learning disorders. Dev. Med. Child Neurol. 19:169-171.

Morley, R., T.J. Cole, R. Powell, and A. Lucas. 1988. Mother's choice to provide breast milk and developmental outcome. Arch. Dis. Child. 63:1382-1385.

Morrow-Tlucak, M., R.H. Haude, and C.B. Ernhart. 1988. Breastfeeding and cognitive development in the first 2 years of life. Soc. Sci. Med. 26:635-639.

Morse, P.F., D.F. Horrobin, M.S. Manku, J.C.M. Stewart, R. Allen, S. Littlewood, S. Wright, J. Burton, D.J. Gould, P.J. Holt, C.T. Jansen, L. Mattila, W. Meigel, T. Dettke, D. Wexler, L. Guenther, A. Bordoni, and A. Patrizi. 1989. Meta-analysis of placebo-controlled studies of the efficacy of Epogam in the treatment of atopic eczema: relationship between plasma essential fatty acid changes and clinical response. Br. J. Dermatol. 121:75-90.

Motohara, K., I. Matsukane, F. Endo, Y. Kiyota, and I. Matsuda. 1989. Relationship of milk intake and vitamin K supplementation to vitamin K status in newborns. Pediatrics 84:90-93.

Mott, G.E., E.M. Jackson, C.A. McMahan, and H.C. McGill, Jr. 1990. Cholesterol metabolism in adult baboons is influenced by infant diet. J. Nutr. 120:243-251.

Mueller, W.H. 1983. The genetics of human fatness. Yearb. Phys. Anthropol. 26:215-230.

Munch-Peterson, S. 1950. On the copper content in mother's milk before and after intravenous copper administration. Acta Paediatr. 39:378-388.

Muñoz, L., C.L. Keen, B. Lönnerdal, and K.G. Dewey. 1986. Coffee intake during pregnancy and lactation in rats: maternal and pup hematological parameters and liver iron, zinc and copper concentration. J. Nutr. 116:1326-1333.

Muñoz, L.M., B. Lönnerdal, C.L. Keen, and K.G. Dewey. 1988. Coffee consumption as a factor in iron deficiency anemia among pregnant women and their infants in Costa Rica. Am. J. Clin. Nutr. 48:645-651.

Murray, M.J., A.B. Murray, N.J. Murray, and M.B. Murray. 1978. The effect of iron status of Nigerien mothers on that of their infants at birth and 6 months, and on the concentration of Fe in breast milk. Br. J. Nutr. 39:627-630.

Myers, M.G., S.J. Fomon, F.P. Koontz, G.A. McGuinness, P.A. Lachenbruch, and R. Hollingshead. 1984. Respiratory and gastrointestinal illnesses in breast and formula-fed infants. Am. J. Dis. Child. 138:629-632.

Naeye, R.L., B. Ladis, and J.S. Drage. 1976. Sudden infant death syndrome: a prospective study. Am. J. Dis. Child. 130:1207-1210.

Nail, P.A., M.R. Thomas, and R. Eakin. 1980. The effect of thiamin and riboflavin supplementation on the level of those vitamins in human breast milk and urine. Am. J. Clin. Nutr. 33:198-204.

Nelson, S.E., R.R. Rogers, E.E. Ziegler, and S.J. Fomon. 1989. Gain in weight and length during early infancy. Early Hum. Dev. 19:223-239.

Newburg, D.S., and R.H. Yolken. 1990. A human-milk fraction inhibits the binding of GP120 to CD4. Pediatr. Res. (abstract) 27:274.

NRC (National Research Council). 1989. Recommended Dietary Allowances, 10th ed. Report of the Subcommittee on the Tenth Edition of the RDAs, Food and Nutrition Board, Commission on Life Sciences. National Academy Press, Washington, D.C. 284 pp.

Nutrition Foundation. 1984. Nutrition Reviews' Present Knowledge in Nutrition, 5th ed. The Nutrition Foundation, Washington, D.C. 900 pp.

O'Connor, P. 1977. Vitamin D-deficiency rickets in two breast-fed infants who were not receiving vitamin D supplementation. Clin. Pediatr. 16:361-363.

Ohtake, M. 1977. Serum zinc and copper levels in healthy Japanese infants. Tohoku J. Exp. Med. 123:265-270.

Oski, F.A., and S.A. Landaw. 1980. Inhibition of iron absorption from human milk by baby food. Am. J. Dis. Child. 134:459-460.

Owen, G.M., C.E. Nelsen, G.I. Baker, and W.E. Connor. 1967. Use of vitamin K_1 in pregnancy. Effect on serum bilirubin and plasma prothrombin in the newborn. Am. J. Obstet. Gynecol. 99:368-373.

Owen, G.M., P.J. Garry, E.M. Hooper, B.A. Gilbert, and D. Pathak. 1981. Iron nutriture of infants exclusively breast-fed the first five months. J. Pediatr. 99:237-240.

Ozsoylu, S. 1977. Breast feeding and rickets. Lancet 2:560.

Palloni, A., and M. Tienda. 1986. The effects of breastfeeding and pace of childbearing on mortality at early ages. Demography 23:31-52.

Palti, H., I. Mansbach, H. Pridan, B. Adler, and Z. Palti. 1984. Episodes of illness in breast-fed and bottle-fed infants in Jerusalem. Isr. J. Med. Sci. 20:395-399.

Pastel, R.A., P.J. Howanitz, and F.A. Oski. 1981. Iron sufficiency with prolonged exclusive breast-feeding in Peruvian infants. Clin. Pediatr. 20:625-626.

Perkins, K.C., and F.A. Oski. 1976. Elevated blood lead in a 6-month-old breast-fed infant: the role of newsprint logs. Pediatrics 57:426-427.

Picciano, M.F., and R.H. Deering. 1980. The influence of feeding regimens on iron status during infancy. Am. J. Clin. Nutr. 33:746-753.

Plank, S.J., and M.L. Milanesi. 1973. Infant feeding and infant mortality in rural Chile. Bull. W.H.O. 48:203-210.

Podratz, R.O., D.D. Broughton, D.H. Gustafson, E.J. Bergstralh, and L.J. Melton. 1986. Weight loss and body temperature changes in breast-fed and bottle-fed neonates. Clin. Pediatr. 25:73-77.

Pomerance, H.H. 1987. Growth in breast-fed children. Hum. Biol. 59:687-693.

Pullan, C.R., G.L. Toms, A.J. Martin, P.S. Gardner, J.K.G. Webb, and D.R. Appleton. 1980. Breast-feeding and respiratory syncytial virus infection. Br. Med. J. 281:1034-1036.

Ravussin, E., S. Lillioja, W.C. Knowler, L. Christin, D. Freymond, W.G. Abbott, V. Boyce, B.V. Howard, and C. Bogardus. 1988. Reduced rate of energy expenditure as a risk factor for body-weight gain. N. Engl. J. Med. 318:467-472.

Rench, M.A., and C.J. Baker. 1989. Group B streptococcal breast abscess in a mother and mastitis in her infant. Obstet. Gynecol. 73:875-877.

Rendle-Short, J., J.R. Tiernan, and S. Hawgood. 1979. Vegan mothers with vitamin B_{12} deficiency. Med. J. Aust. 2:483.

Rivera-Calimlim, L. 1987. The significance of drugs in breast milk: pharmacokinetic considerations. Clin. Perinatol. 14:51-70.

Roberts, C.C., G.M. Chan, D. Folland, C. Rayburn, and R. Jackson. 1981. Adequate bone mineralization in breast-fed infants. J. Pediatr. 99:192-196.

Roberts, S.B., J. Savage, W.A. Coward, B. Chew, and A. Lucas. 1988. Energy expenditure and intake in infants born to lean and overweight mothers. N. Engl. J. Med. 318:461-466.

Roche, A.F., S. Guo, and W.M. Moore. 1989. Weight and recumbent length from 1 to 12 mo of age: reference data for 1-mo increments. Am. J. Clin. Nutr. 49:599-607.

Rocklin, R.E., L. Thistle, L. Gallant, M.S. Manku, and D. Horrobin. 1986. Altered arachidonic acid content in polymorphonuclear and mononuclear cells from patients with allergic rhinitis and/or asthma. Lipids 21:17-20.

Rodgers, B. 1978. Feeding in infancy and later ability and attainment: a longitudinal study. Dev. Med. Child Neurol. 20:421-426.

Rogan, W.J., and B.C. Gladen. 1985. Study of human lactation for effects of environmental contaminants: the North Carolina Breast Milk and Formula Project and some other ideas. Environ. Health Perspect. 60:215-221.

Rogan, W.J., B.C. Gladen, J.D. McKinney, N. Carreras, P. Hardy, J. Thullen, J. Tinglestad, and M. Tully. 1986. Neonatal effects of transplacental exposure to PCBs and DDE. J. Pediatr. 109:335-341.

Rogan, W.J., B.C. Gladen, J.D. McKinney, N. Carreras, P. Hardy, J. Thullen, J. Tingelstad, and M. Tully. 1987. Polychlorinated biphenyls (PCBs) and dichlorodiphenyl dichloroethane (DDE) in human milk: effects on growth, morbidity, and duration of lactation. Am. J. Public Health 77:1294-1297.

Rosenthal, H.L., S. Austin, S. O'Neill, K. Takeuchi, J.T. Bird, and J.E. Gilster. 1964. Incorporation of fallout strontium-90 in deciduous incisors and foetal bone. Nature 203:615-616.

Ruiz-Palacios, G.M., Y. Lopez-Vidal, J. Calva, T.G. Cleary, and L.K. Pickering. 1986. Impact of breast feeding on diarrhea prevention. Pediatr. Res. 20:320A (abstract).

Ryu, J., E.E. Ziegler, and S.J. Fomon. 1978. Maternal lead exposure and blood lead concentrations in infancy. J. Pediatr. 93:476-478.

Saarinen, U.M. 1982. Prolonged breast feeding as prophylaxis for recurrent otitis media. Acta Paediatr. Scand. 71:567-571.

Saarinen, U.M., and M.A. Siimes. 1979a. Iron absorption from breast milk, cow's milk, and iron-supplemented formula: an opportunistic use of changes in total body iron determined by hemoglobin, ferritin, and body weight in 132 infants. Pediatr. Res. 13:143-147.

Saarinen, U.M., and M.A. Siimes. 1979b. Role of prolonged breast feeding in infant growth. Acta Paediatr. Scand. 68:245-250.

Saarinen, U.M., M.A. Siimes, and P.R. Dallman. 1977. Iron absorption in infants: high bioavailability of breast milk iron as indicated by the extrinsic tag method of iron absorption and by the concentration of serum ferritin. J. Pediatr. 91:36-39.

Salmenperä, L., J. Perheentupa, and M.A. Siimes. 1985. Exclusively breast-fed healthy infants grow slower than reference infants. Pediatr. Res. 19:307-312.

Salmenperä, L., J. Perheentupa, P. Pakarinen, and M.A. Siimes. 1986a. Cu nutrition in infants during prolonged exclusive breast-feeding: low intake but rising serum concentrations of Cu and ceruloplasmin. Am. J. Clin. Nutr. 43:251-257.

Salmenperä, L., J. Perheentupa, and M.A. Siimes. 1986b. Folate nutrition is optimal in exclusively breast-fed infants but inadequate in some of their mothers and in formula-fed infants. J. Pediatr. Gastroenterol. Nutr. 5:283-289.

Sandström, B., A. Cederblad, and B. Lönnerdal. 1983. Zinc absorption from human milk, cow's milk, and infant formulas. Am. J. Dis. Child. 137:726-729.

Schaefer, O. 1971. Otitis media and bottle-feeding. An epidemiological study of infant feeding habits and incidence of recurrent and chronic middle ear disease in Canadian Eskimos. Can. J. Public Health 62:478-489.

Schecter, A., and T.A. Gasiewicz. 1987. Health hazard assessment of chlorinated dioxins and dibenzofurans contained in human milk. Chemosphere 16:2147-2154.

Schecter, A.J., J.J. Ryan, and J.D. Constable. 1986. Chlorinated dibenzo-p-dioxin and dibenzofuran levels in human adipose tissue and milk samples from north and south of Vietnam. Chemosphere 15:1613-1620.

Schecter, A., J.J. Ryan, and J.D. Constable. 1987. Polychlorinated dibenzo-p-dioxin and polychlorinated dibenzofuran levels in human breast milk from Vietnam compared with cow's milk and human breast milk from North American continent. Chemosphere 16:2003-2016.

Seward, J.F., and M.K. Serdula. 1984. Infant feeding and infant growth. Pediatrics 74:728-762.

Shannon, W.R. 1921. Demonstration of food proteins in human breast milk by anaphylactic experiments on guinea-pigs. Am. J. Dis. Child. 22:223-231.

Sheard, N.F., and W.A. Walker. 1988. The role of breast-milk in the development of the gastrointestinal tract. Nutr. Rev. 46:1-8.

Shepherd, R.W., D.B. Oxborough, T.L. Holt, B.J. Thomas, and Y.H. Thong. 1988. Longitudinal study of the body composition of weight gain in exclusively breast-fed and intake-measured whey-based formula-fed infants to age 3 months. J. Pediatr. Gastroenterol. Nutr. 7:732-739.

Shukla, A., H.A. Forsythe, C.M. Anderson, and S.M. Marwok. 1972. Infantile over nutrition in the first year of life: a field study in Dudley, Worchestershire. Br. Med. J. 4:507-515.

Siimes, M.A., L. Salmenperä, and J. Perheentupa. 1984. Exclusive breast-feeding for 9 months: risk of iron deficiency. J. Pediatr. 104:196-199.

Sklar, R. 1986. Nutritional vitamin B-12 deficiency in a breast-fed infant of a vegan-diet mother. Clin. Pediatr. 25:219-221.

Smith, A.M., M.F. Picciano, and R.H. Deering. 1983. Folate supplementation during lactation: maternal folate status, human milk folate content, and their relationship to infant folate status. J. Pediatr. Gastroenterol. Nutr. 2:622-628.

Smith, A.M., M.F. Picciano, and R.H. Deering. 1985. Folate intake and blood concentrations of term infants. Am. J. Clin. Nutr. 41:590-598.

Snyderman, S.E., K.C. Ketron, H.B. Burch, O.H. Lowry, O.A. Bessey, L.P. Guy, and L.E. Holt, Jr. 1949. The minimum riboflavin requirement of the infant. J. Nutr. 39:219-232.

Sommer, A. 1982. Nutritional Blindness: Xerophthalmia and Keratomalacia. Oxford University Press, New York. 282 pp.

Specker, B.L., B. Valanis, V. Hertzberg, N. Edwards, and R.C. Tsang. 1985. Sunshine exposure and serum 25-hydroxyvitamin D concentrations in exclusively breast-fed infants. J. Pediatr. 107:372-376.

Specker, B.L., D. Miller, E.J. Norman, H. Greene, and K.C. Hayes. 1988. Increased urinary methylmalonic acid excretion in breast-fed infants of vegetarian mothers and identification of an acceptable dietary source of vitamin B_{12}. Am. J. Clin. Nutr. 47:89-92.

Stagno, S., D.W. Reynolds, R.F. Pass, and C.A. Alford. 1980. Breast milk and the risk of cytomegalovirus infection. N. Engl. J. Med. 302:1073-1076.

Staub, C.P., and G.K. Murphy. 1965. A comparison of Sr 90 component of human and cow's milk. Pediatrics 36:732.

Stunkard, A.J., T.I. Sorensen, C. Hanis, T.W. Teasdale, R. Chakraborty, W.J. Schull, and F. Schulsinger. 1986. An adoption study of human obesity. N. Engl. J. Med. 314:193-198.

Stunkard, A.J., J.R. Harris, N.L. Pedersen, and G.E. McClearn. 1990. The body-mass index of twins who have been reared apart. N. Engl. J. Med. 322:1483-1487.

Sveger, T., H. Linberg, B. Weilbull, V.L. Olsson. 1975. Nutrition, over nutrition and obesity in the first year of life in Malmo, Sweden. Acta Paediatr. Scand. 64:635-640.

Taitz, L.S. 1977. Obesity in pediatric practice: infantile obesity. Pediatr. Clin. North Am. 24:107-115.

Tan, K.L., M.T. Chow, and S.M.M. Karim. 1978. Effect of phototherapy on neonatal riboflavin status. J. Pediatr. 93:494-497.

Taylor, B., and J. Wadsworth. 1984. Breast feeding and child development at five years. Dev. Med. Child Neurol. 26:73-80.

Thapa, S., R.V. Short, and M. Potts. 1988. Breast feeding, birth spacing and their effects on child survival. Nature 335:679-682.

Thiry, L., S. Sprecher-Goldenberg, T. Jonckheer, J. Levy, P. Van de Perre, P. Henrivaux, J. Cogniaux-LeClerc, and N. Clumeck. 1985. Isolation of AIDS virus from cell-free breast milk of three healthy virus carriers. Lancet 2:891-892.

Thomsen, A.C., T. Espersen, and S. Maigaard. 1984. Course and treatment of milk stasis, noninfectious inflammation of the breast, and infectious mastitis in nursing women. Am. J. Obstet. Gynecol. 149:492-495.

Unni, J.C., and J. Richard. 1988. Growth and morbidity of breast-fed and artificially-fed infants in urban south Indian families. J. Trop. Pediatr. 34:179-181.

Vigi, V., R. Chierici, L. Osti, F. Fagioli, and R. Rescazzi. 1984. Serum zinc concentration in exclusively breast-fed infants and in infants fed an adapted formula. Eur. J. Pediatr. 142:245-247.

Vobecky, J.S., J. Vobecky, D. Shapcott, and P.P. Demers. 1983. Nutrient intake patterns and nutritional status with regard to relative weight in early infancy. Am. J. Clin. Nutr. 38:730-738.

Vogt, M.W., D.J. Witt, D.E. Craven, R. Byington, D.F. Crawford, R.T. Schooley, and M.S. Hirsch. 1986. Isolation of HTLV-III/LAV from cervical secretions of women at risk for AIDS. Lancet 1:525-527.

Vuori, E., S.M. Mäkinen, R. Kara, and P. Kuitunen. 1980. The effects of the dietary intakes of copper, iron, manganese, and zinc on the trace element content of human milk. Am. J. Clin. Nutr. 33:227-231.

Weil, W.B., Jr. 1977. Current controversies in childhood obesity. J. Pediatr. 91:175-187.

Weissbluth, M., A.T. Davis, and J. Poncher. 1984. Night waking in 4- to 8-month-old infants. J. Pediatr. 104:477-480.

West, K.P., Jr., M. Chirambo, J. Katz, A. Sommer, and the Malawi Survey Group. 1986. Breast-feeding, weaning patterns, and the risk of xerophthalmia in southern Malawi. Am. J. Clin. Nutr. 44:690-697.

Whitehead, R.G., and A.A. Paul. 1984. Growth charts and the assessment of infant feeding practices in the western world and in developing countries. Early Hum. Dev. 9:187-207.

Whitehead, R.G., M. Lawrence, and A.M. Prentice. 1986. Maternal nutrition and breast feeding. Hum. Nutr.: Appl. Nutr. 40A (Suppl. 1):1-10.

WHO (World Health Organization). 1987. Breast-feeding/breast milk and human immunodeficiency virus (HIV). Weekly Epidemiol. Rec. 62:245-246.

Widdowson, E.M., H. Chan, G.E. Harrison, and R.D.G. Milner. 1972. Accumulation of Cu, Zn, Mn, Cr and Co in the human liver before birth. Biol. Neonate 20:360-367.

Wilson, J.T. 1981. Milk/plasma ratios and contraindicated drugs. Pp. 78-80 in Wilson, J.T., ed. Drugs in Breast Milk. ADIS Press, Balgowlah.

Wilson, D.J., D.J. Locker, C.A. Ritzen, J.T. Watson, and W. Schaffner. 1973. DDT concentrations in human milk. Am. Dis. Child. 125:814-819.

Wilson, J.T., R.D. Brown, D.R. Cherek, J.W. Dailey, B. Hilman, P.C. Jobe, B.R. Manno, J.E. Manno, H.M Redetzki, and J.J. Stewart. 1980. Drug excretion in human breast milk: principles, pharmacokinetics and projected consequences. Clin. Pharmacokinet. 5:1-68.

Wilson, J.T., R.D. Brown, J.L. Hinson, and J.W. Dailey. 1985. Pharmacokinetic pitfalls in the estimation of the breast milk/plasma ratio for drugs. Ann. Rev. Pharmacol. Toxicol. 25:667-689.

Winikoff, B. 1981. Issues in the design of breastfeeding research. Stud. Fam. Plann. 12:177-184.

Wissler, R.W., and H.C. McGill, Jr., chairmen. 1983. Conference on blood lipids in children: optimal levels for early prevention of coronary artery disease. Workshop report: experimental section. Prev. Med. 12:868-902.

Wolff, M.S. 1983. Occupationally derived chemicals in breast milk. Am. J. Ind. Med. 4:259-281.

Wong-Staal, F., and R.C. Gallo. 1985. Human T-lymphocyte retroviruses. Nature 317:395-403.

Woodruff, C.W., C. Latham, and S. McDavid. 1977. Iron nutrition in the breast-fed infant. J. Pediatr. 90:36-38.

Wray, J.D. 1978. Maternal nutrition, breast-feeding and infant survival. Pp. 197-229 in W.H. Mosley, ed. Nutrition and Human Reproduction. Plenum Press, New York.

Wray, J.D. 1990. Breastfeeding: an international and historical perspective. Pp. 62-118 in Falkner, F., ed. Infant and Child Nutrition. Telford Press, Caldwell, N. J.

Wright, P., H.A. MacLeod, and M.J. Cooper. 1983. Waking at night: the effect of early feeding experience. Child Care Health Dev. 9:309-319.

Wright, S. 1985. Atopic dermatitis and essential fatty acids: a biochemical basis for atopy? Acta Dermato-Venereol. Suppl. 114:143-145.

Wright, S., and C. Bolton. 1989. Breast milk fatty acids in mothers of children with atopic eczema. Br. J. Nutr. 62:693-697.

Wyatt, R.G., and L.J. Mata. 1969. Bacteria in colostrum and milk of Guatemalan Indian women. J. Trop. Pediatr. 15:159-162.

Yolken, R., A. Ruff, P. Miotti, B. Clayman, B. Yang, N. Halsey, R. Boulos, R Viscid, and G. Dallabetta. 1990. Measurement of HIV antibodies and nucleic-acids in human milk. Pediatr. Res. (abstract) 27:279.

8

Maternal Health Effects of Breastfeeding

Most studies of human lactation have focused on the quality and quantity of milk produced or on the effects of human milk on infants. Far fewer studies have targeted the effects of lactation on short- or long-term maternal health, and the subcommittee found no studies that evaluated the effects of maternal nutrition on long-term outcomes related to lactation. Reasons for this imbalance are unclear. The perception that the infant's level of risk during breastfeeding may be much higher than that of the mother is a potential factor responsible for a lack of interest in maternal outcomes. From a nutritional standpoint, however, the stress on the mother is substantial relative to the nutritional needs imposed by pregnancy (a condition that has attracted much more attention). The breastfed infant doubles its weight in the first 4 to 6 months after birth and has additional energy demands beyond the gains in energy stores associated with growth. The metabolic adjustments that redirect nutrient use from maternal needs to milk synthesis and secretion involve nearly every maternal organ system.

The decline in breastfeeding from the mid-1940s to the early 1970s (see Chapter 3) also may have been partially responsible for the lack of interest in long-term maternal health outcomes. Socioeconomic and demographic differences between groups that choose to breastfeed and those that choose to feed their infants formula and historical changes in the characteristics of populations who have chosen to breastfeed or formula feed may have discouraged population-based studies of the relationship between long-term maternal outcomes and lactation history.

This chapter focuses on limited examples of maternal health consequences of lactation. Because the focus of this report is on healthy women, the discussion omits the influence of lactation on underlying chronic disease states, such as diabetes mellitus, cardiovascular disease, and cystic fibrosis. The discussion is subdivided into two sections: short-term effects (return of ovulation and maternal sexuality) and long-term effects (obesity, osteoporosis, and breast cancer). The effects of breastfeeding on maternal nutritional status are considered in Chapter 9.

SHORT-TERM HEALTH EFFECTS

Return of Ovulation

Lactation has long been known to increase the length of time between the delivery of a baby and return of regular ovulation. Despite considerable research on this subject, the mechanisms by which lactation exerts this effect on ovarian activity remain incompletely understood (see review by McNeilly et al. [1985]). There is general agreement that suckling suppresses the pulsatile release of gonadotropin-releasing hormone from the hypothalamus and also stimulates the release of prolactin. Gonadotropin-releasing hormone is necessary for the pulsatile release of luteinizing hormone from the pituitary. Luteinizing hormone, in turn, is essential for maturation of the ovarian follicle and, thus, for ovulation. Any direct role prolactin might have in modifying ovarian function remains unresolved.

The characteristics of suckling by the infant appear to be the principal factors that affect the duration of postpartum anovulation (the period of functional importance) or amenorrhea (the length of time that is usually measured) in well-nourished lactating women (McNeilly et al., 1985). Frequency, intensity, and timing of suckling sessions all appear to influence the endocrinologic responses that modulate ovulatory status. These nursing characteristics change as lactation progresses, especially at the time solid foods are added to the infant's diet (Howie et al., 1981).

Maternal nutritional status during lactation may also be an important factor in regulating the duration of postpartum amenorrhea. Observational data show a clear association between poor maternal nutritional status and prolonged postpartum amenorrhea accompanied by persistently elevated prolactin values (see, for example, Hennart et al. [1985]). However, interpretation of this association is not straightforward because there also are differences in suckling characteristics between the infants of well and poorly nourished women.

Several mechanisms have been proposed for the effect of maternal nutritional status on the duration of postpartum amenorrhea. Frisch (1978) hypothesized that a critical proportion of body fat is necessary for the return of normal ovarian function after delivery. Another idea is that the hormonal status that is characteristic of women with chronically inadequate food intake prolongs postpartum amenorrhea (Lunn et al., 1984). Finally, the duration of postpartum amenorrhea might also be a function of (1) characteristics of the milk related to maternal nutritional status (such as volume, composition, and the rate of milk flow) that would lead to changes in the infant's breastfeeding behavior (such as the strength or duration of suckling) or (2) characteristics of the mother's interaction with her infant (number, timing, and duration of breastfeeding sessions) that may vary with her nutritional status (such as would be expected with seasonal agricultural labor and food shortages).

Interventions designed to improve nutritional status among poorly nourished women have consistently produced reductions in the length of postpartum amenorrhea (Bongaarts and Delgado, 1979; Chavez and Martinez, 1973; Lunn et al., 1981). These observations are in accord with the hypothesis proposed by Frisch (1978). However, from this hypothesis one would expect there to be an association between the attainment of a particular body composition and ovulation; this has not been supported by published data (Huffman et al., 1978) and remains controversial (Quandt, 1984).

Plasma concentrations of prolactin, cortisol, insulin, and triiodothyronine decreased in subjects in The Gambia in response to food supplementation during lactation (Prentice et al., 1983b). The authors' interpretation of these results was that supplementation had altered the subjects' state of metabolic adaptation to chronic malnutrition. These women also experienced the most dramatic decrease in the length of postpartum amenorrhea (from 66 to 42 weeks) that has been reported.

However, it is not clear if the consistent decrease in the duration of postpartum amenorrhea results directly from improved maternal nutritional status or from factors that vary with maternal nutritional status, such as the infant's breastfeeding behavior (which may be changed by alterations in milk composition or in the characteristics of the breastfeeding sessions). For example, in the Gambian study, a reduction in the number of daytime breastfeeding sessions (Prentice et al., 1983a) accompanied maternal supplementation, and there was anecdotal evidence of an increase in the women's work activities (Coward et al., 1984). Either of these changes could, in turn, influence maternal endocrinologic status and thereby the duration of postpartum amenorrhea.

Finally, another mechanism by which maternal nutritional status could influence the duration of postpartum amenorrhea is possible but has never been evaluated. In this possibility, enhanced maternal nutritional status would result in improved infant growth that, in turn, would increase the infant's suckling vigor and demand for milk. These differences could result in a lengthening of the duration of postpartum amenorrhea. Testing of this hypothesis requires a demonstrated change in milk volume, composition, or both in response to food supplementation and an appropriate assessment of the amenorrhea outcome.

It is of considerable importance to public health to understand the mechanism by which maternal nutritional status modifies the duration of postpartum anovulation. Worldwide, breastfeeding provides important contraceptive benefits. Its potential usefulness for child spacing on an individual basis has been affirmed (Kennedy et al., 1989) and supported by a clinical trial (M. Labbok, Georgetown University Medical Center, personal communication, 1990; see guidelines used in Labbok et al. [1990]). Thus, it would be wise to examine the time it takes to return to menses and ovulation in experimental studies designed to improve maternal nutritional status during lactation.

Sexuality

Few of the studies examining sexuality in the postpartum period have separated the effects of breastfeeding on sexuality from the changes in sexual receptivity and function that women normally undergo at this time (see the review by Reamy and White [1987]). Because the hormonal changes that accompany lactation are likely modulators of mood and sexuality and because these changes are likely to vary with the intensity of breastfeeding (see Chapter 5), it is reasonable to expect that lactation will affect sexuality but that the effects may vary among lactating women.

In a laboratory study of six women during and after pregnancy, Masters and Johnson (1966) found that such sexual responses to stimulation as genital vasoconstriction and vaginal lubrication were sluggish in the first 3 months post partum and that orgasmic contractions were shorter and weaker. They attributed this to the reduced ovarian function that is normal during this period, and noted that these effects were more frequent among nursing mothers. They also found that the enlarged lactating breast did not consistently increase further in size during sexual arousal. Despite this, 24 nursing mothers queried (as part of a group of 24 nursing and 77 nonnursing women) in the third month after delivery rated their level of sexual interest higher than nonnursing mothers did. In addition to reporting sexual arousal induced by their infants' suckling on some occasions, they expressed interest in returning as soon as possible to sexual relations with their husbands. Masters and Johnson (1966) provide no data on breastfeeding frequency and describe duration only as having successfully nursed for at least 2 months.

These findings are contradicted by those of Alder and Bancroft (1988), who followed women longitudinally from early pregnancy through 6 months post partum. Women who breastfed reported later resumption of sexual intercourse despite antenatal measures of sexual arousal and motivation similar to those of bottle feeders. Within this group of breastfeeding women, the longer women breastfed, the longer they delayed resumption of intercourse. Alder and Bancroft (1988) associated this delay with the more frequent reports of painful intercourse among breastfeeding women, compared with those who bottle fed their infants. The pain has been attributed to poor vaginal lubrication resulting from low estrogen levels, a loss of sexual interest related to low androgen levels, and maternal stress and fatigue associated with the demands of lactation and child care (Alder et al., 1986; Masters and Johnson, 1966).

Similar findings of reduced sexual response were reported by Kayner and Zagar (1983) among a self-selected group of lactating women whose nursing practices were judged to be intensive, based on reports of unrestricted nursing, frequent sleeping with the infant, and delayed introduction of formula or other food supplements for an average of 6.3 $\pm$ 1.99 (standard deviation) months. The period of amenorrhea was found to correlate strongly with the duration of reduced sexual desire.

Positive attitudes toward breastfeeding have been associated with the woman's comfort with her own sexuality (Newton, 1973), whereas negative feelings have been related to a dislike of nudity and sexual feelings (Newton and Newton, 1967). Thus, the positive association of breastfeeding and sexuality found by Masters and Johnson (1966) may be due in part to the highly self-selected nature of the breastfeeding sample used in their research. In addition, some women may meet their sensual and affectional needs by substituting breastfeeding and caretaking of infants for sexual activity (Kayner and Zagar, 1983; Lawrence, 1989; Waletsky, 1979).

The relationship of breastfeeding to female sexuality is therefore complex. The most informative studies thus far have included the collection of antenatal data, a longitudinal approach, and controls for socioeconomic factors. Further research should include those elements as well as controls for nursing intensity and evaluations of both endocrinologic responses and nonhormonal factors as determinants of sexuality.

LONG-TERM HEALTH EFFECTS

Obesity

No comprehensive studies have been conducted in humans to examine the long-term maternal consequences of lactation on the prevalence and severity of, or predisposition toward, obesity. Some studies have been conducted in animals to examine the effects of pregnancy not followed by lactation on maternal body composition. In humans, studies have focused on energy expenditure, adjustments in the metabolism of adipose tissue, and changes in body weight during lactation and on maternal body mass at various times after lactation has ceased. Changes in the pattern of maternal energy expenditure during lactation are reviewed in Chapter 5.

Changes in Adipose Tissue

Studies in rats (Bogart et al., 1940; Jen et al., 1988; Moore and Brasel, 1984) indicate that pregnancy without subsequent lactation results in increased adipose tissue stores and increased fat cell numbers. Conversely, lactation between pregnancies in rats reduces both of these indices of maternal obesity. Major differences between rats and humans in the relative energy costs of lactation, however, limit the inferences that can be made from studies in rats about the long-term health consequences in humans.

Studies of adipose tissue in lactating women (Lafontan et al., 1979; Rebuffe-Scrive et al., 1985) indicate that there are site-specific changes in the metabolism of energy stores during lactation. Basal rates of fat breakdown (lipolysis) are similar in femoral and abdominal adipose tissues in nonpregnant women, but are significantly higher in the femoral depot of lactating women. The lipolytic effect of noradrenaline administration is similar in both tissue sites during lactation but is much less in the femoral region of nonpregnant women and of women during early pregnancy.

In femoral adipose tissue, lipoprotein lipase activity decreases in lactating women; in abdominal adipose tissue, it remains about the same. Levels of adenosine, a locally acting insulin-like effector, have been reported to be lower in femoral than in abdominal adipocytes in lactating women; the lower levels may promote greater lipid mobilization from the femoral site (Stoneham et al., 1988). In nonpregnant and pregnant women, lipid assimilation appears to be favored in femoral sites over abdominal depots, and during lactation, lipid mobilization is favored in femoral adipose tissue.

Changes in Anthropometric Characteristics

Several investigators have followed anthropometric characteristics of well-nourished women (Brewer et al., 1989; Butte et al., 1984; Manning-Dalton and Allen, 1983; Morse et al., 1975; Naismith and Richie, 1975) and marginally nourished women (Adair et al., 1984; Brown et al., 1986; Harrison et al., 1975) during lactation (see also Chapter 4). In a few of those studies, fat stores were estimated. In general, anthropometric changes during lactation were minor. The range of mean daily energy deficits is reported to be 110 to 343 kcal/day in presumably well-nourished women living at home and followed longitudinally during lactation for 4 to 6 months (Brewer et al., 1989; Butte et al., 1984). These deficits could be expected to result in loss of approximately 2.6 to 7.9 kg (~6 to 17 lb) of fat over 6 months.

The wide range of reported values for postpartum weight change among lactating women may be attributable to differences in baseline weight measurements. In some studies (e.g., Butte et al., 1984), baseline weights were obtained at approximately 35 days post partum, whereas others (e.g., Brewer et al., 1989) used maternal body weight on the first postpartum day as the basis for subsequent comparisons. The marked changes in fluid compartments in the early postpartum period most likely result in an overestimation of the net energy deficit when based on early postpartum weights. If the average energy deficit during lactation is closer to 110 than to 343 kcal/day (see above), it is unlikely that adipose tissue stores accumulated during pregnancy will be mobilized fully after 4 to 6 months of lactation, especially with the higher weight gains now recommended during pregnancy (IOM, 1990).

Longitudinal data tend to support the view that the rate of maternal weight loss is higher during the first 4 to 6 months of continued lactation than it is with longer durations of breastfeeding (see Chapter 4). It is more difficult, however, to evaluate longer-term changes in body mass following lactation. Data on 49 women reported by Rookus and coworkers (1987) through 9 months post partum suggest that women who breastfeed for more than 2 months may gain more weight than women whose lactation is purposely suppressed by bromocriptin administration and others who breastfeed for less than 2 months. The analyses were adjusted for age, socioeconomic status, parity, maternal employment status, and smoking; however, only 18 women who breastfed for more than 2 months were studied, and no information was given regarding the extent to which all groups ate until satisfied or the extent to which specific strategies were used by the different groups to achieve weight changes. Data from the late 1940s indicate that weight changes may be similar 24 months post partum among women regardless of the duration of lactation (McKeown and Record, 1957).

Newcomb (1982) estimated the modifying effect of lactation on weight gain associated with increasing parity and found that the positive impact of parity on maternal body weight was 30% greater when parity was associated with subsequent lactation. However, the design of this study was limited: the method of feeding during the index pregnancy was used as a marker for the mode of feeding in previous pregnancies, and the duration and degree of breastfeeding were not defined.

Breastfeeding and the Onset of Obesity

The subcommittee found only two studies addressing the relationship between breastfeeding and the diagnosis of obesity whose onset was associated with pregnancy (Richardson, 1952; Sheldon, 1949). Sheldon (1949) found that approximately 65% of both obese and control women reported positive breastfeeding histories. Richardson (1952) retrospectively studied 40 women who became obese either during or soon after pregnancy and 30 women who became obese several years after their last pregnancy. He found that a significantly greater proportion of women whose obesity onset was related to pregnancy breastfed their infants than did the comparison group (87 and 55%, respectively). Among those in the pregnancy-related obesity group who breastfed, 19% became obese during pregnancy and the remainder became obese following delivery. These observations are limited by the lack of key information, such as maternal socioeconomic characteristics and the duration and degree of lactation.

There is little doubt that major physiologic adjustments influence energy stores during lactation. Animal data support the view that excess fat is more likely to accumulate in women who do not breastfeed after pregnancy and who have adequate food intakes. The consequences of lactation on long-term maternal energy balance, however, are less clear in humans than in animals and require detailed investigation.

Osteoporosis

The calcium content in humans is approximately 23 g/kg of fat-free body mass (Avioli, 1980). In a 55-kg (121-lb) woman with approximately 25% body fat, the calcium content is approximately 900 to 1,000 g. A lactating woman with a milk output of 750 ml/day for 6 months loses approximately 50 g of calcium in milk, or about 5% of total body calcium. If one assumes that there are no changes in the efficiency of calcium absorption during lactation, approximately 660 mg of dietary calcium is needed, on average, to replace the 262 mg lost through milk per day. However, there is evidence from animal studies that calcium absorption rates may increase during lactation (Halloran and DeLuca, 1980). One should also consider that approximately 30 g of calcium is transferred to the fetus during gestation. Therefore, the rebuilding of maternal calcium stores, especially over successive pregnancies and lactations, is of potential concern in populations at risk of osteoporosis.

Bone Metabolism

Bone metabolism during and after lactation is understood incompletely. Several mechanisms may act during pregnancy and lactation to ameliorate the impact of lactational demands for calcium. Serum osteocalcin levels are higher in lactating women early in the postpartum period compared with those of pregnant and of nonpregnant, nonlactating control women (osteocalcin is a hormone released at rates proportional to the formation of new bone). However, serum calcium and serum immunoreactive parathyroid hormone (iPTH) levels are unchanged, and no correlations have been reported between calcium and iPTH serum concentrations and osteocalcin serum concentrations (Cole et al., 1987). The higher osteocalcin levels nonetheless suggest that lactating women have higher bone turnover than those of the other groups studied. Data from a rat model suggest that osteoclast and osteocyte responses during pregnancy result in significantly greater bone mechanical strength (Currey, 1973). These responses and the decreased lacunar volume observed during lactation suggest that osteocytes are mobilized to deposit bone during pregnancy and serve as an effective buffer during lactation (Mercer and Crenshaw, 1985).

Bone Mineralization

Few studies have been conducted to measure bone mineralization at distinct periods of the reproductive cycle of women who have breastfed. In general, published studies suggest that bone mineralization decreases acutely in lactating women but that remineralization occurs in the postlactation period. Chan et al. (1982, 1987), Hayslip et al. (1989), Wardlaw and Pike (1986), and Tylavsky et al. (1989) reported acute bone loss among lactating women. Those studies have used single- or dual-photon absorptiometry to measure bone mineralization.

Studies in which bone mineralization has been examined at intervals following the cessation of lactation have shown either no effects or positive effects of lactation on bone mineralization. No effect was found when bone mineral content was measured by single- or dual-beam absorptiometry in women aged 25 to 37 (Koetting and Wardlaw, 1988) and in older women (mean age, 49 years) (Johnell and Nilsson, 1984). A preliminary report of a longitudinal study of women followed from before conception to 4 months after the cessation of lactation found a loss of bone mineralization with pregnancy and lactation and a recovery of losses in the postlactation period (Tylavsky et al., 1989).

In other studies, no effect was attributable to lactation when assessments were made by radiography in women aged 30 to 44 subdivided into two groups that had breastfed for relatively long periods (presumably more than 6 months): those who had one or two children, and those who had seven or more children (Walker et al., 1972). Similarly, no effect was found in investigations by Alderman and coworkers (1986) of the relation between reproductive history and the occurrence of hip and forearm fractures in postmenopausal women (over age 50).

In contrast to those studies, Aloia and colleagues (1983) reported that 80 white, postmenopausal women (mean age, 52 years) who had breastfed had a higher bone mass than those who had not breastfed. Bone mass was measured by total body neutron activation analysis and photon absorptiometry of the distal radius. Breastfeeding and pregnancy were associated with higher bone mass. In a subsequent comparison of 58 women with postmenopausal osteoporosis and 58 age-matched normal women, osteoporotic women were found to have undergone an earlier menopause (age 46 years versus 49 years, respectively), smoked cigarettes more (59 versus 30%, respectively), and breastfed less (16 versus 35%, respectively), than controls (Aloia et al., 1985).

Hreshchyshyn et al. (1988) examined the relationship between parity, breastfeeding, and bone densities of the lumbar spine and femoral neck. Measurements were obtained by dual-photon absorptiometry in 588 ambulatory white women aged 21 to 95. No statistically significant differences in lumbar spine bone mineral density were detected between women who had breastfed compared with those who had not; however, parous women who breastfed longer than 2 weeks had higher bone mineral density than those who had not. Breastfeeding was reported to increase lumbar spine density by 1.5% per breastfed child. Femoral neck density was not related to lactation history.

These data suggest that acute bone loss is likely to occur during lactation;

however, the magnitude of the losses is difficult to estimate from the few published data. Assessments in older women suggest either that calcium repletion occurred more effectively among women who had lactated or that other behavioral characteristics among that group promoted enhanced bone mass over the long term. The data are not conclusive. Future studies should focus greater attention on the definition of breastfeeding, the estimation of calcium intakes, and an improved definition of the interval between measurements of interest and timing of breastfeeding.

Breast Cancer

The association of lactation history with a variety of cancer risks has been examined sporadically (Kvåle and Heuch, 1987). Breast cancer has received the most attention, but the biologic plausibility of a relationship between a positive lactation history and reduced risk of breast cancer has not been well described (deWaard and Trichopoulos, 1988; Henderson et al., 1985; Kelsey and Berkowitz, 1988; Korenmon, 1980; Yuan et al., 1988). In general, the link to breast cancer is believed to be the modifying effect of lactation on the potential exposure of the breast to estrogen and other steroids during the reproductive period.

Factors usually related to breast cancer have been age, country of birth, socioeconomic class, place of residence, race, age at first full-term pregnancy, oophorectomy, body build, age at menarche, age at menopause, family history of premenopausal bilateral breast cancer, history of cancer in one breast, fibrocystic disease, primary cancer in an ovary or in the endometrium, radiation to the chest, or first-degree relatives with breast cancer (Kelsey and Berkowitz, 1988). Lactation history was not listed. MacMahon et al. (1970) reported that although nulliparous women had a greater risk of breast cancer than parous women did, neither parity nor lactation had an effect on risk after controlling for the age at the first full-term pregnancy.

Byers and colleagues (1985) summarized the findings of 17 epidemiologic studies of the relationship between lactation and breast cancer risk reported between 1966 and 1983. Relative risks associated with "ever" having breastfed were calculated for women of all ages in 15 of the studies; in 10 of those studies, the relative risk was less than 1.00, denoting a protective effect. Relative risk associated with "ever" having breastfed among women younger than age 50 was less than 1.00 in 11 of the 13 studies in which this estimate was made. Among women over age 50, the relative risk was less than 1.00 in only 5 of the 12 studies that estimated risk for that population.

Byers et al. (1985) also reported the results of a case-control study of 453 white women with breast cancer and 1,365 white women without breast cancer selected randomly from the same geographical area. A negative association between lactation and breast cancer risk (which implies a protective effect of lactation) was reported among premenopausal women and was not accounted for by other associated variables, namely, age, parity, age at menarche, age at first pregnancy, years of education, or stopping lactation because of insufficient milk.

Several other investigators (Layde et al., 1989; McTiernan and Thomas, 1986; Tao et al., 1988; Yuan et al., 1988) also reported a protective effect of breastfeeding against cancer. In some studies, protection was found in both premenopausal and postmenopausal women. In all, the protection appeared to increase with increasing duration of lactation. The degree of protection afforded by various durations of breastfeeding, however, was highly variable among studies, even though analyses were adjusted for parity, age at first full-term pregnancy, age at interview, and other potentially confounding or modifying variables. The wide range of protection (odds ratios varied from 0.4 to 0.8) is probably due to nonreproductive risk factors related to breast cancer.

Other reports present less consistent findings or conclude that breastfeeding is not protective. Kvåle and Heuch (1987) evaluated relationships between previous lactation experience and risk of breast cancer in 50,274 parous Norwegian women (approximate age range, 20 to 69 years) studied prospectively between 1961 and 1980. A nonlinear relationship was reported between duration of lactation per birth and risk of breast cancer: that is, for the first, second, and third births the highest risk was observed for those with an intermediate duration of breastfeeding (4 to 10 months), and the lowest risk was observed for those with short (less than 4 months) or long (greater than 12 months) durations. The total duration of breastfeeding for all children showed significant inverse associations with breast cancer, but no consistent relationship was detected when results were adjusted for parity.

London and colleagues (1990) examined the relationship between breast cancer and lactation in a cohort of 89,413 parous women (age range, 30 to 55 years) who were free from cancer in 1976 and provided retrospective information on the total duration of lactation through 1986. No relationship between the risk of breast cancer and the duration of lactation (≤ 23 months) was observed in this study after adjustments for age and parity.

The reasons for the discrepancies among studies are not clear. Disagreement among studies may be due to different methods and designs (e.g., variations among methods used to ascertain lactation duration, selection and characterization of controls, and retrospective compared with prospective approaches), diverse lactation practices among distinct cohorts, differences in diets or other nonreproductive factors among various populations, or any combination of these.

A better understanding of breastfeeding's effects could be expected from increased knowledge of mammary gland functions that modulate the risk of breast cancer and from more detailed consideration of nursing histories, duration of breastfeeding for each child, extent of breastfeeding, intervals between pregnancies, maternal diet and body composition, and other factors appropriate to individual environments (Byers et al., 1985).

CONCLUSIONS

• Lactation normally delays the return to regular ovulation. The effect of maternal nutritional status on this delay is not understood. Although lactation provides important contraceptive benefits on a worldwide basis, it is not a dependable method of contraception for individuals.

• Lactation appears to have a negative impact on sexuality; however, the relationship between both functions is complex and requires further study to understand the factors that modulate this relationship.

• There are insufficient data to determine whether lactation influences maternal risk of adult-onset obesity.

• There are insufficient data to determine whether lactation influences maternal risk of osteoporosis.

• Most recent epidemiologic evaluations suggest that breastfeeding may be protective against breast cancer, but there is conflicting evidence.

REFERENCES

Adair, L.S., E. Pollitt, and W.H. Mueller. 1984. The Bacon Chow study: effect of nutritional supplementation on maternal weight and skinfold thicknesses during pregnancy and lactation. Br. J. Nutr. 51:357-369.

Alder, E., and J. Bancroft. 1988. The relationship between breast feeding persistence, sexuality and mood in postpartum women. Psychol. Med. 18:389-396.

Alder, E.M., A. Cook, D. Davidson, C. West, and J. Bancroft. 1986. Hormones, mood and sexuality in lactating women. Br. J. Psychiatry 148:74-79.

Alderman, B.W., N.S. Weiss, J.R. Daling, C.L. Ure, and J.H. Ballard. 1986. Reproductive history and postmenopausal risk of hip and forearm fracture. Am. J. Epidemiol. 124:262-267.

Aloia, J.F., A.N. Vaswani, J.K. Yeh, P. Ross, K. Ellis, and S.H. Cohn. 1983. Determinants of bone mass in postmenopausal women. Arch. Intern. Med. 143:1700-1704.

Aloia, J.F., S.H. Cohn, A. Vaswani, J.K. Yeh, K. Yuen, and K. Ellis. 1985. Risk factors for postmenopausal osteoporosis. Am. J. Med. 78:95-100.

Avioli, L.V. 1980. Major minerals. Pp. 294-309 in R.S. Goodhart and M.E. Shils, eds. Modern Nutrition in Health and Disease. Lea and Febiger, Philadelphia.

Bogart, R., G. Sperling, L.L. Barnes, and S.A. Asdell. 1940. The influence of reproductive condition upon growth in the female rat. Am. J. Physiol. 128:355-371.

Bongaarts, J., and H. Delgado. 1979. Effects of nutritional status on fertility in rural Guatemala. Pp 107-133 in Leridon, H., and J. Menken, eds. Natural Fertility: Patterns and Determinants of Natural Fertility; Proceedings of a Seminar in Natural Fertility, Paris, 1977. Liege, Ordina Editions.

Brewer, M.M., M.R. Bates, and L.P. Vannoy. 1989. Postpartum changes in maternal weight and body fat depots in lactating vs nonlactating women. Am. J. Clin. Nutr. 49:259-265.

Brown, K.H., A.D. Robertson, and N.A. Akhtar. 1986. Lactational capacity of marginally nourished mothers: infants' milk nutrient consumption and patterns of growth. Pediatrics 78:920-927.

Butte, N.F., C. Garza, J.E. Stuff, E.O. Smith, and B.L. Nichols. 1984. Effect of maternal diet and body composition on lactational performance. Am. J. Clin. Nutr. 39:296-306.

Byers, T., S. Graham, T. Rzepka, and J. Marshall. 1985. Lactation and breast cancer: evidence for a negative association in premenopausal women. Am. J. Epidemiol. 121:664-674.

Chan, G.M., N. Ronald, P. Slater, J. Hollis, and M.R. Thomas. 1982. Decreased bone mineral status in lactating adolescent mothers. J. Pediatr. 101:767-770.

Chan, G.M., M. McMurry, K. Westover, K. Engelbert-Fenton, and M.R. Thomas. 1987. Effects of increased dietary calcium intake upon the calcium and bone mineral status of lactating adolescent and adult women. Am. J. Clin. Nutr. 46:319-323.

Chavez, A., and C. Martinez. 1973. Nutrition and development of infants from poor rural areas. III. Maternal nutrition and its consequences on fertility. Nutr. Rep. Int. 7:1-8.

Cole, D.E.C., C.M. Gundberg, L.J. Stirk, S.A. Atkinson, D.A. Hanley, L.M. Ayer, and L.S. Baldwin. 1987. Changing osteocalcin concentrations during pregnancy and lactation: implications for maternal mineral metabolism. J. Clin. Endocrinol. Metab. 65:290-294.

Coward, W.A., A.A. Paul, and A.M. Prentice. 1984. The impact of malnutrition on human lactation: observations from community studies. Fed. Proc., Fed. Am. Soc. Exp. Biol. 43:2432-2437.

Currey, J.D. 1973. Interactions between age, pregnancy and lactation, and some mechanical properties, of the femora of rats. Calcif. Tissue Res. 13:99-112.

de Waard, F., and D. Trichopoulos. 1988. A unifying concept of the aetiology of breast cancer. Int. J. Cancer 41:666-669.

Frisch, R.E. 1978. Population, food intake, and fertility: there is historical evidence for a direct effect of nutrition on reproductive ability. Science 199:22-30.

Halloran, B.P., and H.F. DeLuca. 1980. Calcium transport in small intestine during pregnancy and lactation. Am. J. Physiol. 239:E64-E68.

Harrison, G.A., A.J. Boyce, C.M. Platt, and S. Serjeantson. 1975. Body composition changes during lactation in a New Guinea population. Ann. Hum. Biol. 2:395-398.

Hayslip, C.C., T.A. Klein, H.L. Wray, and W.E. Duncan. 1989. The effects of lactation on bone mineral content in healthy postpartum women. Obstet. Gynecol. 73:588-592.

Henderson, B.E., R.K. Ross, H.L. Judd, M.D. Krailo, and M.C. Pike. 1985. Do regular ovulatory cycles increase breast cancer risk? Cancer 56:1206-1208.

Hennart, P., Y. Hofvander, H. Vis, and C. Robyn. 1985. Comparative study of nursing mothers in Africa (Zaire) and in Europe (Sweden): breastfeeding behaviour, nutritional status, lactational hyperprolactinaemia and status of the menstrual cycle. Clin. Endocrinol. 22:179-187.

Howie, P.W., A.S. McNeilly, M.J. Houston, A. Cook, and H. Boyle. 1981. Effect of supplementary food on suckling patterns and ovarian activity during lactation. Br. Med. J. 283:757-759.

Hreshchyshyn, M.M., A. Hopkins, S. Zylstra, and M. Anbar. 1988. Associations of parity, breast-feeding, and birth control pills with lumbar spine and femoral neck bone densities. Am. J. Obstet. Gynecol. 159:318-322.

Huffman, S.L., A.K.M.A. Chowdhury, and W.H. Mosley. 1978. Postpartum amenorrhea: how is it affected by maternal nutritional status? Science 200:1155-1157.

IOM (Institute of Medicine). 1990. Nutrition During Pregnancy: Weight Gain and Nutrient Supplements. Report of the Subcommittee on Nutritional Status and Weight Gain During Pregnancy, Subcommittee on Dietary Intake and Nutrient Supplements During Pregnancy, Committee on Nutritional Status During Pregnancy and Lactation, Food and Nutrition Board. National Academy Press, Washington, D.C. 468 pp.

Jen, K.L.C., N. Juuhl, and P.K.H. Lin. 1988. Repeated pregnancy without lactation: effects on carcass composition and adipose tissue cellularity in rats. J. Nutr. 118:93-98.

Johnell, O., and B.E. Nilsson. 1984. Life-style and bone mineral mass in perimenopausal women. Calcif. Tissue Int. 36:354-356.

Kayner, C.E., and J.A. Zagar. 1983. Breast-feeding and sexual response. J. Fam. Pract. 17:69-73.

Kelsey, J.L., and G.S. Berkowitz. 1988. Breast cancer epidemiology. Cancer Res. 48:5615-5623.

Kennedy, K., R. Rivera, and A. McNeilly. 1989. Consensus statement on the use of breastfeeding as a family planning method. Contraception. 39:477-496.

Koetting, C.A., and G.M. Wardlaw. 1988. Wrist, spine, and hip bone density in women with variable histories of lactation. Am. J. Clin. Nutr. 48:1479-1481.

Korenman, S.G. 1980. The endocrinology of breast cancer. Cancer 46:874-878.

Kvåle, G., and I. Heuch. 1987. Lactation and cancer risk: is there a relation specific to breast cancer? J. Epidemiol. Commun. Health 42:30-37.

Labbok, M., P. Koniz-Booher, J. Shelton, and K. Krasovec. 1990. Guidelines for Breastfeeding in Family Planning and Child Survival Programs. Institute for International Studies in Natural Family Planning, Georgetown University, Washington, D.C.

Lafontan, M., L. Dang-Tran, and M. Berlan. 1979. Alpha-adrenergic antilipolytic effect of adrenaline in human fat cells of the thigh: comparison with adrenaline responsiveness of different fat deposits. Eur. J. Clin. Invest. 9:261-266.

Lawrence, R.A. 1989. Breastfeeding: A Guide for the Medical Profession, 3rd ed. C.V. Mosby, St. Louis. 652 pp.

Layde, P.M., L.A. Webster, A.L. Baughman, P.A. Wingo, G.L. Rubin, and H.W. Ory. 1989. The independent associations of parity, age at first full term pregnancy, and duration of breastfeeding with the risk of breast cancer. Cancer and Steroid Hormone Study Group. J. Clin. Epidemiol. 42:963-973.

London, S.J., G.A. Colditz, M.J. Stampfer, W.C. Willett, B.A. Rosner, K. Corsano, and F.E. Speizer. 1990. Lactation and risk of breast cancer in a cohort of US women. Am. J. Epidemiol. 132:17-26.

Lunn, P.G., M. Watkinson, A.M. Prentice, P. Morrell, S. Austin, and R.G. Whitehead. 1981. Maternal nutrition and lactational amenorrhoea. Lancet 1:1428-1429.

Lunn, P.G., S. Austin, A.M. Prentice, and R.G. Whitehead. 1984. The effect of improved nutrition on plasma prolactin concentrations and postpartum infertility in lactating Gambian women. Am. J. Clin. Nutr. 39:227-235.

MacMahon, B., T.M. Lin, C.R. Lowe, A.P. Mirra, B. Ravnihar, E.J. Salber, D. Trichopoulos, V.G. Valaoras, and S. Yuasa. 1970. Lactation and cancer of the breast: a summary of an international study. Bull. W.H.O. 42:185-194.

Manning-Dalton, C., and L.H. Allen. 1983. The effects of lactation on energy and protein consumption, postpartum weight change and body composition of well nourished North American women. Nutr. Res. 3:293-308.

Masters, W.H., and V.E. Johnson. 1966. Human Sexual Response. Little, Brown, Boston. 366 pp.

McKeown, T., and R.G. Record. 1957. The influence of reproduction on body weight in women. J. Endocrinol. 15:393-409.

McNeilly, A.S., A. Glasier, and P.W. Howie. 1985. Endocrine control of lactational infertility. I. Pp. 1-24 in J. Dobbing, ed. Maternal Nutrition and Lactational Infertility. Nestle Nutrition Workshop Series, Vol. 9. Raven Press, New York.

McTiernan, A., and D.B. Thomas. 1986. Evidence for a protective effect of lactation on risk of breast cancer in young women: results from a case-control study. Am. J. Epidemiol. 124:353-358.

Mercer, R.R., and M.A. Crenshaw. 1985. The role of osteocytes in bone resorption during lactation: morphometric observations. Bone 6:269-274.

Moore, B.J., and J.A. Brasel. 1984. One cycle of reproduction consisting of pregnancy, lactation or no lactation, and recovery: effects on fat pad cellularity in ad libitum-fed and food-restricted rats. J. Nutr. 114:1560-1565.

Morse, E.H., R.P. Clarke, S.B. Merrow, and B.E. Thibault. 1975. Comparison of the nutritional status of pregnant adolescents with adult pregnant women. II. Anthropometric and dietary findings. Am. J. Clin. Nutr. 28:1422-1428.

Naismith, D.J., and C.D. Ritchie. 1975. The effect of breast-feeding and artificial feeding on body-weights, skinfold measurements and food intakes of forty-two primiparous women. Proc. Nutr. Soc. 34:116A-117A.

Newcombe, R.G. 1982. Development of obesity in parous women. J. Epidemiol. Comm. Health 36:306-309.

Newton, N. 1973. Interrelationships between sexual responsiveness, birth, and breast feeding. Pp. 77-98 in J. Zubin and J. Money, eds. Contemporary Sexual Behavior: Critical Issues in the 1970s. Johns Hopkins University Press, Baltimore, Md.

Newton, N., and M. Newton. 1967. Psychologic aspects of lactation. N. Engl. J. Med. 277:1179-1188.

Prentice, A.M., S.B. Roberts, A. Prentice, A.A. Paul, M. Watkinson, A.A. Watkinson, and R.G. Whitehead. 1983a. Dietary supplementation of lactating Gambian women. I. Effect on breast-milk volume and quality. Hum. Nutr.: Clin. Nutr. 37C:53-64.

Prentice, A.M., P.G. Lunn, M. Watkinson, and R.G. Whitehead. 1983b. Dietary supplementation of lactating Gambian women. II. Effect on maternal health, nutritional status and biochemistry. Hum. Nutr.: Clin. Nutr. 37C:65-74.

Quandt, S.A. 1984. Nutritional thriftiness and human reproduction: beyond the critical body composition hypothesis. Soc. Sci. Med. 19:177-182.

Reamy, K.J., and S.E. White. 1987. Sexuality in the puerperium: a review. Arch. Sex. Behav. 16:165-186.

Rebuffe-Scrive, M., L. Enk. N. Crona, P. Lönnroth, L. Abrahamsson, U. Smith, and P. Björntorp. 1985. Fat cell metabolism in different regions in women: effect of menstrual cycle, pregnancy, and lactation. J. Clin. Invest. 75:1973-1976.

Richardson, J.S. 1952. The treatment of maternal obesity. Lancet 262:525-528.

Rookus, M.A., P. Rokebrand, J. Burema, and P. Deurenberg. 1987. The effect of pregnancy on the body mass index 9 months postpartum in 49 women. Int. J. Obesity 11:609-618.

Sheldon, J.H. 1949. Maternal obesity. Lancet 257:869-873.

Stoneham, S., T. Kiviluoto, L. Keso, and J.J. Ohisalo. 1988. Adenosine and the regional differences in adipose tissue metabolism in women. Acta Endocrinol. 118:327-331.

Tao, S.C., M.C. Yu, R.K. Ross, and K.W. Xiu. 1988. Risk factors for breast cancer in Chinese women of Beijing. Int. J. Cancer 42:495-498.

Tylavsky, F.A., R.C. Curtis, J.J.B. Anderson, and J.A. Metz. 1989. Changes in radial and vertebral bone mass due to pregnancy and lactations in humans. J. Bone Mineral Res. 4:S414.

Waletsky, L.R. 1979. Breastfeeding and weaning: some psychological considerations. Prim. Care 6:341-355.

Walker, A.R.P., B. Richardson, and F. Walker. 1972. The influence of numerous pregnancies and lactations on bone dimensions in South African Bantu and Caucasian mothers. Clin. Sci. 42:189-196.

Wardlaw, G.M., and A.M. Pike. 1986. The effect of lactation on peak adult shaft and ultra-distal forearm bone mass in women. Am. J. Clin. Nutr. 44:283-286.

Yuan, J.M., M.C. Yu, R.K. Ross, Y.T. Gao, and B.E. Henderson. 1988. Risk factors for breast cancer in Chinese women in Shanghai. Cancer Res. 48:1949-1953.

9
Meeting Maternal Nutrient Needs During Lactation

In this chapter, the subcommittee synthesizes information presented in earlier chapters, especially that concerning maternal nutritional status, milk volume and composition, infant nutrition, and health effects of lactation on the mother later in life. It then examines estimated nutrient needs in relation to realistic dietary patterns for lactating women.

WHAT ARE THE NUTRITIONAL DEMANDS OF LACTATION?

Nutrient Secretion in Milk

Nutrient needs during lactation depend primarily on the volume and composition of milk produced and on the mother's initial nutrient needs and nutritional status. Among women exclusively breastfeeding their infants, the energy demands of lactation exceed prepregnancy demands by approximately 640 kcal/day during the first 6 months post partum compared with 300 kcal/day during the last two trimesters of pregnancy (NRC, 1989). In contrast, the demand for some nutrients, such as iron, is considerably less during lactation than during pregnancy.

Table 9-1 provides the estimated daily output of various nutrients in human milk compared with the increments in nutrient intakes for lactating women as specified in the *Recommended Dietary Allowances* (RDAs) (NRC, 1989). Each nutrient output is given as a range, reflecting milk volumes from 600 to 1,000 ml/day and the average concentration of each nutrient in human milk, as described in Chapter 6 (Table 6-1). Because there is variability in the milk

213

concentrations of some nutrients, both between women and in the same woman at different stages of lactation, the estimates in Table 9-1 are provided primarily as an illustration of the relative levels of secretion in milk. They reflect the nutrient output by women exclusively breastfeeding a single infant; therefore, they are *underestimates* for those women breastfeeding twins or triplets and *overestimates* for those whose infants are given substantial amounts of other milks or solid foods.

Previous editions of *Recommended Dietary Allowances* (e.g., NRC, 1980) presented RDAs for lactating women as increments to be added to the RDAs for nonpregnant, nonlactating women. In contrast, the 1989 RDAs for lactating women are presented as absolute amounts. This provides convenient numbers that apply to all lactating women regardless of age and reflects the limited precision of the published data. The absolute values in the 1989 RDAs represent the RDAs for nonpregnant, nonlactating women aged 25 to 50 plus increments, which are shown in Table 9-1. For many nutrients, it is evident that the RDA increments were designed to exceed the estimated daily output during lactation. The RDAs for lactating women are the same for mothers of all ages, but some of the RDAs for nonpregnant, nonlactating women differ for women of different age groups. The difference is most notable for vitamin D and calcium. For those two nutrients, no increment for lactation is included for women younger than 25. Their prepregnancy RDAs are considerably higher than those of the older group (10 μg compared with 5 μg for vitamin D, and 1,200 mg compared with 800 mg for calcium), and they are identical to the older women's RDAs for these nutrients during lactation.

Daily outputs of energy, vitamin A, vitamin B_{12}, iron, and iodine in milk tend to exceed the recommended increments. The allowance for energy is based on the assumption that lactating women can draw on fat stores deposited during pregnancy to help support milk production. Thus, gradual weight loss is expected during lactation. For women who are underweight or whose weight gain during pregnancy was low, a 650-kcal/day increase in energy intake during the first 6 months of lactation is recommended. Total energy needs during lactation depend greatly on the level of physical activity, as described in Chapter 5.

In estimating output for several nutrients, the subcommittee used values for milk concentrations that were higher than from those used in deriving the RDAs. These are identified in Table 9-1, along with other comments regarding the rationale for the RDA increments for lactation.

Long-Term Nutrient Output During Lactation

In addition to examining the daily output of nutrients in milk, it is useful to estimate the overall nutrient outputs resulting from various durations of lactation. Obviously, these estimates depend on the timing and degree to which

TABLE 9-1 Estimated Secretion of Nutrients in Mature Human Milk Compared with Increments in Recommended Dietary Allowances (RDAs) for Lactating Women

A. Energy, Protein, and Fat-Soluble Vitamins

Measure	Energy, kcal	Protein, g	Vitamin A, μg RE[a]	Vitamin D, μg	Vitamin E, mg of α-TE[b]	Vitamin K, μg
Estimated secretion in milk[c]	420–700	6.3–10.5	400–670	0.3–0.6	1.4–2.3	1.3–2.1
Increment in RDAs[d,e] for the following periods of lactation:						
0–6 mo	500	15	500	5	4	0
6–12 mo	500	12	400	5	3	0
Comments	Estimated 80% efficiency in conversion to milk energy	Estimated 70% efficiency in conversion to milk protein	None	Increment advised in part to maintain calcium balance	Estimated 75% absorption	No increment listed because usually intakes usually exceed RDA

Table 9-1 continues

TABLE 9-1—Continued

B. Water-Soluble Vitamins

Measure	Vitamin C, mg	Thiamin, mg	Riboflavin, mg	Niacin, mg of NE[f]	Vitamin B$_6$, mg	Folate, μg	Vitamin B$_{12}$, μg
Estimated secretion in milk[c]	24–40	0.13–0.21	0.21–0.35	0.9–1.5	0.06–0.09	50–83	0.6–1.0
Increment in RDAs[d,e] for the following periods of lactation:							
0–6 mo	35	0.5	0.5	5	0.5	100	0.6
6–12 mo	30	0.5	0.4	5	0.5	80	0.6
Comments	Estimated 85% absorption	Increment higher than secretion due to increased energy needs	Estimated 70% utilization for milk production	Increment higher than secretion due to increased energy needs	The milk concentration used by the subcommittee is for unsupplemented women	Estimated 50% absorption; RDA based on 50 rather than 83 μg/liter	RDA based on 0.6 rather than 1.0 μg/liter

C. Minerals

Measure	Calcium, mg	Phosphorus, mg	Magnesium, mg	Iron, mg	Zinc, mg	Iodine, μg	Selenium, μg
Estimated secretion in milk[c]	168–280	84–140	21–35	0.18–0.30	0.9–1.5[g] 0.3–0.5[h]	66–110	12–20
Increment in RDAs[d,e] for the following periods of lactation:							
0–6 mo	400	400	75	0	7	50	20
6–12 mo	400	400	60	0	4	50	20
Comments	None	Based on a desired ratio of 1 to 1 for calcium to phosphorus intake	Estimated 50% absorption	Secretion during lactation is less than menstrual loss	Estimated 20% absorption	Based on need of infant, not maternal loss in milk	Estimated 80% absorption

[a] RE = Retinol equivalents.
[b] α-TE = α-Tocopherol equivalents.
[c] At volumes of 600–1,000 ml/day, based on milk composition shown in Table 6-1.
[d] From NRC (1989).
[e] Women aged 25 to 50.
[f] NE = Niacin equivalents.
[g] 0 to 6 months; see Chapter 6.
[h] 6 to 12 months; see Chapter 6.

human milk is replaced with other foods over the period of weaning. If the mother ingests lower amounts of a nutrient than she requires to meet her own needs and to cover nutrients secreted in the milk, she can draw upon body stores. To illustrate the possible impact of inadequate intake on the mother, Table 9-2 lists the estimated total body content of protein, calcium, and folate; the average amounts of iron and vitamin A stored by women; and the estimated outputs during partial or exclusive breastfeeding for various durations. Energy output in milk is not listed: changes in maternal body stores cannot be easily computed since energy-supplying nutrients could originate in either fat or lean tissue.

As shown in Table 9-2, protein output in milk during 6 months of exclusive breastfeeding totals approximately 1,500 g (1.5 kg). For a 60-kg woman with 25% body fat, lean body mass is 45 kg, or about 11 kg of protein. Assuming that the efficiency of conversion of body protein to milk protein approximately equals the conversion of dietary protein to milk protein (~70% [NRC, 1989]), a woman consuming only the RDA for protein for a nonpregnant, nonlactating woman would need to mobilize about 19% of her lean tissue to support 6 months of milk production. In the absence of adequate calcium intake, calcium output in milk represents 2 to 8% of total body calcium, as described in Chapter 8. Although iron losses in milk during 6 months of exclusive breastfeeding are equivalent to approximately 14% of the average woman's iron stores, this is only about half of what is ordinarily lost through menstruation (NRC, 1989). Thus, unless there was excessive blood loss at delivery, the total demand for iron during lactation is reduced while the woman is still amenorrheic compared with the demand when the woman is nonpregnant and nonlactating. When menstruation resumes, the combined demands of milk production and menstruation could draw heavily on iron reserves if dietary iron intake is low.

Vitamin A reserves vary greatly among women and may be precariously low in women whose habitual intake of the vitamin is marginal. In the U.S. population, on average, women are expected to have vitamin A stores of approximately 200 mg (NRC, 1989)—more than the total output of many women over usual periods of lactation (see Table 9-2). However, for a woman with much smaller stores whose diet barely meets her own vitamin A requirement, the loss of the vitamin in milk could theoretically deplete vitamin A stores within a few months.

Since folate tends to be excreted in the urine if intake exceeds demand, body stores of folate are not large. Thus, with limited dietary sources of folate, reserves would be depleted after only a few months of lactation.

The estimates discussed above are meaningful only in the context of dietary information. For example, total protein output in milk during 6 months of exclusive breastfeeding is high compared with total body protein, but this is not of great concern in the United States, where protein intake is usually

TABLE 9-2 Estimated Long-Term Demand of Lactation for Selected Nutrients

	Nutrient Output				
Source of Demand	Protein, g (% of total body content[a])	Calcium, g (% of total body content[a])	Iron, mg (% of stores[a])	Vitamin A, mg (% of stores[a])	Folate, mg (% of stores[a])
Estimated body content[b,c]	11,250	1,035	300	209	6–7
Partial breastfeeding for 6 mo	756 (10)	20 (2)	22 (7)	48 (23)	6 (~100)
Exclusive breastfeeding for 6 mo	1,512 (19)	40 (4)	43 (14)	96 (46)	12 (~100)
Exclusive breastfeeding for 6 mo, plus partial breastfeeding for 6 mo	2,268 (29)	60 (6)	65 (22)	144 (69)	18 (>100)
Exclusive breastfeeding for 6 mo, plus partial breastfeeding for 12 mo	3,024 (38)	80 (8)	87 (29)	192 (92)	24 (>100)

[a]Based on average milk composition values from Table 6-1 and a volume of 800 ml/day for exclusive breastfeeding and 400 ml/day for partial breastfeeding, assuming that none of the demand is met by the maternal diet.
[b]For a 60-kg (132-lb) woman, based on values provided by the NRC (1989).
[c]Percentage of total body content or stores not applicable.

generous. Calcium output during lactation may be of greater concern for reasons discussed in Chapter 8.

CAN NUTRIENT NEEDS DURING LACTATION BE MET BY USUAL DIETARY INTAKE ALONE?

Predicted Average Intakes by U.S. Women During Lactation

One approach recommended for estimating the likelihood of nutrient deficiencies is to compare the distribution of intakes of each nutrient with the hypothetical distribution of requirements in a given population (NRC, 1986). If this method could be used, it would avoid the use of arbitrary cutoff values to define deficient intakes. As noted in Chapter 4, however, data on the usual dietary intakes of lactating women are not sufficient for this method to be applied, and the data that are available were generally obtained from relatively affluent groups, who are unlikely to be representative of the population as a whole.

For these reasons, and because energy needs are highly variable and energy intake is difficult to quantify, the subcommittee opted to evaluate the likelihood of nutrient shortfalls during lactation based on the *nutrient density* (nutrient intake per 1,000 kcal) of the average woman's diet in the United States. Total energy intakes by women are generally underestimated in national surveys; the nutrient density approach avoids this potential bias. However, the calculated nutrient densities could also be biased if underreporting is greater for certain foods than for others. No data are available to evaluate this possibility.

Table 9-3 provides nutrient densities for protein, minerals, and vitamins as determined from nationally representative samples of U.S. women aged 19 to 50 and the total nutrient intakes that would be predicted from those densities at three different levels of energy intake (nutrient density × kcal of energy = total intake). The three levels of energy intake chosen for the calculations are 2,700 kcal (the estimated energy needs for lactation listed in *Recommended Dietary Allowances* [NRC, 1989]), 2,200 kcal (a value closer to the average reported intakes of lactating women, as described in Chapter 4), and 1,800 kcal (a level that might occur if a lactating woman were actively restricting food intake in order to lose weight). Intakes of specific nutrients at these three levels of energy intake can be compared with the RDAs for lactation, also listed in Table 9-3.

Comparisons of Estimated and Recommended Intakes

Several patterns become apparent when comparing estimated intakes with the RDAs shown in Table 9-3. At an intake of 2,700 kcal, average predicted intakes are below the RDAs for only two nutrients: calcium and zinc. At an intake of 2,200 kcal, however, predicted intakes of calcium, magnesium,

TABLE 9-3 Estimated Mean Nutrient Intakes by U.S. Women at Three Energy Levels Compared with the Recommended Dietary Allowances (RDAs) for Lactation

A. Protein and Fat-Soluble Vitamins

Measure	Protein, g	Vitamin A, µg of RE[a]	Vitamin D, µg	Vitamin E, mg of α-TE[b]	Vitamin K, µg
Average nutrient density of diets of U.S. women aged 19 to 50 yr[d] (nutrient content per 1,000 kcal)	40	805	NR[c]	5	NR
Nutrient intake assuming average nutrient density at:					
2,700 kcal	108	2,174	NA[e]	14	NA
2,200 kcal	88	1,771	NA	11	NA
1,800 kcal	72	1,449	NA	9	NA
RDA for lactation[f]					
0–6 mo	65	1,300	10	12	65
6–12 mo	62	1,200	10	11	65

Table 9-3 continues

TABLE 9-3—Continued

B. Water-Soluble Vitamins

Measure	Vitamin C, mg	Thiamin, mg	Riboflavin, mg	Niacin, mg of NE	Vitamin B$_6$, mg	Folate, μg	Vitamin B$_{12}$, μg
Average nutrient density of diets of U.S. women aged 19 to 50 yr^d (nutrient content per 1,000 kcal)	56	0.7	0.9	11.2	0.8	13.7	2.9
Nutrient intake assuming average nutrient density at:							
2,700 kcal	151	1.9	2.4	30.2	2.2	370	7.8
2,200 kcal	123	1.5	2.0	24.6	1.8	301	6.4
1,800 kcal	101	1.3	1.6	20.2	1.4	247	5.2
RDA for lactation^f							
0–6 mo	95	1.6	1.8	20	2.1	280	2.6
6–12 mo	90	1.6	1.7	20	2.1	260	2.6

C. Minerals

Measure	Calcium, mg	Phosphorus, mg	Magnesium, mg	Iron, mg	Zinc, mg	Iodine, µg	Selenium, µg
Average nutrient density of diets of U.S. women aged 19 to 50 yr[d] (nutrient content per 1,000 kcal)	397	645	143	7.0	5.8	145[g]	3.5[g]
Nutrient intake assuming average nutrient density at:							
2,700 kcal	1,072	1,742	386	18.9	15.7	392	95
2,200 kcal	873	1,419	315	15.4	12.8	319	77
1,800 kcal	715	1,161	257	12.6	10.4	261	63
RDA for lactation[f]							
0–6 mo	1,200	1,200	355	15	19	200	75
6–12 mo	1,200	1,200	340	15	16	200	75

[a]RE = Retinol equivalents.
[b]α-TE = α-Tocopherol equivalents.
[c]NR = Not reported.
[d]From Continuing Survey of Food Intake by Individuals, Wave I, USDA (1987).
[e]NA = Not applicable.
[f]Assumes 2,700 kcal of energy per day, from NRC (1989).
[g]Estimated from the Total Diet Study, Pennington et al. (1989).

zinc, thiamin, vitamin B_6, and vitamin E fall below the RDA. At 1,800 kcal, predicted intakes fall below the RDAs for all the nutrients listed above plus riboflavin, folate, phosphorus, and iron.

Several cautions are necessary in interpreting these patterns:

- The RDAs for most nutrients include a wide margin of safety, so intakes below the RDAs do not necessarily indicate inadequacy. Of the nutrients for which predicted average intake is below the RDA, most intake estimates range from 73 to 97% of the RDA, except intakes for zinc, which are 67 and 55% of the RDA (at 2,200 and 1,800 kcal, respectively) and for calcium and vitamin B_6, which are 60 and 67%, respectively (each at 1,800 kcal). There is also a wide range in the nutrient densities used to generate the averages shown in Table 9-3. Even if the average predicted intake of a given nutrient is at or above the RDA, the intakes of a substantial proportion of the population would fall below that level.

- The margin of safety in the RDA varies by nutrient. As shown in Table 9-1, for example, the increment in the RDA for vitamin B_6 for lactation is more than five times the estimated secretion of this vitamin in milk. In contrast, the increment for folate is less than two times the estimated secretion.

- Overt signs of deficiency are extremely rare in the United States, even for nutrients with small safety margins.

- Nutrient densities of diets consumed by lactating women are likely to differ from those for U.S. women as a whole. Inspection of data for lactating women shown in Chapter 4 indicates that densities of calcium and vitamin A, for example, are 40 to 50% higher in the diets of the lactating women surveyed than the values shown in Table 9-3, possibly because greater quantities of milk products are consumed. It could be argued either that women who choose to breastfeed are women who ordinarily have high nutrient intakes, or that women consume more nutrient-rich foods when breastfeeding. Whatever the case, higher than average densities of some nutrients in diets of the few lactating women studied to date are not grounds for complacency, because the samples in these studies were generally not randomly selected. There is no evidence that the same nutrient intakes would pertain to breastfeeding women in less affluent or less educated groups.

Keeping these cautions in mind, this subcommittee attempted to determine which nutrients are most likely to be in short supply in the diets of lactating women, relative to the RDAs, and the consequences of any such shortfalls.

Calcium

Calcium is clearly a concern because it is difficult for many lactating women to consume the RDA of 1,200 mg/day, especially if milk products are not a major part of the diet. This may be even more relevant for women younger than age 25 who breastfeed, since the calcium content of bones is ordinarily expected to increase until age 25. As discussed in Chapter 6, a low calcium intake will not affect the concentration of calcium in human milk, but its effect on the mother's long-term bone density is uncertain, especially if the duration of breastfeeding is long. The evidence reviewed in Chapter 8 does not indicate a higher prevalence of osteoporosis in women who breastfed their children, but there is little information on the bone health of breastfeeding women with low calcium intakes. Lactating women in Nepal with low calcium intakes maintained milk calcium levels similar to those of U.S. women, but levels of urinary hydroxyproline were more than twice as high, indicating greater bone resorption (Moser et al., 1988). There is some evidence from animal studies that calcium absorption is enhanced during lactation (Halloran and DeLuca, 1980), but the degree to which this can compensate for low intakes is unclear. Although it is evident that calcium status is only one of many possible factors in the etiology of osteoporosis, dietary guidance for lactating women should include recommendations for good sources of calcium.

Zinc

There is no generally accepted indicator to use for evaluating the adequacy of zinc intakes. The RDA increment for zinc during lactation is 4 to 13 times higher than the estimated zinc secretion in milk to allow for poor absorption of dietary zinc (estimated at 20% for nonpregnant, nonlactating adults). However, stable isotope studies of seven lactating women in Brazil whose zinc intake averaged only 8.4 mg/day indicate that zinc absorption may be as high as 59 to 84% (Jackson et al., 1988).

The difference between the RDA increment and estimated zinc secretion is especially large during the second 6 months of lactation, when zinc concentrations in milk decline substantially, regardless of the woman's zinc intake (Krebs et al., 1985). Low intakes are not generally reflected in low zinc concentrations in milk, and no major health risks have been associated with zinc intakes lower than the RDA. However, maternal zinc status might be jeopardized by low intake: zinc levels in plasma were found to be lower among lactating women than among nonlactating controls in Nigeria (Mbofund and Atinmo, 1985) but not in the United States (Moser and Reynolds, 1983), despite relatively low zinc intakes in both studies. Given the importance of adequate zinc status to immune function and other outcomes, further research on maternal zinc status during lactation is warranted.

Magnesium

Magnesium is the only other mineral for which intake by lactating women may often be marginal, when compared with the RDA. Again, however, the increment recommended during lactation is two to three times the estimated daily secretion in milk, to account for an estimated absorption of 50% (NRC,

1989). The effect of lactation on magnesium absorption is not known. Despite the relatively large difference between recommended and actual magnesium intakes, the only evidence of maternal magnesium deficiency during lactation appears in two anecdotal reports of extraordinary cases: in a wet nurse whose milk output was estimated to be 1,700 ml/day for 3 months (Greenwald et al., 1963) and in a woman who secreted three times the normal level of magnesium in her milk (Kamble and Ookalkar, 1989). Women in Ghana who breastfed for up to 12 months post partum had levels of serum magnesium lower than those of nonlactating controls (Fenuku and Earl-Quarcoo, 1978), but in lactating U.S. women whose mean magnesium intake was 248 mg/day, neither plasma magnesium nor erythrocyte magnesium differed from values for nonlactating women (Moser et al., 1983). Magnesium intake from diet or supplements has not been associated with maternal plasma or erythrocyte magnesium (Moser et al., 1983), nor is it likely to influence magnesium concentrations in milk (see Chapter 6). The long-term impact of low magnesium intake on the mother's well-being has not been studied.

Vitamin B_6

The vitamins most likely to occur in low levels (relative to the RDAs) in the diets of lactating women are B_6, E, thiamin, and folate. Vitamin B_6 levels in milk are strongly influenced by dietary intake: levels in the milk of women supplemented with 2.5 mg/day are twice as high as those of unsupplemented women (192 compared with 93 μg/liter) (Styslinger and Kirksey, 1985), but the RDA increment for lactation appears generous even if based on the vitamin B_6 content of the milk of supplemented women. On the other hand, protein intakes by lactating women in the United States are high (average predicted intakes range from 111 to 166% of the RDA; Table 9-3); thus, the RDA increment allows for the increase in vitamin B_6 requirement that accompanies increases in protein intake.

Low vitamin B_6 intakes during lactation may adversely affect both the infant and the mother, although evidence of overt deficiencies is rare in the United States. Kirksey and Roepke (1981) reported three cases of breastfed infants with central nervous system disorders, which they attributed to vitamin B_6 deficiency. The mothers of all three infants had been long-term (4- to 12-year) users of oral contraceptives prior to pregnancy at a time when the estrogen content of such preparations was much higher than it is currently; these mothers were considered to have inadequate vitamin B_6 status. Levels of plasma pyridoxal 5-phosphate (PLP) tend to be lower in breastfed infants than in formula-fed infants, and there is a correlation between vitamin B_6 levels in human milk and infant plasma PLP (Andon et al., 1989; McCoy et al., 1985). However, none of the infants in two studies of unsupplemented lactating women in the United States ($N = 6$ in Styslinger and Kirksey [1985] and $N =$

30 in Andon et al. [1989]) had any clinical symptoms of vitamin B_6 deficiency. Women in the study by Andon and colleagues generally had adequate vitamin B_6 status; none had used oral contraceptives in the preceding 5 years.

Chang and Kirksey (1990) measured maternal plasma PLP and milk vitamin B_6 levels in 47 lactating women who received daily pyridoxine supplements containing 2.5, 4.0, 7.5, or 10 mg. Combined with the women's usual diets, the 4.0-mg supplements resulted in maternal PLP concentrations reportedly similar to those of nonlactating women (although no data for nonlactating women were provided) and in milk vitamin B_6 concentrations that were nearly as high as those of the women receiving the higher-dose supplements. The influence of maternal supplementation on infant vitamin B_6 status was not evaluated. In an earlier study (Borschel et al., 1986), two of five breastfed infants whose mothers were supplemented with 2.5 mg of vitamin B_6 per day had plasma PLP levels of less than 25 nmol/liter (6.18 ng/ml), which the authors described as relatively low. However, Reynolds and colleagues (1990) have questioned whether plasma PLP is an adequate index of vitamin B_6 status, especially in infants, and suggest that some individuals may have low PLP values without any clinical evidence of vitamin B_6 deficiency.

Taken all together, and without indices of vitamin B_6 status other than plasma PLP, the above studies do not provide sufficient evidence to warrant routine vitamin B_6 supplementation of lactating women.

Vitamin E

Although average predicted vitamin E intakes may fall somewhat below the RDA, this is generally not cause for concern for two reasons. First, the allowance for vitamin E is based primarily on estimates of customary intakes from food sources in the United States, rather than on minimum requirements. Second, the calculated nutrient density of vitamin E shown in Table 9-3 may be an underestimate, since there may be selective underreporting of fat intake (and thus vitamin E) in the surveys on which the calculation is based. Although maternal vitamin E intake can influence the levels of this vitamin in milk, there is no evidence of vitamin E deficiency in individuals with normal fat absorption (NRC, 1989).

Thiamin

The RDA increment for thiamin during lactation is considerably higher than thiamin losses in milk—in part because the need for thiamin depends on energy intake, which is expected to be higher during lactation. The predicted average thiamin intakes shown in Table 9-3 are less than the RDA only at lower than recommended energy intakes, suggesting that low thiamin intake is seldom a problem. Low maternal thiamin intake can result in low thiamin levels in milk, however. Therefore, in the judgment of the subcommittee, intakes of at least 1.3 mg/day (the RDA for nonpregnant, nonlactating women of 1.1 mg/day plus an increment for milk secretion of 0.2 mg/day [Table 9-1]) are desirable among women consuming 2,200 kcal/day or less.

Folate

Predicted average folate intakes fall below the RDA only when energy intake is less than 2,000 kcal/day. However, the margin of safety between the folate output in milk and the RDA is quite narrow (Table 9-1). The RDA is based on an average folate concentration of 50 μg/liter in human milk, but a well-conducted study using an accurate method (Brown et al., 1986) suggests that average concentrations are approximately 85 μg/liter. This higher value was used as the basis for estimating the daily secretion of folate in Table 9-1. If absorption of folate from a mixed diet is estimated to be 50%, the desired increment would be about 140 μg of folate per day. At this level, folate needs during lactation would be approximately 320 μg/day (the sum of 180 μg/day for nonpregnant, nonlactating women plus 140 μg/day for lactation). At an energy intake of 2,200 kcal/day, the average predicted maternal folate intake is lower than this amount—301 μg/day (Table 9-3). Approximately 10% of the U.S. population is believed to have low folate stores (LSRO, 1984), and poor folate status of women post partum is not uncommon (Butte et al., 1981; Martinez, 1980; Qvist et al., 1986).

In a study of 91 middle-class lactating women in Norway who did not receive supplemental folate, Ek (1983) observed that folate levels in the red blood cells of women breastfeeding for more than 6 months declined 30% during the first 2 months, and increased thereafter, slightly exceeding levels observed at parturition. The folate levels in their milk did not reflect these changes, and there were no signs of folate deficiency in the mothers. The folate levels in red blood cells of women who breastfed for less than 1 month changed very little during the first 12 months post partum. This and other studies (Metz, 1970; Tamura et al., 1980) indicate that maternal reserves of folate may be depleted to maintain folate levels in milk. If dietary intake and maternal reserves of folate have been chronically low, milk folate levels will increase in response to increased folate intake (see Chapter 6). Thus, adequate folate intake is important to protect the health of both the mother and the infant.

Nutrient Concerns for Selected Groups of Lactating Women

The discussion above focuses on nutrients likely to be consumed by lactating women in the United States in amounts lower than the RDAs. Within certain age, income, and ethnic groups, however, the diet may be characterized by nutrient densities higher or lower than the averages shown in Table 9-3. Intake data from national surveys are available by age, race (white, black, and other) (e.g., USDA, 1987), and income (above and below the poverty level) (e.g., NCHS, 1983; USDA, 1988). Such data may be useful in identifying potential nutrient inadequacies in selected groups.

Following are four examples of groups whose diets, on average, have nutrient densities lower than the values shown in Table 9-3. An energy intake of 2,200 kcal was assumed when calculating recommended nutrient densities.

• Diets of adolescents (aged 15 to 17) typically contain less iron (an average of 5.7 mg/1,000 kcal) (NCHS, 1983) than recommended during lactation (6.8 mg/1,000 kcal).

• Diets of adolescents with family incomes below the poverty level have a low vitamin A content (1,500 IU/1,000 kcal) (NCHS, 1983) compared with a desired density of 1,950 IU/1,000 kcal.

• On average, the diets of black women contain about 30% less calcium, 20% less magnesium, and 20% less vitamin A than average diets consumed by white women (USDA, 1987).

• Diets of low-income adult women are characterized by lower densities of calcium and vitamin A than are typical of diets of women above the poverty level (NCHS, 1983).

Thus, special care should be taken to ensure that breastfeeding women in such groups have access to a nutrient-dense diet.

Women with restricted eating patterns will have undesirably low intakes of certain nutrients. This applies to those whose total food and energy intake is low (unless nutrient density is unusually high) and to those who avoid foods that are major sources of nutrients, such as calcium-rich dairy products, vitamin D-fortified milk, animal foods (for vitamin B_{12}), or fruits and vegetables (for folate and vitamin C).

In some cultural groups, beliefs regarding foods that should not be consumed by lactating women may affect dietary patterns (Baumslag, 1986), but the influence of restrictive food beliefs on nutrient intake is not well documented.

FOOD GUIDANCE FOR LACTATING WOMEN

Numerous food guides for lactating women have been developed by various state and national agencies concerned with maternal nutrition. There is considerable variability in the dietary recommendations provided in these guides, as illustrated by the number of daily servings they recommend from each of the food groups (Table 9-4). For example, the recommended amount of protein-rich foods ranges from 4 to 12 oz/day, suggested servings of milk vary from three to six per day, and servings from the bread and cereals group range from four to eight per day. Some of the guides specify subcategories of fruits and vegetables, such as "vitamin C-rich," "dark green leafy," and "other," whereas other guides lump all fruits and vegetables together and specify three to six servings.

The foods selected from within each food group can strongly influence the

230

TABLE 9-4 Recommended Numbers of Servings[a] During Lactation, by Publication

Reference	Protein	Milk, Dairy — Intake by Adults of All Ages	Milk, Dairy — Intake by Teens	Breads, Cereals	All Fruits and Vegetables	All Fruits	All Vegetables	Vitamin C Rich	Dark Green, Leafy or Vitamin A Rich	Starchy Vegetables	Other Vegetables	Unsaturated Fat
DHHS, 1980	8–12	5	NR[b]	4	NR[c]	NR[c]	NR[c]	1	1	NR	1	NR
USDA, 1988a	4–6	4	NR	4	4	NR[c]	NR[c]	NR[c]	NR[c]	NR	NR[c]	NR
Virginia Department of Health, 1981	6–9	3–4[d]	NR	4	NR[c]	NR[c]	NR[c]	1	1	NR	2	NR
American Red Cross, 1984	6–7	3	4	>8	NR[c]	3–4	3–5[c]	NR[c]	NR[c]	NR	NR[c]	NR
Michigan Department of Public Health, 1984	6	4	6	6	6[f]	NR[c]	NR[c]	2	1	NR	NR[c]	NR
USDA, 1984	6–7	3	4	>8	NR[c]	2–4	3–5	NR[c]	1	1	1	NR
Bouden, 1985	8–12	5	NR	4	3	NR[c]	NR[c]	NR[c]	NR[c]	NR	NR[c]	NR
Alabama Department of Public Health, 1987	4–6	4–6	6	>6	>5	NR[c]	NR[c]	NR[c]	NR[c]	NR	NR[c]	NR
California Department of Health Services, 1990	7	3	NR	7	3[g]	NR[c]	NR[c]	1	1	NR	NR[c]	3

[a]Protein servings refers to ounces of meat, poultry, or fish or the equivalent amount of protein from other sources. Serving sizes for other food groupings differed somewhat among the publications but were generally as follows: milk, 1 cup or the equivalent in calcium content; breads and cereals, 1 piece or 30 g (1 oz) dry; fruits and vegetables, 1 piece or 1/2 cup; unsaturated fat, 1 teaspoon or the equivalent amount of fat from selected sources.
[b]NR = No recommendation.
[c]See related columns in the row.
[d]Take five to six servings frequently.
[e]Include all types regularly.
[f]Include at least one raw fruit or vegetable.
[g]Exclusive of other fruits and vegetables specified in this row.

nutrient density of the total diet. Guides that specify many servings from some food groups may be difficult to follow if they depart greatly from typical eating patterns of the U.S. population. Although most food guides were developed to help individuals make food selections that would approach the RDAs, following them does not guarantee that the RDAs will be met. Only one of the food guides—the *Daily Food Guide for Women* (California Department of Health Services, 1990)—has been accompanied by an analysis demonstrating that following the guide will lead to nutrient intakes close to the RDAs (Newman and Lee, in press).

In providing food guidance, foods that are important sources of the nutrients most likely to be in short supply should be identified. A selection of important food sources of the key nutrients identified in this chapter is listed below. Many more foods contain smaller but still important amounts of these nutrients.

- *Calcium*: milk; cheese; yogurt; fish with edible bones; tofu processed with calcium sulfate; bok choy; broccoli; kale; collard, mustard, and turnip greens; breads made with milk.
- *Zinc*: meat, poultry, seafood, eggs, seeds, legumes, yogurt, whole grains (bioavailability from this source is variable).
- *Magnesium*: nuts, seeds, legumes, whole grains, green vegetables, scallops, and oysters (in general, this mineral is widely distributed in food rather than concentrated in a small number of foods).
- *Vitamin B_6*: bananas, poultry, meat, fish, potatoes, sweet potatoes, spinach, prunes, watermelon, some legumes, fortified cereals, and nuts.
- *Thiamin*: pork, fish, whole grains, organ meats, legumes, corn, peas, seeds, nuts, fortified cereal grain (widely distributed in foods).
- *Folate*: leafy vegetables, fruit, liver, green beans, fortified cereals, legumes, and whole-grain cereals.

CONCLUSIONS

- The total amounts of nutrients that the lactating mother secretes in her milk are directly related to the extent and duration of lactation.
- Lactating women who meet the RDA for energy are likely to meet the RDA for all nutrients except calcium and zinc if the nutrient density of their diets is close to the average for young U.S. women. If nutrient intake is lower than the total demand for both maternal maintenance needs and milk production (because of low energy intake, low nutrient density of the diet, or both), the mother's body will mobilize available nutrients from body tissues during lactation. The level of nutrient intake needed to prevent net mobilization is not known for individual women, but because the RDAs include a generous safety margin, it is likely to be below the RDA. At energy intakes less than 2,700 kcal/day, the nutrients for which intake is most likely to be low, relative to need, include calcium, magnesium, zinc, vitamin B_6, and folate.

TABLE 9-5   Suggested Measures for Improving Nutrient Intake of
Women with Restrictive Eating Patterns

Type of Restrictive Eating Pattern	Corrective Measures
Excessive restriction of food intake, i.e., ingestion of <1,800 kcal of energy per day, which ordinarily leads to unsatisfactory intake of nutrients compared with the amounts needed by lactating women	Encourage increased intake of nutrient-rich foods to achieve an energy intake of at least 1,800 kcal/day; if the mother insists on curbing food intake sharply, promote substitution of foods rich in vitamins, minerals, and protein for those lower in nutritive value; in individual cases, it may be advisable to recommend a balanced multivitamin-mineral supplement; discourage use of liquid weight loss diets and appetite suppressants
Complete vegetarianism, i.e., avoidance of all animal foods, including meat, fish, dairy products, and eggs	Advise intake of a regular source of vitamin B_{12}, such as special vitamin B_{12}-containing plant food products or a 2.6-μg vitamin B_{12} supplement daily
Avoidance of milk, cheese, or other calcium-rich dairy products	Encourage increased intake of other culturally appropriate dietary calcium sources, such as collard greens for blacks from the southeastern United States; provide information on the appropriate use of low-lactose dairy products if milk is being avoided because of lactose intolerance; if correction by diet cannot be achieved, it may be advisable to recommend 600 mg of elemental calcium per day taken with meals
Avoidance of vitamin D-fortified foods, such as fortified milk or cereal, combined with limited exposure to ultraviolet light	Recommend 10 μg of supplemental vitamin D per day

• To help them maintain satisfactory nutritional status, lactating women should be given sound nutrition information and encouraged to follow eating patterns that include frequent consumption of nutrient-rich foods, especially those that supply the minerals and vitamins listed above. Women who continue to breastfeed after return of their menses may benefit by increased consumption of iron-rich foods. Continued consumption of nutrient-rich diets after lactation may help to replenish body reserves of nutrients utilized during pregnancy and lactation.

• Selected groups of lactating women may need special attention to avoid nutritional problems in either themselves or their infants. These include groups with restricted eating patterns (such as complete vegetarians, women who diet to lose weight, and those who avoid dairy products), adolescents, and low-income women.

RECOMMENDATIONS FOR CLINICAL PRACTICE

● Encourage lactating women to follow dietary guidelines that promote a generous intake of nutrients from fruits and vegetables, whole-grain breads and cereals; calcium-rich dairy products; and protein-rich foods such as meats, fish, and legumes (see also Table 9-5). The evidence does not warrant recommending routine vitamin-mineral supplementation of lactating women.

● If dietary evaluation suggests that one or more nutrients may be provided in lower than recommended amounts by the diet of an individual woman, promote selection and consumption of more food choices that are rich in these nutrients.

● For women whose eating patterns lead to a very low intake of one or more nutrients, provide individualized diet counseling (preferred) or recommend nutrient supplementation as described in Table 9-5.

REFERENCES

Alabama Department of Public Health. 1987. Foods for the Nursing Mother: Food Plan for the Nursing Mother. WIC Program, Alabama Department of Public Health, Montgomery, Ala.

American Red Cross. 1984. Better Eating for Better Health: Participant's Guide. What Should I Feed My Baby? American Red Cross, Washington, D.C. 15 pp.

Andon, M.B., R.D. Reynolds, P.B. Moser-Veillon, and M.P. Howard. 1989. Dietary intake of total and glycosylated vitamin B-6 and the vitamin B-6 nutritional status of unsupplemented lactating women and their infants. Am. J. Clin. Nutr. 50:1050-1058.

Baumslag, N. 1986. Breastfeeding: Cultural practices and variations. Pp. 621-642 in Human Lactation 2. Hamosh, M. and A.S. Goldman, eds. Plenum Press, New York.

Borschel, M.W., A. Kirksey, and R.E. Hannemann. 1986. Effects of vitamin B-6 intake on nurtiture and growth of young infants. Am. J. Clin. Nutr. 43:7-25.

Bouden, E.S. 1985. Health Practices to Improve Pregnancy Outcomes: A Guide for the Primary Care Practitioner. Pennsylvania Department of Health, Harrisburg, Pa. 237 pp.

Brown, C.M., A.M. Smith, and M.F. Picciano. 1986. Forms of human milk folacin and variation patterns. J. Pediatr. Gastroenterol. Nutr. 5:278-282.

Butte, N.F., D.H. Calloway, and J.L. Van Duzen. 1981. Nutritional assessment of pregnant and lactating Navajo women. Am. J. Clin. Nutr. 34:2216-2228.

California Department of Health Services, Maternal and Child Health Branch and WIC Supplemental Foods Branch. 1990. Dietary guidelines and daily food guide. Pp. 59-92 in Nutrition During Pregnancy and Postpartum Period: A Manual for Health Care Professionals. Department of Health Services, Sacramento, Calif.

Chang, S., and A. Kirksey. 1990. Pyridoxine supplementation of lactating mothers: relation to maternal nutrition status and vitamin B-6 concentrations in milk. Am. J. Clin. Nutr. 51:826-831.

DHHS (Department of Health and Human Services). 1980. Breast Feeding. DHHS Publ. No. (HSA) 80-5109. Health Services Administration, Public Health Service, U.S. Department of Health and Human Services, Rockville, Md. 22 pp.

Ek, J. 1983. Plasma, red cell, and breast milk folacin concentrations in lactating women. Am. J. Clin. Nutr. 38:929-935.

Fenuku, R.I., and S.N. Earl-Quarcoo. 1978. Serum calcium, magnesium and inorganic phosphate during lactation. Trop. Geogr. Med. 30:495-498.

Greenwald, J.H., A. Dubin, and L. Cardon. 1963. Hypo-magnesium tetany due to excessive lactation. Am. J. Med. 35:854-860.

Halloran, B.P., and H.F. DeLuca. 1980. Calcium transport in small intestine during pregnancy and lactation. Am. J. Physiol. 239:E64-E68.

Jackson, M.J., R. Giugliano, L.G. Giugliano, E.F. Oliveira, R. Shrimpton, and I.G. Swainbank. 1988. Stable isotope metabolic studies of zinc nutrition in slum-dwelling lactating women in the Amazon valley. Br. J. Nutr. 59:193-203.

Kamble, T.K., and D.S. Ookalkar. 1989. Lactational hypomagnesaemia. Lancet 2:155-156.

Kirksey, A., and J.L.B. Roepke. 1981. Vitamin B_6 nutriture of mothers of three breast-fed neonates with central nervous system disorders. Fed. Proc., Fed. Am. Soc. Exp. Biol. 40:864.

Krebs, N.F., K.M. Hambidge, M.A. Jacobs, and J.O. Rasbach. 1985. The effects of dietary zinc supplement during lactation on longitudinal changes in maternal zinc status and milk zinc concentrations. Am. J. Clin. Nutr. 41:560-570.

LSRO (Life Sciences Research Office). 1984. Assessment of the Folate Nutritional Status of the U.S. Population Based on Data Collected in the Second National Health and Nutrition Examination Survey, 1976-1980. Federation of American Societies for Experimental Biology, Bethesda, Md. 96 pp.

Martinez, O.B. 1980. Red cell folate values of a group of non pregnant mothers. Can. J. Public Health 71:163-169.

Mbofung, C.M.F., and T. Atinmo. 1985. Zinc, copper and iron concentrations in the plasma and diets of lactating Nigerian women. Br. J. Nutr. 53:427-439.

McCoy, E., K. Strynadka, and K. Brunet. 1985. Vitamin B_6 intake and whole blood levels of breast and formula fed infants: serial whole blood vitamin B_6 levels in premature infants. Curr. Top. Nutr. Dis. 13:79-96.

Metz, J. 1970. Folate deficiency conditioned by lactation. Am. J. Clin. Nutr. 23:843-847.

Michigan Department of Public Health. 1984. Breastfeeding: A Special Gift. H-828. Bureau of Health Promotion and Disease Prevention, Michigan Department of Public Health, Lansing, Mich. 36 pp.

Moser, P.B., and R.D. Reynolds. 1983. Dietary zinc intake and zinc concentrations of plasma, erythrocytes, and breast milk in antepartum and postpartum lactating and nonlactating women: a longitudinal study. Am. J. Clin. Nutr. 38:101-108.

Moser, P.B., C.F. Issa, and R.D. Reynolds. 1983. Dietary magnesium intake and the concentration of magnesium in plasma and erythrocytes of postpartum women. J. Am. Coll. Nutr. 4:387-396.

Moser, P.B., R.D. Reynolds, S. Acharya, M.P. Howard, M.B. Andon, and L.A. Lewis. 1988. Copper, iron, zinc, and selenium dietary intake and status of Nepalese lactating women and their breast-fed infants. Am. J. Clin. Nutr. 47:729-734.

NCHS (National Center for Health Statistics). 1983. Dietary Intake Source Data: United States, 1976-80. Vital and Health Statistics, Series 11, No. 231. DHHS Publ. No. (PHS) 83-1681. National Center for Health Statistics, Public Health Service, U.S. Department of Health and Human Services, Hyattsville, Md. 483 pp.

Newman, V., and D. Lee. In press, 1991. Developing a Daily Food Guide for Women. J. Nutr. Educ. 23(2).

NRC (National Research Council). 1980. Recommended Dietary Allowances, 9th ed. Report of the Committee on Dietary Allowances, Food and Nutrition Board, Division of Biological Sciences, Assembly of Life Sciences. National Academy Press, Washington, D.C. 185 pp.

NRC (National Research Council). 1986. Nutrient Adequacy: Assessment Using Food Consumption Surveys. Report of the Subcommittee on Criteria for Dietary Evaluation, Coordinating Committee on Evaluation of Food Consumption Surveys, Food and Nutrition Board, Commission on Life Sciences. National Academy Press, Washington, D.C. 146 pp.

NRC (National Research Council). 1989. Recommended Dietary Allowances, 10th ed. Report of the Subcommittee on the Tenth Edition of the RDAs, Food and Nutrition Board, Commission on Life Sciences. National Academy Press, Washington, D.C. 284 pp.

Pennington, J.A.T., B.E. Young, and D.B. Wilson. 1989. Nutritional elements in U.S. diets: results from the Total Diet Study, 1982 to 1986. J. Am. Diet. Assoc. 89:659-664.

Qvist, I., M. Abdulla, M. Jägerstad, and S. Svensson. 1986. Iron, zinc and folate status during pregnancy and two months after delivery. Acta Obstet. Gynecol. Scand. 65:15-22.

Reynolds, R.D., M.B. Andon, and P.B. Moser-Veillon. 1990. Reply to M.W. Borschel and A. Kirksey (letter). Am. J. Clin. Nutr. 51:1116-1117.

Styslinger, L., and A. Kirksey. 1985. Effects of different levels of vitamin B_6 supplementation on vitamin B_6 concentrations in human milk and vitamin B_6 intakes of breastfed infants. Am. J. Clin. Nutr. 41:21-31.

Tamura, T., Y. Yoshimura, and T. Arakawa. 1980. Human milk folate and folate status in lactating mothers and their infants. Am. J. Clin. Nutr. 33:193-197.

USDA (U.S. Department of Agriculture). 1984. Promoting Breastfeeding: A Guide for Health Professionals Working in the WIC and CSF Programs. FNS-247. Food and Nutrition Service, U.S. Department of Agriculture, Alexandria, Va. 51 pp.

USDA (U. S. Department of Agriculture). 1987. Nationwide Food Consumption Survey. Continuing Survey of Food Intakes by Individuals. Women 19-50 Years and Their Children 1-5 Years, 1 Day, 1986. Report No. 86-1. Nutrition Monitoring Division, Human Nutrition Information Service, U.S. Department of Agriculture, Hyattsville, Md. 98 pp.

USDA (U.S. Department of Agriculture). 1988a. How WIC Helps: Eating for You and Your Baby. Program Aid No. 1198. Food and Nutrition Service, U.S. Department of Agriculture, Alexandria, Va. 6 pp.

USDA (U.S. Department of Agriculture). 1988b. Nationwide Food Consumption Survey. Continuing Survey of Food Intakes by Individuals. Low-Income Women 19-50 Years and Their Children 1-5 Years, 4 Days, 1985. Report No. 85-5. Nutrition Monitoring Division, Human Nutrition Information Service, U.S. Department of Agriculture, Hyattsville, Md. 220 pp.

Virginia Department of Health. 1981. Breastfeeding: The Best Feeding for Your Baby. WIC Program, Bureau of Nutrition, Virginia Department of Health, Richmond, Va. 7 pp.

10

Research Recommendations

Throughout this report, many unanswered questions were encountered concerning the nutritional status of lactating women and links between maternal nutrition and both infant and maternal health. The subcommittee concluded that research is needed to develop indicators of nutritional status during lactation, to identify groups at risk of nutritional problems, and to determine effects of maternal nutritional status on various measures of lactation performance (such as the volume and composition of milk, the duration of lactation, and infant growth and health).

In the process of reviewing data concerning the nutrition of breastfeeding women, the subcommittee could not ignore the very different likelihood of breastfeeding given race or ethnic group, income, and region of residence in the United States. Indeed, the most disadvantaged groups, which would be the groups most likely to benefit from breastfeeding, were found to have the lowest breastfeeding rates. Many factors other than maternal nutrition influence both a woman's desire to breastfeed and her success in doing so. To implement the subcommittee's recommendations for breastfeeding, it is desirable to know much more about the determinants of breastfeeding. To investigate the effects of maternal nutrition on the milk, the infant, and the mother herself, much more information is needed on the interactions between milk production, infant demand, and maternal nutrient intake and stores, as well as on the transfer of nutrients from mother to milk and the factors regulating this process.

The following recommendations are not listed in order of priority.

RECOMMENDATIONS THAT FOCUS PRIMARILY ON NUTRITION

Following are the subcommittee's research recommendations that concern mainly the nutrition of the lactating woman or of her breastfed infant.

Indicators of Maternal Nutritional Status

• **Research is needed to develop indicators of nutritional status for lactating women.**

First, the identification of normative values for nutritional status should be based on observations of representative, healthy, lactating women in the United States. In addition, indicators are needed both of (1) risks of adverse outcomes related to the mother's dietary intake and (2) the potential of the mother or her nursing infant to benefit from interventions designed to improve their nutritional status or health.

Identification of Groups of Mothers Who Need Nutritional Intervention

• **Research is needed to identify groups of lactating women in the United States who are at nutritional risk or who could benefit from nutrition intervention programs.**

In general, it has been difficult to identify groups of mothers and infants in the United States with nutritional deficits that are severe enough to have measurable functional consequences. Priority should be given to the study of lactating women in subpopulations believed to be at risk of inadequate intake of certain nutrients, such as calcium (black women) and vitamin A (low-income women). The potential influence of culture-specific food beliefs on nutrient intake of lactating women should be included in any such investigations.

Maternal Nutrition and Lactation Performance

• **Intervention studies of improved design and technical sophistication are needed to investigate the effects of maternal diet and nutritional status on milk volume; milk composition; infant nutritional status, growth, and health; and maternal health.**

The nursing dyad (the mother and her infant) has seldom been the focus of studies. Thus, a key aspect of this recommendation is concurrent examination of the mother, the volume and composition of the milk, and the infant. The design of such research should be adequate for causal inference; thus, if possible, it should include random assignment of lactating subjects to treatment groups. Appropriate sampling and handling of milk for the valid assessment of energy density, nutrient concentration, and total milk volume are essential, as is accurate measurement of nutrient concentrations.

With regard to energy balance of lactating women, the threshold below which energy intake is insufficient to support adequate milk production has not yet been identified. Resolution of this question will probably require supplementation studies of women in developing countries whose diets are chronically energy deficient. Although such deficient diets are not common in the United States, identification of the level of energy intake that is too low to support lactation will be useful in establishing guidelines for women who want to breastfeed but also want to restrict their energy intake to lose weight. Although chronically low energy intakes by women in disadvantaged populations may not be completely analogous to acute energy restriction among otherwise well-nourished women, ethical considerations limit the kinds of investigations that could directly address the influence of energy restriction. In supplementation studies, measurements should be made of lactation performance and of any impact on the mother's nutritional status and health, including the period of lactation amenorrhea.

With regard to specific nutrients, the impact of relatively low intakes of folate, vitamin B_6, calcium, zinc, and magnesium during lactation on the mother's nutritional status and health needs to be assessed in more detail. As a part of this assessment, studies of the absorption of calcium, zinc, and magnesium during lactation will be useful. There is also a need to identify a reliable indicator of vitamin B_6 status of infants and to document the relationships between this indicator, maternal vitamin B_6 intake, and vitamin B_6 content in milk. Finally, resolution of the conflicting findings concerning the impact of maternal protein intake on milk volume would be desirable.

Physical Activity, Energy Intake, and Lactation

- **The impact of high levels of physical activity on milk volume, milk composition, and duration of lactation requires further study, especially in populations in which energy intake is low relative to total need. Such research should be designed to identify the relative energy deficit imposed by high levels of physical activity.**

With greater numbers of women involved in physically demanding work and with increased interest in physical fitness, an increased number of women in the United States may need or want to resume heavy physical activity post partum. The potential impact of such activity on lactation is unknown.

Maternal Nutrition and the Infant's Immune Function

- **Studies should be conducted to determine relationships, if any, between the nutritional status of the mother, the concentrations and functions of the components of the immunologic system in human milk, and the susceptibility of the recipient infant to common infectious agents.**

Desirable design features of these studies include categorization of sufficient numbers of breastfeeding women according to their nutritional status, measurement of the levels and functions of key immunologic agents in human milk, monitoring of the immune system of the infants, and determination of the incidence and severity of common infections in the nursing dyad during the study periods.

Currently, there are conflicting reports concerning the effects of maternal nutritional status upon the immunologic system in human milk. If the nutritional status of the mother alters the levels or functions of those defense agents in human milk, it would be important to investigate how low dietary intake by the mother influences the recipient infant's risk for infectious diseases compared with that of breastfed infants of well-nourished mothers, as well as that of formula-fed infants. If relationships between maternal diet and infant risk are found, studies are warranted to investigate whether nutritional supplementation of the mother corrects the problem.

Indices of Nutritional Status of Infants

• **Improved indices are needed for the evaluation of specific nutrient status.**

Most estimates of nutrient requirements of infants are based on measurements of specific nutrient intakes of exclusively breastfed infants. This approach often is the result of inadequate alternatives for the assessment of the status of specific nutrients (e.g., vitamin B_6, folate, and zinc). Improved indices of nutrient status depend upon a better understanding of the role of specific nutrients in the normal development of functional capacities. The need for population-based studies and more detailed metabolic approaches is evident for both practical purposes (clinical recommendations and management) and an improved understanding of the physiology of normal development.

Absorption and Utilization of Nutrients from Human Milk

• **The bioavailability of specific nutrients (especially folate and iron) in human milk merits study, as does the biological basis for the high efficiency of nutrient utilization by breastfed infants.**

Reviews of the composition of human milk and the general nutritional status of breastfed infants indicate that nutrients in human milk are highly bioavailable and that they are utilized with a high degree of efficiency. Mechanisms that account for these observations are not understood. An improved understanding of these observations should lead to knowledge of normal nutrient needs, better human milk substitutes, and more effective nutritional management of high-risk infants, such as very-low-birth-weight infants and infants with impaired gastrointestinal and renal function.

RECOMMENDATIONS THAT FOCUS ON NONNUTRITIONAL FACTORS INFLUENCING BREASTFEEDING

Determinants of Breastfeeding

• **Given the decrease since 1982 in the percentage of mothers who breastfeed, further research is needed to identify the determinants of the decision to both initiate and continue breastfeeding among U.S. women in general and, in particular, among adolescents, those with limited education, and black, Hispanic, and other minority women.**

Such research should use methods designed to elucidate maternal beliefs and values, as well as situational factors related to infant-feeding practices. Special attention should be given to the beliefs and attitudes women hold regarding the interaction of maternal diet and nutritional status with breastfeeding.

Current data are limited to a few very small studies. Knowledge of beliefs, attitudes, and situational factors is necessary for both breastfeeding promotion and effective nutritional counseling of lactating women.

Health Care in Support of Lactation

• **Research is needed to study how various approaches to the health care of lactating women (and those who plan to breastfeed) affect their lactation performance.**

Such care would include nutritional screening or evaluation of the mother, nutritional guidance based on this screening, and guidance in establishing breastfeeding. It would be useful to compare approaches used prenatally, at an early (1 to 2 weeks post partum) office or home visit, and during the usual visit at 4 to 6 weeks post partum.

Since mothers are routinely discharged from the hospital within 24 to 48 hours after delivery, little time is available to encourage lactation or to cover other aspects of health education. Breastfeeding problems such as engorgement, sore nipples, delayed milk supply, and weak suck are most common in the first week post partum; they usually occur after the mother has left the hospital and is no longer in direct contact with health care providers. The first week post partum is also a useful time for checking the neonate's weight and for monitoring the neonate for health problems such as jaundice. After delivery, the mother is likely to be highly receptive to educational messages regarding her food intake during lactation and the overall health and nutrition of her infant. Home visits provide opportunities for assessment of resources and environmental conditions that could affect the mother's nutrition or her overall health and ability to breastfeed.

Maternal Anxiety, Stress, and Illness

• **Studies are needed to investigate the potential influence of maternal anxiety, stress, and illness on milk volume and composition.**

Such research would need to include various measures of anxiety and stress—acute and chronic, as well as physical and emotional.

Although certain types of acute physical stress have been associated with impairment of the milk-ejection reflex, there is no information on effects of the more common emotional stresses of caring for a newborn and coping with other demands of family, with work, or with either lack or loss of income.

RECOMMENDATIONS THAT FOCUS PRIMARILY ON GROWTH AND HEALTH

Infant Growth

• **Growth charts are needed that characterize the growth of breastfed infants.**

Acceptable approaches for developing such charts include either (1) the collection of longitudinal data, preferably monthly, on length, weight, extent of breastfeeding, and demographic variables from a large, representative sample of infants or (2) the application of appropriate statistical methods to data from a smaller sample of healthy infants who are breastfed throughout the first year of life. Development of the charts should be accompanied by studies designed to distinguish between normal and faltering growth of breastfed infants, using functional outcomes such as physical activity, mental and motor development, and morbidity.

Current infant growth charts were developed using data derived from infants who were primarily formula fed during a period when infant-feeding practices differed considerably from those in use today. Evidence from several studies suggests that growth rates of infants breastfed on demand differ from those illustrated on available growth charts.

Data on normative growth have been recently published for infants followed in Iowa between 1965 and 1987 (Nelson et al., 1989). They are not fully appropriate for constructing growth charts for breastfed infants since those infants were followed only just past the third month of age, the breastfed infants were allowed up to 240 ml of formula per day, and, before 1979, all infants were permitted to receive solid foods beginning at age 1 month.

To interpret the growth charts developed, criteria are needed for identifying a cutoff below which growth rates are unsatisfactory.

Psychological Health of Mother and Infant

• **Studies should be conducted to investigate the psychological benefits of breastfeeding to the mother and infant.**

It is widely believed that breastfeeding has powerful psychological benefits for the mother and infant. Nonetheless, there is relatively little scientific evidence to support that belief. If this belief is correct, the public health implications would be profound. Some of the specific points that should be addressed are the effects of breastfeeding upon the self-esteem of the mother, the mother's concerns with parenting, the ability of the mother to deal with social problems in her family, social interactions between the mother and the infant, the social development of the infant, the ability of the child to adapt to new environmental circumstances, and the possibility that observed effects are related to the transfer of substances to the infant through the milk.

Infant Mortality

• **It is essential to determine whether and to what extent breastfeeding protects against infant and early child mortality in populations with generally low rates of infant mortality, and especially in subpopulations with higher than usual infant and child mortality rates.**

The rates of infant and early childhood mortality are at or near their historically lowest levels in the industrialized countries; nevertheless, there is every reason to believe that breastfeeding would still confer some benefit on survival. It is unknown at the moment whether infant and early childhood mortality rates are lower among breastfed infants in situations in which death rates are generally low. This information is particularly important among subpopulations, such as ethnic minorities, many of which have higher mortality rates than the population at large.

Use of Substances

• **The potential influence of maternal smoking and moderate alcohol and coffee consumption on milk production, composition, and infant health requires further investigation.**

Data are needed on the direct effects of smoking on milk volume, not just on plasma prolactin levels. Studies should include consideration of dose-related effects.

At present, there is no clear basis for determining the level of cigarette smoking or alcohol consumption that could harm the infant. Although the recommendation is not to smoke at all and to drink alcoholic beverages in moderation, if at all, many women may not follow this advice. Furthermore, preliminary evidence from Costa Rica (Muñoz et al., 1988) suggests that coffee intake may affect milk iron concentration and infant iron status, but studies of women in other populations and with lower coffee intakes (<3 cups/day) are needed.

Human Immunodeficiency Virus

• **Investigations should be performed to ascertain whether human immunodeficiency virus (HIV) infection is transmitted to the recipient infant via breastfeeding, whether there are other health effects of breastfeeding upon infants who are otherwise infected with HIV, and whether breastfeeding has harmful or beneficial effects on the health of the mother infected with HIV.**

Current public health policies concerning breastfeeding and HIV are based upon a very limited, somewhat anecdotal data base. Moreover, the two principal public health pronouncements are at odds with each other: the first precludes breastfeeding (CDC, 1985), whereas the second encourages breastfeeding in the case of HIV-infected mothers (WHO, 1987). Systematic studies are therefore required to determine the following:

—To what extent is HIV excreted in the milk of HIV-positive women?

—Is the excretion of HIV in human milk limited to mothers who have received HIV-contaminated blood during the perinatal period?

—If HIV is present in human milk, does it present a risk to the recipient infant who was not exposed prenatally, does it increase the risk for an infant who was infected prenatally, or does it immunize against the infection?

—Does human milk inhibit the growth of or kill HIV?

—Does breastfeeding have a salutary effect upon the HIV-infected infant by defending the recipient against complicating opportunistic agents?

—Does the increased nutritional burden of lactation decrease the resistance of HIV-infected women to the infection?

—Do other changes during lactation, such as the secretion of lactogenic hormones, affect the ability of the immunologic system of the woman to deal with this retrovirus?

Long-Term Health of the Recipient of Human Milk

• **Long-term studies should be conducted to determine whether breastfeeding protects against chronic conditions that first become apparent in later life.**

These conditions include atopic disorders; type I diabetes mellitus; obesity; atherosclerosis, hypertension, and other chronic cardiovascular diseases; inflammatory bowel disease; and lymphoma and other malignancies. Research on these issues should include measures of the duration of exclusive and partial breastfeeding, timing of introduction of other foods, and family history of the condition, among other variables.

There are a number of retrospective studies that suggest that breastfeeding may reduce the risks of developing certain chronic conditions later in life. If that is the case, then the public health advantages of breastfeeding transcend the immediate period of breastfeeding. Possible benefits are great since these conditions are not readily amenable to definitive therapy, and their related health care costs are very high. Thus, more definitive prospective studies and more detailed retrospective cohort and case-control studies of groups at high risk for the condition are warranted. If long-term protective effects are confirmed, studies should be conducted to ascertain whether the effects are modified by maternal nutrition. If the positive findings are borne out or extended, they would provide a further indication for promoting breastfeeding among the entire U.S. population.

Health Effects of Lactation on Women with Chronic Diseases

• **Investigations are needed of the effects of lactation on the health of women who have specific chronic diseases (such as type I diabetes mellitus, cystic fibrosis, and hypertriglyceridemias).**

The subcommittee's review indicates that information on women with underlying chronic diseases is particularly limited. Consequently, there is incomplete understanding of adjustments that may be necessary during lactation in the clinical management of those conditions. Surveys and detailed metabolic studies of specific populations are indicated to determine the extent to which current infant feeding recommendations apply to this group of women.

Effects of Chronic Diseases on Lactation

• **Investigations of the effects of specific chronic diseases (such as diabetes mellitus and cystic fibrosis) on the process of lactation are needed.**

Improved understanding of lactation in healthy women provides a basis for investigations of the impact of underlying chronic diseases on that physiologic process. The metabolic adjustments made during lactation involve nearly every maternal organ system. Knowledge of changes in lactation resulting from relevant pathophysiologies will enhance the understanding of normal lactation and provide a basis for the improved management of the lactating woman and her breastfed infant.

Short-Term and Long-Term Health of the Mother

- **Studies are required that investigate short-term effects (changes in body weight, sexuality, and behavior, as well as incidence of infectious disease) and long-term effects (such as obesity, osteoporosis, and specific cancers) of lactation on the health of women.**

Breastfeeding recommendations usually are based on the expected effects on the infant's nutritional status, the infant's decreased susceptibility to infectious illnesses, and improved maternal-infant bonding. Benefits and risks to the mother are considered less often. As reviewed in Chapter 8, there are reasons to suspect that lactation may decrease the mother's risk of developing breast cancer and osteoporosis. Lactation's effects on maternal weight status is of particular short- and long-term interest. Given current recommendations regarding breastfeeding and the physiologic changes associated with lactation, a more thorough examination of maternal outcomes is central to the implementation of current policy and to helping women make fully informed choices.

REFERENCES

CDC (Centers for Disease Control). 1985. Recommendations for assisting in the prevention of perinatal transmission of human T-lymphotropic virus type III/lymphadenopathy-associated virus and acquired immunodeficiency syndrome. Morbid. Mortal. Wkly. Rep. 34:721-732.

Muñoz, L.M., B. Lönnerdal, C.L. Keen, and K.G. Dewey. 1988. Coffee consumption as a factor in iron deficiency anemia among pregnant women and their infants in Costa Rica. Am. J. Clin. Nutr. 48:645-651.

Nelson, S.E., R.R. Rogers, E.E. Ziegler, and S.J. Fomon. 1989. Gain in weight and length during early infancy. Early Hum. Dev. 19:223-239.

WHO (World Health Organization). 1987. Breast-feeding/breast milk and human immunodeficiency virus (HIV). Weekly Epidemiol. Rec. 62:245-246.

Appendixes

Appendix
A

Appendix A presents a compilation of abstracts of studies that address relationships of the mode of infant feeding with the infant's subsequent survival. Abstracts are presented in either tabular or narrative form and are arranged chronologically by type of study (mortality rates, relative risk, or both; case fatality; and miscellaneous). Table A-1 presents a chronological listing of the data and indicates the location of each abstract.

TABLE A-1 Chronological Listing of Estimated Relative Risk (RR) of Mortality in Industrialized Countries Among Children Fed Formula Only or Formula Plus Human Milk Compared with Breastfed Infants and Children[a]

Period and Site of Study	RR[b] Bottle	RR[b] Mixed	Type of Study and Abstract Providing Detailed Description	Reference
1869–1910, Three German states	NA[c]	NA	Correlation, A-21	Knodel and van de Walle, 1967
1885–1886 Berlin, Germany	4.0– 10.8[d]	NA	Mortality rates, A-1	Thiemich and Bessau, 1930; reviewed in Mannheimer, 1955
1895–1896 Berlin, Germany	4.1– 14.2[d]	NA	Mortality rates, A-1	Thiemich and Bessau, 1930; reviewed in Mannheimer, 1955
1900–1903, Derby, England	2.83	1.41	Mortality rates, A-2	Howarth, 1905
1900–1904, Kingdom of Bavaria, Germany	NA	NA	Correlation, A-22	Greenwood and Brown, 1912
1901–1905, Finsbury, London	27.5	9.8	Case-control, A-3	Newman, 1906
NR[e] Liverpool, England	2.71[f], 2.49[g]	1.59[f], 0.92[g]	Mortality rates, A-4	Armstrong, 1904
1903–1905, Brighton, England	35.1	3.1	Case-control, A-5	Newsholme, 1906, reviewed in Newman, 1906
1906, Berlin, Germany	2.6– 10.9[d]	NA	Mortality rates, A-1	Thiemich and Bessau, 1930; reviewed in Mannheimer, 1955
1910, Boston, Mass.	6.06	NA	Mortality rates, A-6	Davis, 1913
1924–1929, Chicago, Ill.	5.6	4.6	Mortality rates, A-7	Grulee et al., 1934, 1935
NR, Birmingham, England	4.59	1.55	Case-fatality, A-17	Smellie, 1939
NR, Toronto, Canada	0.89	0.65	Case-fatality, A-18	Ebbs and Mulligan, 1942
1936–1942, Liverpool, England	5.62	2.52	Mortality rates, A-8	Robinson, 1951
1941–1942, Belfast, Ireland	5.15– 13.72[d]	NA	Mortality rates, A-9	Deeny and Murdock, 1944
1943–1947, Stockholm, Sweden	1.34– 1.75[f]	0.63– 0.66[f]	Mortality rates, A-10	Mannheimer, 1955
1942 and 1943, Isleworth, England	1.96	NA	Case-fatality, A-19	Gairdner, 1945

Table A-1 continues

TABLE A-1 Continued

1943–1946, Louisville, Ky.	NA	NA	Case-fatality, A-20	Prince and Bruce, 1948
1946, Great Britain	1.7^h	NA	Mortality rates, A-11	Douglas, 1950
1956–1971, Copenhagen, Denmark	NA	NA	Case-control, A-12	Biering-Sorensen et al., 1978
1959–1966, United States	NA	NA	Mortality rates, A-13	Naeye et al., 1976
1962, Canada	2.03	NA	Mortality rates, A-14	Department of National Health and Welfare, Canada, 1963, as quoted in Gerard and Tan (1978)
1973–1979, Sheffield, England	NA	NA	Postnatal intervention, A-15	Carpenter et al., 1983
NR, United States	NA	NA	Case-control, A-16	Arnon et al., 1982

[a]The bases for the estimates of relative risk are shown in Abstracts A-1 through A-19. Relative risks computed for these studies represent somewhat different comparisons. For example, mortality might be compared for infants at different ages or for infants hospitalized with diarrhea.

[b]Relative risk for breastfed infants = 1.0.

[c]NA = Data not available for estimating relative risk.

[d]Range covers values from 1 to 12 months of age.

[e]NR = Period not reported.

[f]To age 1 year.

[g]To age 2 weeks.

[h]To age 2 years, comparison of infants breastfed for 8 weeks or longer with those breastfed for less than 8 weeks.

MORTALITY RATES AND RELATIVE RISK OF MORTALITY

ABSTRACT A-1   Infant Deaths/1,000 Births and Relative Risk (RR) of Death, by Feeding Method and Month of Age, Berlin, Germany, Between 1885 and 1906[a,b]

Years	Age of Mortality, mo	Number of Infant Deaths/1,000 Births by Feeding Method		RR[c]
		Breast	Bottle	
1885–1886	1	22.4	142.0	6.3
	2	9.0	82.7	9.2
	3	6.8	72.2	10.6
	4	6.4	61.8	9.7
	5	5.3	57.1	10.8
	6	4.9	50.7	10.3
	7	4.7	46.5	9.9
	8	4.5	40.8	9.1
	9	5.3	33.3	6.3
	10	5.4	29.5	5.5
	11	6.3	24.9	4.0
	12	NA[d]	NA	NA
1895–1896	1	19.6	111.9	5.7
	2	7.3	58.7	8.0
	3	4.3	49.7	11.6
	4	3.6	46.6	12.9
	5	2.6	37.0	14.2
	6	2.5	31.0	12.4
	7	2.5	27.7	11.1
	8	2.3	24.1	10.5
	9	2.0	21.3	10.7
	10	3.8	19.1	5.0
	11	3.1	16.7	5.4
	12	3.6	14.6	4.1
1906	1	22.4	59.1	2.6
	2	7.9	31.3	4.0
	3	4.3	27.3	6.3
	4	2.4	22.1	9.2
	5	1.7	18.5	10.9
	6	2.2	16.1	7.3
	7	1.4	14.1	10.1
	8	1.8	12.2	6.8
	9	2.1	10.2	4.9
	10	1.5	9.2	6.1
	11	1.3	8.0	6.2
	12	1.5	8.0	5.3

[a]From Thiemich and Bessau (1930), as quoted in Mannheimer (1955).
[b]Data on feeding practices were collected for all deaths and during census for survivors.
[c]Relative risk for breastfed infants = 1.0.
[d]NA = Not available.

ABSTRACT A-2   Infant Deaths/1,000 Births and Relative Risk (RR) of Mortality by Feeding Method, Derby, England, 1900 to 1903[a]

Specific Causes of Mortality	Number of Infant Deaths/1,000 Births (RR) by Feeding Method		
	Breast	Bottle	Mixed
All causes	69.8	197.5 (2.83)[b]	98.7 (1.41)
Respiratory diseases	14.1	26.5 (1.84)	12.6 (0.88)
Gastrointestinal diseases	9.9	57.8 (5.84)	25.0 (2.53)
Marasmus	12.5	39.4 (3.15)	18.8 (1.50)
Tuberculosis	3.4	13.5 (3.97)	5.6 (1.65)
Convulsions	15.0	25.9 (1.73)	20.9 (1.39)

[a]From Howarth (1905).
[b]Relative risk for breastfed infants = 1.

COMMENTS: Feeding history was obtained during infant's life; of the 8,343 infants studied, 63.3% were breastfed, 27.3% were mixed fed, and 19.5% were formula fed.

ABSTRACT A-3   Feeding Practices and Relative Risk (RR) of Death from Diarrhea in a Case-Control Study of Infants Aged 0 to 3 Months, Finsbury, London, England, 1901 to 1905[a]

Feeding Method	Infants Fed by Each Method, %		RR
	Infants Who Died (N = 118)	Surviving Infants (N = 1,822)	
Breast	22.0	80.8	1.0
Bottle	52.5	7.0	27.5
Mixed	25.4	9.5	9.8

[a]From Newman (1906).

COMMENTS: Fascinating review of evidence to 1906, including lowered infant mortality during closing of Lancashire mills secondary to cutoff of cotton during American Civil War.

ABSTRACT A-4   Infant Deaths/1,000 Births and Relative Risk (RR) of Mortality by Feeding Method, Liverpool, England[a,b]

Specific Ages of Mortality	Number of Infant Deaths/1,000 Births (RR), by Feeding Method		
	Breast	Bottle	Mixed
Up to age 1 yr	84	228 (2.71)[b]	134 (1.59)
Age 1–2 yr	40	99 (2.49)	36 (0.92)

[a]From Armstrong (1904). Period of study not reported.
[b]Relative risk for breastfed infants = 1.

COMMENTS: Data from 1,000 children of 224 mothers attending the Infirmary for Children; 68.9% were breastfed, 18.4% were bottle fed, and 12.7% were mixed fed to age 6 months.

ABSTRACT A-5   Feeding Practices and Relative Risk (RR) of Epidemic Diarrhea Infant Death in a Case-Control Study in Brighton, England, 1903 to 1905[a]

	Infants Fed by Each Method, %		
Feeding Method	Infants Who Died (N = 121)	Surviving Infants (N = 1,259)	RR
Breast	6.5	62.3	1.0
Bottle	80.3	21.9	35.1
Mixed	5.0	15.3	3.1
Unknown	8.2	0.5	NA[b]

[a]From Newsholme (1906), as reviewed in Newman (1906).
[b]NA = Not applicable.

ABSTRACT A-6   Deaths/1,000 Births and Relative Risk (RR) of Mortality for Infants Aged 2 Weeks to 1 Year, by Feeding Method, Boston, 1910[a]

	Number of Infant Deaths/ 1,000 Births, by Feeding Method		
Cause of Mortality	Breast	Bottle	RR[b]
All causes	36	218	6.06
Diarrhea	9	98	12.25

[a]From Davis (1913). A case-control study of 1,600 deaths, plus mail questionnaires from mothers of 736 controls. It was unclear how mixed feeding was classified.
[b]Relative risk for breastfed infants = 1.

ABSTRACT A-7   Death Rates/1,000 Births and Relative Risk (RR) of Death for 20,061 Infants up to 1 Year of Age Served by Welfare Clinics in Chicago, 1924 to 1929[a]

Feeding Method	Death Rate/ 1,000 Births	RR
Breast	1.5	1.0
Bottle	8.4	5.6
Mixed	6.9	6.9

[a]From Grulee et al. (1934, 1935).

ABSTRACT A-8 Death Rates/1,000 Births and Relative Risk (RR) of Death for 3,266 Infants Aged 7 Months or Less, Liverpool, England, 1936 to 1942[a]

Feeding Method	Mortality/1,000 to Age 7 Months	RR
Breast	10.2	1.0
Bottle	57.3	5.62
Mixed	25.7	2.52

[a]From Robinson (1951).

COMMENTS: Excludes infants with birthweights of <2 kg (4.4 lb) who were "weakly" or whose clinic visits were discontinued before age 7 months. Mortality was attributed almost entirely to infections.

ABSTRACT A-9 Infant Deaths/1,000 Births and Relative Risk (RR) of Death, by Feeding Method and Age, Belfast, Ireland, June 1941 to June 1942[a]

Age of Mortality, mo	Number of Infant Deaths/1,000 Births by Feeding Method		RR[b]
	Breast	Bottle	
<1	7.5	103.0	13.72
1–2	5.0	38.0	7.68
2–3	3.4	43.5	12.76
3–6	5.7	43.4	7.57
6–12	7.1	36.8	5.15

[a]From Deeny and Murdock (1944). Results were estimated from authors' data. Based on 554 infant deaths plus 477 survivors (every fifth child during first 6 months of age).
[b]Relative risk for breastfed infants = 1.0.

ABSTRACT A-10   Deaths/1,000 Births and Relative Risk (RR) of Death for 67,738 Infants Who Survived the First Month, by Feeding Method, Age, and Cause of Death, 1943 to 1947, Stockholm, Sweden[a]

Age or Cause of Mortality	Death Rate/1,000 Births (RR) by Feeding Method		
	Breast[b]	Bottle	Mixed
Age 2–12 mo	4.63	8.12 (1.75)	3.08 (0.66)
Age 3–12 mo	3.19	6.48 (2.03)	2.90 (0.91)
Congenital disease	NR[c]	NR (1.73)	NR
Infections	NR	NR (1.28)	NR
Respiratory disease	NR	NR (2.55)	NR
Intestinal disease	NR	NR (6.79)	NR
Other causes	NR	NR (4.79)	NR

[a]From Mannheimer (1955).
[b]Relative risk for breastfed infants = 1.0.
[c]NR = Not reported.

COMMENTS: RRs were 3.66 and 4.32 for infants fed cow's milk exclusively from age 2 months. The apparent advantage of mixed feeding lasted less than 4 months. The apparent disadvantage of bottle feeding decreased after 6 months and was gone after 9 months. Compared with breastfed infants, a smaller proportion of bottle-fed infants received care at child welfare centers (64 and 48%, respectively). Rates were lower for mixed-fed than for breastfed infants in all categories except intestinal disease, for which they were equal. Excess deaths in the bottle-fed group were observed only among infants weighing >2,500 g at birth. Feeding method was unrelated to income.

ABSTRACT A-11   Death Rates/1,000 Births for 4,669 Infants Aged 8 Weeks to 2 Years and Relative Risk (RR) of Death by Duration of Breastfeeding, Great Britain, March 1946[a]

Duration of Breastfeeding, wk	Death Rate/1,000	RR
<8	18.5	1.7
≥8	10.9	1.0

[a]From Douglas (1950). Excludes infants from the upper classes.

COMMENTS: Among the upper classes, mortality was only slightly increased among those breastfed <8 weeks.

ABSTRACT A-12   Case-Control Study of Feeding Methods of Infants Developing Sudden Infant Death Syndrome (SIDS) and Control Infants, Copenhagen, 1956 to 1971[a]

Study Group	Feeding Method,[b] % (no.) of Infants		
	Breast	Bottle	Mixed
Cases	60.2 (74)	20.3 (25)	19.5 (24)
Controls	79.2[c] (412)	7.7 (40)	13.1 (68)

[a]From Biering-Sørensen et al. (1978).
[b]Feeding histories were derived from the notes of health visitors for both the sudden infant deaths and a selection of infants used as controls.
[c]$p < .0005$.

COMMENTS: Odds ratio for bottle feeding versus any breastfeeding at 2 weeks of age = 3.06. Authors review past work on SIDS and breastfeeding. Given that breastfeeding rates declined from 1956 to 1971, but SIDS incidence did not, authors conclude relationship is not causal.

ABSTRACT A-13   Naeye and colleagues (1976) investigated feeding methods in a study of 125 infants with sudden infant death syndrome (SIDS) and 375 controls, using data from the Collaborative Perinatal Project of the National Institute of Neurological and Communicative Disorders and Stroke, 1959 to 1966. The odds ratio for bottle feeding compared with breastfeeding was 1.30. Infants with SIDS had frequent neonatal problems, including abnormal suck, need for gavage feeding, and late initiation of bottle feeding, suggesting that the choice of feeding method may have been secondary to neonatal problems.

ABSTRACT A-14   Deaths/1,000 Births and Relative Risk (RR) of Death for 3,684 Infants Aged 1 to 12 Months, by Feeding Method, American Indians in Canada, 1962[a]

Cause of Death	Deaths/1,000 Births, by Feeding Method		RR[b]
	Breast	Bottle	
All causes	26.6	53.8	2.03
Gastrointestinal or respiratory disease	3.9	32.7	8.29

[a]From Department of National Health and Welfare Canada (1963), as quoted in Gerard and Tan (1978).
[b]Relative risk for breastfed infants = 1.0.

ABSTRACT A-15   Carpenter and colleagues (1983) used a complex analytic method in their investigation of infant death rates between 1973 and 1979 in Sheffield, England. During that time there was a program of postnatal intervention by health visitors for high-risk infants in Sheffield. Postneonatal mortality (deaths to infants 28 days to 1 year of age) fell far more steeply in the study group than it did in all of England and Wales. Among "preventable" deaths, rates fell from 5.2 to 1.9 per 1,000 births. (Among the study group, intention to breastfeed rose from 40 to 70%.) The authors attributed 24% of the fall in the death rate, or 0.8 deaths/1,000 births, to increased rates of breastfeeding.

ABSTRACT A-16   Feeding Methods of Infants Hospitalized with Infant Botulism, Infants with Sudden Infant Death Syndrome (SIDS), and Control Infants in California (1976 to 1979) and Elsewhere in the United States Through 1978[a]

Condition	Subject	Feeding Methods in Study Population, %		
		Breast	Formula	Mixed
Infant	Cases ($N = 50$)	66.0[b]	24.0[c]	10.0[d]
botulism	Controls ($N = 125$)	43.2[b]	33.6[c]	23.2[d]
SIDS	Cases ($N = 10$)	0	80.0	20.0
	Controls ($N = 20$)	30.0	35.0	35.0

[a]From Arnon et al. (1982).
[b]Current breastfeeding.
[c]Never breastfed.
[d]Past breastfeeding.

CASE FATALITY STUDIES

ABSTRACT A-17   Case Fatality and Relative Risk (RR) of Death by Method of Infant Feeding Among Infants Hospitalized with Diarrhea, Birmingham, England[a]

Feeding Method	Number of Infants Hospitalized	Number of Infant Deaths/1,000 Cases	RR
Breast	12	167	1.0
Bottle	209	766	4.59
Mixed	154	259	1.55

[a]From Smellie (1939). Of the 500 hospitalized infants, 375 were younger than 9 months of age.

ABSTRACT A-18 Case Fatality and Relative Risk (RR) of Death Among 1,500 Infants Hospitalized with Infections, by Method of Infant Feeding, Toronto, Canada[a]

Feeding Method	Number of Infants Hospitalized	Infant Deaths/ 1,000 Cases	RR
Breast	227	185	1.0
Bottle[b]	836	164	0.89
Mixed	437	121	0.65

[a]From Ebbs and Mulligan (1942).
[b]Never breastfed.

COMMENTS: This study is exceptional, given that higher case-fatality rates were observed among breastfed infants. The reported results may imply lower case fatalities in bottle- and mixed-fed infants but could have arisen in other ways. For example, severity of infection was lower among breastfed infants: only the most severe cases might have been hospitalized. Furthermore, the results do not imply that death rates were higher among breastfed infants: if the incidence among them was lower, the opposite could have been true. Finally, the attending clinician may have been loathe to hospitalize breastfed infants, and this also would have possibly selected for higher severity among the breastfed infants.

ABSTRACT A-19 Case Fatality and Relative Risk (RR) of Death of 216 Infants Hospitalized with Diarrhea, by Duration of Breastfeeding, Isleworth, England, 1942 and 1943[a]

Duration of Breastfeeding, mo	No. of Infant Deaths/1,000 Cases	RR
>1	300	1.00
<1	550	1.86

[a]From Gairdner (1945).

ABSTRACT A-20 Prince and Bruce (1948) investigated case fatalities among 570 infants hospitalized with diarrhea in Louisville, Ky., from 1943 to 1946. Although the overall case fatality was 11%, there were no deaths among infants still breastfed at the time of admission.

MISCELLANEOUS STUDIES

ABSTRACT A-21   Indices of Breastfeeding Correlated with Infant
Mortality in Three German States, by Location, 1869 to 1910[a]

Breastfeeding Index	Period of Breastfeeding Index	Period of Infant Mortality	Correlation Coefficients Between Infant Mortality and the Breastfeeding Index (number of cases)			
			State	Rural	Urban	Total
Proportion ever breastfed	1904–1906	1869–1878	Bavaria	− .80 (88)	− .87 (15)	− .81
		1901–1905	Bavaria	− .76 (91)	− .7 (17)	− .76
		1878–1882	Baden	− .54 (47)	NR[b]	− .54 (52)
Proportion breastfed ≥6 mo	1911	1873–1875	Hessen	− .59 (19)	NR	− .55 (24)
		1906–1910	Hessen	− .62 (19)	NR	− .61 (24)
Duration of breastfeeding	1904–1906	1869–1878	Bavaria	− .83 (76)	− .92 (14)	− .83
		1901–1905	Bavaria	− .71 (79)	− .68 (16)	− .70

[a]From Knodel and van de Walle (1967).
[b]NR = Not reported.

ABSTRACT A-22   In a reanalysis of data of Groth and Hahn (1910), Greenwood and Brown (1912) reported a correlation of .76 ± 0.03 between the
bottle-feeding rates and infant death rates from 92 districts of the Kingdom
of Bavaria, Germany, between 1900 and 1904.

REFERENCES

Armstrong, H. 1904. A note on the comparative mortality of breast-fed and hand-reared infants. Br. J. Child. Dis. 1:115-116.

Arnon, S.S., K. Damus, B. Thompson, T.F. Midura, and J. Chin. 1982. Protective role of human milk against sudden death from infant botulism. J. Pediatr. 100:568-573.

Biering-Sørensen, F., T. Jørgensen, and J. Hilden. 1978. Sudden infant death in Copenhagen 1956-1971. I. Infant feeding. Acta Paediatr. Scand. 67:129-137.

Carpenter, R.G., A. Gardner, M. Jepson, E.M. Taylor, A. Salvin, R. Sunderland, J.L. Emery, E. Pursall, and J. Roe. 1983. Prevention of unexpected infant death: evaluation of the first seven years of the Sheffield Intervention Programme. Lancet 1:723-727.

Davis, W.H. 1913. Statistical comparison of the mortality of breast-fed and bottle-fed infants. Am. J. Dis. Child. 5:234-247.

Deeny, J., and E.T. Murdock. 1944. Infant feeding in relation to mortality in the city of Belfast. Br. Med. J. 1:146-148.

Department of National Health and Welfare, Canada. 1963. Survey of Maternal and Child Health of Canadian Registered Indians 1962. Cited in Gerard, J.W., and K.K.T. Tan. 1978. Hazards of formula feeding. Keeping Abreast, Journal of Human Nurturing. 3:20-25.

Douglas, J.W.B. 1950. The extent of breast feeding in Great Britain in 1946, with special reference to the health and survival of children. J. Obstet. Gynecol. Br. Emp. 57:335-361.

Ebbs, J.H., and F. Mulligan. 1942. The incidence and mortality of breast- and artificially-fed infants admitted to hospital with infections. Arch. Dis. Child. 17:217-219.

Gairdner, P. 1945. Infantile diarrhoea: an analysis of 216 cases with special reference to institutional outbreaks. Arch. Dis. Child. 20:22-27.

Gerard, J.W., and K.K.T. Tan. 1978. Hazards of formula feeding. Keeping Abreast, Journal of Human Nurturing. 3:20-25.

Greenwood, M., Jr., and J.W. Brown. 1912. An examination of some factors influencing the rate of infant mortality. J. Hyg. 12:5-45.

Groth and Hahn. 1910. Die Säuglingsverhältnisse in Bayern. München (Lindauer) (Sonderabdr. a.d. Zeitschr. d. K. Bayer. Stat. Landesamts. Jahrg). Cited in Greenwood, M., Jr., and J.W. Brown. 1912. An examination of some factors influencing the rate of infant mortality. J. Hyg. 12:5-45.

Grulee, C.G., H.N. Sanford, and P.H. Herron. 1934. Breast and artificial feeding: influences on morbidity and mortality of twenty thousand infants. J. Am. Med. Assoc. 103:735-739.

Grulee, C.G., H.N. Sanford, and H. Schwartz. 1935. Breast and artificially fed infants: a study of the age incidence in the morbidity and mortality in twenty thousand cases. J. Am. Med. Assoc. 104:1986-1988.

Howarth, W.J. 1905. The influence of feeding on the mortality of infants. Lancet 2:210-213.

Knodel, J., and E. van de Walle. 1967. Breast feeding, fertility and infant mortality: an analysis of some early German data. Popul. Stud. 21:109-131.

Mannheimer, E. 1955. Mortality of breast fed and bottle fed infants: a comparative study. Acta Genet. Stat. Med. 5:134-163.

Naeye, R.L., B. Ladis, and J.S. Drage. 1976. Sudden infant death syndrome: a prospective study. Am. J. Dis. Child. 130:1207-1210.

Newman, G. 1906. Infant Mortality: A Social Problem. Methuen & Co, London. 356 pp.

Newsholme, A. 1906. Domestic infection in relation to epidemic diarrhoea. J. Hyg. 6:139-148.

Prince, G.E., and J.W. Bruce. 1948. Mortality of acute infantile diarrhea at the Louisville General Hospital from 1943 to 1947. J. Pediatr. 33:342-345.

Robinson, M. 1951. Infant morbidity and mortality: a study of 3266 infants. Lancet 1:788-794.

Smellie, J.M. 1939. Infantile diarrhoea. Lancet 236:969-973.

Thiemich, M., and G. Bessau. 1930. Allgemeiner Teil. Pp. 1-100 in E. Feer, ed. Lehrbuch der Kinderheilkunde, 10th ed. Fischer, Jena, Germany.

Appendix
B

Appendix B presents a compilation of abstracts of studies that address relationships of the mode of infant feeding with the infant's subsequent survival in developing countries. Abstracts are presented in either tabular or narrative form and are arranged chronologically.

ABSTRACT B-1A Death Rate and Relative Risk (RR) of Death by Feeding Method from Birth Among Infants Born in 11 Villages of the Ludhiana District, Punjab, India, 1955 to 1959[a]

| | | Death Rate/1,000 and RR, During First Year of Life | | | |
| | | 0–28 days | | 2–11 mo | |
Feeding Method at Birth	Sample Size	Number of Deaths/1,000	RR	Number of Deaths/1,000	RR
Breast	739	46	1.00	74	1.00
Bottle	20	750	16.30	200	2.70

[a]From Gordon et al. (1963).

ABSTRACT B-1B Mortality from Diarrheal Disease Among Children Breastfed at Birth[a]

Age, mo	Breastfed Only			Weaned During This Period			Previously Weaned		
	Sample Size	Cases of Diarrhea/100/yr[b]	Diarrheal Deaths/1,000/yr	Sample Size	Cases of Diarrhea/100/yr	Diarrheal Deaths/1,000/yr	Sample Size	Cases of Diarrhea/100/yr	Diarrheal Deaths/1,000/yr
0–2	524	136		3	267		NA[c]	NA	NA
3–5	380	124		4	100		3	267	
6–8	196	184		8	350		4	100	
9–11	91	128		11	291		7	171	
0–11			23.5			0			(~1,000.0)[d]
12–14	31	90		3	240		11	218	
15–17	17	118		31	168		40	150	
18–20	3	133		79	213		61	230	
21–23	1	NR[e]		39	154		138	151	
12–23			153.8			0			48
24–26	1	NR		34	165		87	138	
27–29	0	NR		21	133		120	87	
24–29			NA			0			10

[a]From Gordon et al. (1963).
[b]The same child may have diarrhea more than one time during the year.
[c]NA = Not applicable.
[d]Four deaths occurred during 3.5 person-years of observation.
[e]NR = Not reported.

COMMENTS: Deaths for partially breastfed infants were not presented. Diarrhea increased with the initiation of supplemental foods among breastfed infants in 11 villages in Punjab, India, from 1955 to 1959. "No deaths occurred among cases in the immediate weaning period; fatalities occurred in cases of the late post weaning period. . . . The explanation would appear to be in the nutritional state of the child" (Gordon et al., 1963, p. 368).

ABSTRACT B-2 Comparison of Feeding Methods Used for Jamaican Children Who Died Between the Ages of 6 and 36 Months, 1962 to 1963[a]

	Deaths[b]		Random Controls[c]	
Feeding Method	Number	% of Total	Number	% of Total
Never fully breastfed	4	2.9	7	5.2
Fully breastfed <3 mo	37	27.0	24	17.9
Fully breastfed 3–6 mo	73	53.3	69	51.5
Fully breastfed >6 mo	23	16.8	34	25.4
Unknown	11	[d]	14	[d]

[a]From McKenzie et al. (1967).
[b]Random sample of deaths ($N = 285$); completed questionnaires concerning infant feeding were available for 72%.
[c]Random sample of controls ($N = 275$); completed questionnaires were available for 56%.
[d]Children whose feeding method was unknown were excluded from the analysis.

COMMENTS: Relative risk of death was 1.42 for infants breastfed less than 3 months compared with those breastfed longer. Relative risk was calculated from authors' data.

ABSTRACT B-3 Ratios of Observed to Expected Deaths Among 8,456 Births in Rural Senegal, 1962 to 1968, by Breastfeeding Status and Age[a]

	Currently Breastfeeding			Weaned		
Age, mo	Number of Observed Deaths	Number of Expected Deaths	Ratio	Number of Observed Deaths	Number of Expected Deaths	Ratio
0–11	455	460	0.99	9	4	2.25
12–23	360	351	1.03	36	45	0.80
24–35	64	59	1.08	181	186	0.97

[a]From Cantrelle and Leridon (1971).

ABSTRACT B-4 Death Rates and Relative Risk (RR) Among 1,283 Infants in 15 Rural Communities in Chile, by Feeding Method[a]

	Death Rate/1,000[b] and RR, by Feeding Method				
	Breast,	Bottle		Mixed	
Age, mo	Number of Deaths/1,000	Number of Deaths/1,000	RR[c]	Number of Deaths/1,000	RR
1	29.2	60.5	2.07	56.0	1.92
3	13.8	38.7	2.80	37.5	2.72
6	10.0	19.9	1.99	14.0	1.40

[a]From Plank and Milanesi (1973), obtained in a survey of 1,712 women aged 15 to 44 in 1969 and 1970.
[b]Death rate for infants between specified age and age 1 year.
[c]Relative risk for breastfeeding = 1.0.

COMMENTS: The increase in mortality associated with bottle feeding was less than when supplemental foods were given (but was not lower when infants were partially breastfed).

ABSTRACT B-5 Percentage of Infants Breastfeeding in Total Study Sample and Among Those Who Died, and the Relative Risk (RR) of Death for Short-Term Breastfeeding[a]

	Percentage of Infants Breastfed, by Study Population and Breastfeeding Duration				RR[b] of Death for Breastfeeding for <6 mo
	All Infants		Infants Who Died		
Study Area	<6 mo	≥6 mo	<6 mo	≥6 mo	
El Salvador	20	80	78.0	22.0	14.2
Kingston, Jamaica	51	49	87.4	12.6	7.1
Medellin, Colombia	61.8	31.2	91.3	8.8	6.4
Sao Paolo, Brazil	77.2	22.8	95.9	4.1	6.8

[a]From Wray (1978), who analyzed data for deaths from Puffer and Serrano (1973) and for rate of breastfeeding among survivors in El Salvador (Menchu et al., 1972), Kingston (Grantham-MacGregor and Back, 1970), Medellin (Oberndorfer and Mejia, 1968), and Sao Paolo (Iunes et al., 1975).
[b]Relative risk for breastfeeding for ≥6 mo = 1.0.

ABSTRACT B-6 Mortality and Relative Risk (RR) of Death Among Breastfed and Bottle-Fed Infants in One Australian Aboriginal Settlement, 1953 to 1972[a]

Age, mo	Breastfed Infants[b]			Bottle-Fed Infants			RR[c]
	Number of Deaths	Sample Size	Mortality Rate/1,000	Number of Deaths	Sample Size	Mortality Rate/1,000	
1-3	3	547	5.5	4	525	7.6	1.38
4-6	0	99	0	11	705	15.6	d
7-12	0	20	0	9	1,588	5.7	d

[a]From Dugdale (1980).
[b]It was unclear whether breastfeeding included mixed feeding.
[c]Relative risk for breastfed infants = 1.0.
[d]Cannot be estimated.

ABSTRACT B-7   Case Fatality and Relative Risk (RR) for Death from Measles Among 602 Breastfed and Weaned Children in Guinea-Bissau (West Africa), 1979[a]

| Age, mo | Breastfed Infants | | Weaned Infants | | RR[b] |
	Number of Cases	Case Fatality, %	Number of Cases	Case Fatality, %	
0–11	71	28	1	0	c
12–23	43	37	16	25	0.68
24–35	14	14	42	26	1.86
36–71	2	0	112	11	e

[a]From Aaby et al. (1981). Data on feeding were obtained 2 months before a measles epidemic.
[b]Relative risk for breastfed infants = 1.0.
[c]Cannot be estimated.

ABSTRACT B-8   Postneonatal Mortality[a] and Relative Risk (RR) Among Breastfed and Never Breastfed Infants in Six Guatemalan Villages, 1960 to 1974[b]

| Period of Birth | Sample Size | Never Breastfed Infants, %[c] | Postneonatal Mortality Rates/1,000, by Feeding Method | | RR[d] |
			Ever Breastfed Infants	Never Breastfed Infants	
Before 1960	1,128	6.3	75	375	5.0
1960–1968	1,985	6.5	47	193	4.1
1969–1974	1,442	4.9	39	189	4.8

[a]Postneonatal mortality = number of deaths between ages 28 days and 1 year per 1,000 live births.
[b]Based on unpublished data from del Pinal (1981).
[c]The low proportions of infants never breastfed suggest that illness may have prevented breastfeeding.
[d]Relative risk for ever breastfed infants = 1.0.

ABSTRACT B-9   Relative Risk (RR) of Survival by
Duration of Breastfeeding Among the Last Child
Born to Each of 2,907 Women at Three Hospitals in
Cairo, Egypt, 1977 to 1978[a]

Duration of Breastfeeding, mo	RR of Survival (rather than mortality)
>12	1.0
9–12	0.99
6–9	0.87[b]
3–6	0.85[b]
1–3	0.71[b]
0–1	0.71[b]

[a]From Janowitz et al. (1981).
[b]$p \leq .05$.

COMMENTS: It is unclear to what age results refer or whether ages
of all groups were equivalent. Results were adjusted for maternal
education, parity, age, and past infant death (results therefore are
probably overcontrolled).

ABSTRACT B-10   Case-Fatality Rates and Relative Risk (RR) Among
2,339 Young Breastfeeding and Weaned Children Hospitalized with
Measles, Diarrhea, or Acute Lower Respiratory Disease, by
Breastfeeding Status in Kigali, Rwanda[a]

| Age, mo | Case Fatality Rate, % | | RR[b] |
	Breastfed Infants	Weaned Infants	
0–5	11.2	20.7	1.85
6–11	13.5	26.8	1.99[c]
12–17	17.3	31.5	1.82
18–23	15.1	23.7	1.57[d]

[a]Based on data from Lepage et al. (1981).
[b]Relative risk for breastfed infants = 1.0.
[c]$p < .001$ for entire first year.
[d]$p < .001$ for entire second year.

ABSTRACT B-11   Mortality Rates and Relative Risk (RR) of Death Among Very Low and Low Birth Weight Infants in the Special Care Nursery, Bombay, India, by Feeding Method and Birth Weight[a,b]

| Birth Weight, kg | Mortality, % | | RR[d] |
	Breastfed Infants	Bottle-Fed Infants[c]	
1.00–1.30	35.0	59.1	1.69
1.31–1.50	30.0[e]	50.0	1.67
1.51–1.80	20.0[e]	40.0	2.02
Total	23.0[e]	47.0	2.04

[a]From Patel et al. (1981).

[b]Age of the infants was not provided. There were 100 infants in each feeding group.

[c]The number of "breastfed" infants who were fed human milk by tube or bottle was not stated.

[d]Relative risk for breastfed infants in each weight group = 1.0.

[e]$p < .01$.

ABSTRACT B-12   Infant Deaths Resulting from Diarrhea in 12 Villages in Egypt, by Age and Feeding Method, 1979 to 1980[a]

| Age, mo | Percentage of All Deaths Due to Diarrhea | | |
	Breastfed Infants (N [deaths] = 150)	Exclusively Bottle-Fed Infants (N [deaths] = 19)	Mixed-Fed Infants (N [deaths] = 33
0–5	28	60	63
6–11	76	86	71

[a]Based on data from Tekçe (1982).

ABSTRACT B-13 Reduction of Infant Death Rate in Malaysia Attributed to Breastfeeding (Compared with Never Breastfeeding), by Age, 1976 and 1977[a]

| Age[b] | Adjusted Impact of Breastfeeding Throughout the Preceding Period, Reduction in Deaths/1,000 | |
	Exclusive Breastfeeding	Mixed Feeding
8–28 days	16.0	5.1
1–5 mo	23.2	10.5
6–12 mo	20.6	10.0

[a]From Butz et al. (1984), DaVanzo et al. (1983), DaVanzo and Habicht (1986), and Habicht et al. (1986, 1988). Data from the Malaysian Family Life Survey, which included 1,262 households, 5,573 singleton live births, and 270 infant deaths.
[b]Age period to which the feeding method applies.

COMMENTS: Neither death rates of nonbreastfed infants nor numbers of breastfed infants were presented. Effects were much smaller in households with a toilet and piped water. The authors' conclusion of a declining association of breastfeeding and mortality with age is not obviously supported by the data presented. The same data set was used by Holland (1987) and Millman and Cooksey (1987). The data do not allow estimation of relative risks.

ABSTRACT B-14 Death Rates and Relative Risk (RR) Among Breastfed, Bottle-Fed, and Mixed-Fed Infants Delivered to More Than 15,000 Women in One Hospital in Tehran, Iran, by Feeding Method, 1977 and 1978[a]

Feeding Method	Sample Size	Number of Deaths	Death Rate/1,000	RR
Breast or mixed	12,004	307	25.6	1.0
Bottle	2,379	868	364.8	14.3

[a]From Janowitz and Nichols (1983).

ABSTRACT B-15 Schmidt (1983) reported on a collaborative study among urban poor in eight Latin American countries and Portugal involving 7,659 children in 1981 and 1982. The infant mortality rate for formula-fed infants was 18.6/1,000 live births, but the results were not presented in a form that allows calculation of mortality rates for those infants who were breastfed or mixed fed or for those whose feeding method was unknown. Furthermore, results were not stratified by site or age of child. The group that was breastfed only was probably much younger (and more susceptible to higher death rates) than the weaned group.

ABSTRACT B-16   Adjusted Relative Risk (RR) of Mortality Among 1- to 12-Month-Old Breastfed and Never Breastfed Infants Living in Urban and Rural Areas of Brazil, 1980[a]

Characteristic of Residence	RR	
	Breastfed	Never Breastfed (CI)[b]
Urban	1.0	1.53 (0.97–2.41)[c]
Rural	1.0	2.31 (1.41–3.78)[d]

[a]From Goldberg et al. (1984). Data obtained from a survey in four states in northeastern Brazil, including 7,852 women and 3,457 children.
[b]CI = 95% confidence interval.
[c]$p = .07$.
[d]$p < .01$.

COMMENTS: Results were adjusted for mother's education, employment, age at the time of delivery, parity, time since birth, and use of health services. Adjusting for use of health services may not be appropriate in that it might make real differences between the groups less apparent.

ABSTRACT B-17   Adjusted Relative Risk (RR) of Mortality Associated with Bottle Feeding of Infants in the Near East[a]

Country	Year of Survey	Total Sample Size	RR of Mortality of Bottle-Fed Infants, by Age[b]	
			1–5 mo	1–11 mo
Jordan	1976	8,458	3.35	2.95
Tunisia	1978	7,060	3.35	2.95
Yemen	1979	3,889	NS[c]	NR[d]
Egypt	1980	11,961	8.39	6.38

[a]From Adlakha and Suchindran (1985). Data were obtained in world fertility surveys.
[b]Relative risk for infants breastfed during the ages specified = 1.0 for each country.
[c]NS = Not significantly different.
[d]NR = Not reported.

COMMENTS: Infants had been breastfed at least until the end of month 1 after delivery. There were very few nonbreastfed infants (4 to 8%) during the first month, suggesting that these infants were aberrant.

ABSTRACT B-18   Percent Mortality and Relative Risk (RR) of Mortality
Associated with Replacement of Formula by Human Milk for Low-
Birth-Weight Infants in a Special Care Nursery in Bombay, India, 1978
to 1980[a]

| Birth Weight, g | Mortality,[b] % (sample size) | | RR[c] |
	Human Milk	Formula	
≤1,250	77.0 (74)	84.3 (102)	1.09
1,251–1,499	40.2 (102)	59.6 (104)	1.48
≥1,500	18.5 (157)	34.4 (186)	1.86
Total sample	38.1 (333)	54.1 (392)	1.42

[a]From Daga and Daga (1985).
[b]Mortality differences were observed primarily after 72 h of age; diarrhea and sepsis were
the principal causes of death.
[c]Relative risk of death for breastfed infants = 1.0.

ABSTRACT B-19   Barros and colleagues (1982) conducted a study involving
all 5,914 births in the hospital in Pelotas, Brazil, in 1982. The children
were followed up at age 2 years. Of the infants born weighing less than
2,000 g, 42% were never breastfed (compared with less than 10% of all
others). The children who were small at birth were also more likely to be
weaned. The authors reported that even if breastfeeding (either partial or
exclusive) had no protective effect, nonbreastfed babies appeared to be at
30% increased risk of death. The duration of breastfeeding was unrelated
to birthweight in the highest two (of five) socioeconomic groups.

ABSTRACT B-20   Relative Risk (RR) of Mortality Among Breastfed
Infants in Peru, 1977 and 1978, Based on the First and Next-to-Last
Births of 5,640 Women Aged 15 to 49 Years[a]

Age, mo[b]	RR[c] of Mortality, Breastfed Compared with Other Infants	p Value
1–2	0.37	<.01
3–5	0.57	<.01
6–11	0.44	<.01
12–23	0.88	NR[d]
24–59	0.67	NR

[a]From Palloni and Tienda (1986). Based on data from the World Fertility Survey.
[b]Period of breastfeeding was up to the lower age bound in each category.
[c]Relative risk was based on a risk of 1.0 for infants not breastfed, using multivariate analysis.
[d]NR = Not reported.

COMMENTS: The total number of births included was not reported. Results were controlled
for previous birth interval; birth order; gender; mother's age, education, and region; and
father's occupation.

ABSTRACT B-21   Infant Deaths from Diarrhea or Measles by Feeding
Method Among Infants Attending a Clinic in Benin, Nigeria, 1981[a]

Feeding Method	Number of Deaths	Sample Size	Infant Deaths/1,000
Breast	0	65	0
Mixed	20	282	70.9
Bottle	9	67	134.3
Total	29	414	70.0

[a]From Scott-Emuakpor and Okafor (1986). Relative risks not calculable, given that there were no deaths in the breastfed group.

ABSTRACT B-22   Relative Risk (RR) of Infant Death in Malaysia by
Duration of Breastfeeding and Infant Age, 1976[a]

Duration of Breastfeeding, mo	RR[b] by Age of Infant, mo			
	0–1	2–3	4–6	7–12
Never	1.00	1.00	1.00	1.00
Ever	0.82	NA[c]	NA	NA
<1	NA	0.89	0.61	NA
1	NA	0.41	0.64	0.87
2–3	NA	NA	0.14	
4–6	NA	NA	NA	0.54

[a]From Holland (1987).
[b]Relative risk was derived from the author's log-linear models based on data from the Malaysian Family Life Survey, which included 1,262 households and 5,593 births. This is the same data set as that used by Butz et al. (1984) and Millman and Cooksey (1987).
[c]NA = Not applicable.

ABSTRACT B-23   Logit Coefficient and Relative Risk (RR) of Increased
Mortality Among Infants in Malaysia, by Feeding Method, 1976[a]

Period of Measuring Mortality	Feeding Method	Logit Coefficient	RR[b]
Through 1 mo	All others versus ever breastfed	1.82^c–$2.06^{c,d}$	6.11–7.85
Through 1 yr	Bottle only	1.10^c–$1.47^{c,d}$	3.00–4.35
1–12 mo	Breastfed <1 mo versus longer breastfeeding	0.69–$0.85^{c,d}$	1.99–2.34

[a]From Millman and Cooksey (1987). Based on data from the Malaysian Family Life Survey.
[b]Range of relative risks associated with range of logit coefficients.
[c]$p < .01$.
[d]Range depends on logistic model used.

ABSTRACT B-24   Relative Risk (RR) of Mortality Among Guatemalan Children by Duration of Breastfeeding and Age, 1974 to 1976[a]

Age, mo	RR^b by Duration of Breastfeeding			
	0	1–5 mo	6–11 mo	11–23 mo
1–5	6.1^c	NA^d	NA	NA
6–11	3.7^c	2.3^e	NA	NA
12–23	0.8	1.3	1.3	NA
24–59	0.4	0.4	0.5	0.6

[a]From Pebley and Stupp (1987), who obtained data on approximately 2,880 children in four villages that had health and nutrition intervention and from two urban communities.
[b]Relative risk for exclusively breastfed infants = 1.0.
[c]$p < 0.05$.
[d]NA = Not applicable.
[e]$p < 0.01$.

ABSTRACT B-25   Adjusted Relative Risk (RR) of Infant Mortality, by Disease and Method of Feeding, Among Infants in Urban Southern Brazil, 1985[a]

Method of Feeding	RR of Death, by Disease		
	Diarrhea	Respiratory Infections	Other Infections
Breast only	1.0	1.0	1.0
Breast plus formula	4.5^b	2.1	0.1^b
Breast plus cow's milk	3.4^b	1.2	1.4
Formula only	16.3^b	3.9^b	2.3
Cow's milk only	11.6^b	3.3^b	2.6

[a]From Victora et al. (1987, 1989).
[b]Significantly different from the risk for those breastfeeding only.

ABSTRACT B-26   Infant and Child Mortality/1,000 in Rural Sierra Leone
and Beta Coefficients from Regression Analysis, by Duration of
Breastfeeding, 1979[a,b]

Duration of Breastfeeding, mo	Infant and Child Mortality/1,000[c]	Beta Coefficients from Regression Analysis
<6	356	Reference group
6–12	253	-0.094^d
13–24	194	-0.162^d
≥25	286	-0.080^d

[a]From Bailey (1988). Based on data obtained from a probability survey of 2,000 women aged 15 to 49.

[b]In regression analysis "Dependent variable is . . . ratio of infant and child deaths to live births corresponding to each mother in the sample" (Bailey, 1988, p. 165).

[c]No statistical test presented.

[d]$p < .001$.

COMMENTS: Results are open to circularity: death could *cause* a shorter period of breast-feeding. It is unclear to what age death rates refer and how infants less than age 3 years at the time of the survey were handled in the analysis.

ABSTRACT B-27   Mortality and Relative Risk (RR) of Mortality Within
1 Month of Interview Among Children in Bangladesh, by Breastfeeding
Status and Age, 1985 and 1986[a]

Age, mo	Breastfed Infants[b]		Weaned Infants		
	Number of Deaths	Period, Child-Months[c]	Number of Deaths	Period, Child-Months	RR[d]
12–17	11	6,622	0	176	[e]
18–23	8	5,108	3	753	3.39
24–29	7	5,267	12	2,611	3.45
30–36	3	3,035	7	4,103	1.73
Total	29	20,032	22	7,643	2.83

[a]From Briend et al. (1988).

[b]Includes infants partially or exclusively breastfed.

[c]Child-months refers to the number of months of observation summed across all children.

[d]Relative risk for breastfed infants = 1.0.

[e]Cannot be estimated.

COMMENTS: An effect was observed only among those with the smallest arm circumferences. Incidence of diarrhea was not affected, but the case fatality rate was higher among weaned children. The possibility of a spurious association of diarrhea causing weaning was ruled out.

REFERENCES

Aaby, P., J. Bukh, I.M. Lisse, A.J. Smits, L. Smedman, O. Jeppsson, and A. Lindeberg. 1981. Breastfeeding and measles mortality in Guinea-Bissau. Lancet 2:1231.

Adlakha, A.L., and C.M. Suchindran. 1985. Factors affecting infant and child mortality. J. Biosoc. Sci. 17:481-496.

Bailey, M. 1988. Factors affecting infant and child mortality in rural Sierra Leone. J. Trop. Pediatr. 34:165-168.

Barros, F.C., C.G. Victora, J.P. Vaughan, P.G. Smith. 1986. Birth weight and duration of breast-feeding: Are the beneficial effects of human milk being overestimated? Pediatrics 78:656-661.

Briend, A., B. Wojtyniak, and M.G. Rowland. 1988. Breast feeding, nutritional state, and child survival in rural Bangladesh. Br. Med. J. 296:879-882.

Butz, W.P., J.-P. Habicht, and J. DaVanzo. 1984. Environmental factors in the relationship between breastfeeding and infant mortality: the role of sanitation and water in Malaysia. Am. J. Epidemiol. 119:516-525.

Cantrelle, P., and H. Leridon. 1971. Breast feeding, mortality in childhood and fertility in a rural zone of Senegal. Popul. Stud. 25:505-533.

Daga, S.R., and A.S. Daga. 1985. Impact of breast milk on the cost-effectiveness of the special care unit for the newborn. J. Trop. Pediatr. 31:121-123.

DaVanzo, J., and J.-P. Habicht. 1986. Infant-mortality decline in Malaysia, 1946-1975: the roles of changes in variables and changes in the structure of relationships. Demography 23:143-160.

DaVanzo, J., W.P. Butz, and J.-P. Habicht. 1983. How biological and behavioural influences on mortality in Malaysia vary during the first year of life. Popul. Stud. 37:381-402.

del Pinal, J.H. 1981. Breastfeeding and Infant Mortality: Retrospective Evidence from Six Communities in Guatemala. Paper Presented at the Annual Meeting of the Population Association of America, March 25-27, 1981. Population Association of America, Washington, D.C. 25 pp.

Dugdale, A.E. 1980. Infant feeding, growth and mortality: a 20-year study of an Australian Aboriginal community. Med. J. Aust. 2:380-385.

Goldberg, H.I., W. Rodrigues, A.M.T. Thome, B. Janowitz, and L. Morris. 1984. Infant mortality and breast-feeding in North-Eastern Brazil. Popul. Stud. 38:105-115.

Gordon, J.E., I.D. Chitkara, and J.B. Wyon. 1963. Weanling diarrhea. Am. J. Med. Sci. 245:345-377.

Grantham-McGregor, S.M., and E.H. Back. 1970. Breast feeding in Kingston, Jamaica. Arch. Dis. Child. 45:404-409.

Habicht, J.-P., J. DaVanzo, and W.P. Butz. 1986. Does breastfeeding really save lives, or are apparent benefits due to biases? Am. J. Epidemiol. 123:279-290.

Habicht, J.-P., J. DaVanzo, and W.P. Butz. 1988. Mother's milk and sewage: their interactive effects on infant mortality. Pediatrics 81:456-461.

Holland, B. 1987. Breast-feeding, social variables, and infant mortality: a hazards model analysis of the case of Malaysia. Soc. Biol. 34:78-93.

Iunes, M., D. Sigulem, and A.C. Campino. 1975. Estado Nutricional de Criances de 6 a 60 Meses no Municipio de Sao Paolo. 11. Analise de Dados, Sao Paolo: Escola Poaulista de Medicina.

Janowitz, B., and D.J. Nichols. 1983. Child survivorship and pregnancy spacing in Iran. J. Biosoc. Sci. 15:35-46.

Janowitz, B., J.H. Lewis, A. Parnell, F. Hefnawi, M.N. Younis, and G.A. Serour. 1981. Breast-feeding and child survival in Egypt. J. Biosoc. Sci. 13:287-297.

Lepage, P., C. Munyakazi, and P. Hennart. 1981. Breastfeeding and hospital mortality in children in Rwanda. Lancet 2:409-411.

McKenzie, H.I., H.G. Lovell, K.L. Standard, and W.E. Miall. 1967. Child mortality in Jamaica. Milbank Mem. Fund Q. 45:303-321.

Menchu, M.A., M. Flores, M.Y. Lara, and M. Behar. 1972. Lactancia y destete en el area rural de Centro America y Panama. Arch. Latinoam. Nutr. 22:83-99.

Millman, S.R., and E.C. Cooksey. 1987. Birth weight and the effects of birth spacing and breastfeeding on infant mortality. Stud. Fam. Plann. 18:202-212.

Oberndorfer, L., and W. Mejia. 1968. Statistical analysis of the duration of breast-feeding. A study of 200 mothers of Antioquia Province, Colombia. J. Trop. Pediatr. 14:27-42.

Palloni, A., and M. Tienda. 1986. The effects of breastfeeding and pace of childbearing on mortality at early ages. Demography 23:31-52.

Patel, R.B., S.A. Khanna, K. Lahiri, and G.V. Kulkarni. 1981. Breast milk in low birth weight babies. Indian J. Pediatr. 48:195-196.

Pebley, A.R., and P.W. Stupp. 1987. Reproductive patterns and child-mortality in Guatemala. Demography 24:43-60.

Plank, S.J., and M.L. Milanesi. 1973. Infant feeding and infant mortality in rural Chile. Bull. W.H.O. 48:203-210.

Puffer, R.R., and C.V. Serrano. 1973. Patterns of Mortality in Childhood. Report of the Interamerican Investigation of Mortality in Childhood. Scientific Publ. No. 262. Pan American Health Organization, Washington, D.C. 470 pp.

Schmidt, B.J. 1983. Breast-feeding and infant morbidity and mortality in developing countries. J. Pediatr. Nutr. 2:S127-S130.

Scott-Emuakpor, M.M., and U.A. Okafor. 1986. Comparative study of morbidity and mortality of breast-fed and bottle-fed Nigerian infants. East Afr. Med. J. 63:452-457.

Tekçe, B. 1982. Oral rehydration therapy: an assessment of mortality effects in rural Egypt. Stud. Fam. Plann. 13:315-327.

Victora, C.G., P.G. Smith, J.P. Vaughan, L.C. Nobre, C. Lombardi, A.M. Teixeira, S.M. Fuchs, L.B. Moreira, L.P. Gigante, and F.C. Barros. 1987. Evidence for protection by breast-feeding against infant deaths from infectious diseases in Brazil. Lancet 2:319-322.

Victora, C.G., P.G. Smith, J.P. Vaughan, L.C. Nobre, C. Lombardi, A.M. Teixeira, S.C. Fuchs, L.B. Moreira, L.B. Gigante, and F.C. Barros. 1989. Infant feeding and deaths due to diarrhea: a case-control study. Am. J. Epidemiol. 129:1032-1041.

Wray, J.D. 1978. Maternal nutrition, breast-feeding and infant survival. Pp. 197-229 in W.H. Mosley, ed. Nutrition and Human Reproduction. Plenum Press, New York.

Appendix
C

Appendix C presents data from a complete literature survey of data on human milk composition conducted by Margaret C. Neville (University of Colorado Health Sciences Center, personal communication, 1990). References were included if they presented data for milk composition by actual duration of lactation, but the data vary in accuracy. Nutrients included are those analyzed by Dr. Neville and colleagues.

TABLE C-1 Summary of Composition Data for Macronutrients of Human Milk. Data compiled by Neville, University of Colorado, personal communication, 1990

Nutrient, Analytic Method	Days Post Partum								Reference
	21	30	45	60	90	120	150	180	
Lactose, mmol/liter									
NR[a]	200	200	202	NR	NR	NR	NR	NR	Hytten, 1954
NR	NR	225	NR	222	227	227	227	227	Prentice et al., 1983
"Agricultural method"	NR	199	NR	199	200	203	197	200	Nagra, 1989
Colorimetric	NR	223	NR	226	225	232	242	234	Brown et al., 1986
Enzymatic	156	137	NR	NR	NR	NR	NR	NR	Hibberd et al., 1982
Enzymatic, lactase by Somgyi	NR	206	NR	211	222	223	223	227	Dewey and Lönnerdal, 1983
β-galactosidase, then glucose	NR	205	193	213	234	205	208	213	Morriss et al., 1986
Folin	NR	205	NR	211	225	222	222	222	Kader et al., 1972
Gas chromatography	210	202	196	NR	NR	NR	NR	NR	Lemons et al., 1982
Hartmann and Kulski, 1978	NR	NR	NR	NR	225	NR	NR	206	Saint et al., 1986
HPLC[b]	NR	178	NR	NR	NR	NR	NR	NR	Butte and Calloway, 1981
Method of Conetta on Technicon	NR	205	NR	NR	214	NR	223	NR	Lönnerdal et al., 1976
Technicon	NR	208	212	NR	NR	NR	NR	NR	Gross et al., 1980
Technicon	199	NR	NR	NR	NR	NR	NR	NR	Gross et al., 1981
YSI analyzer	NR	189	NR	192	194	195	NR	NR	Butte et al., 1984
YSI analyzer	177	NR	182	NR	188	NR	NR	191	Neville, University of Colorado, personal communication, 1990

Protein, g/dl

Method									Reference
NR	NR	1.30	NR	1.09	1.05	1.02	1.03	1.04	Prentice et al., 1983
"Agricultural method"	NR	1.05	NR	0.99	1.01	0.99	0.98	1.01	Nagra, 1989
BCA[c] assay with human milk standard	1.20	NR	1.09	NR	0.94	NR	NR	1.00	Neville, University of Colorado, personal communication, 1990
Biuret	NR	1.30	NR	1.00	1.00	1.30	0.95	0.90	Lauber and Reinhardt, 1979
Kjeldahl	1.23	0.97	0.93	NR	NR	NR	NR	NR	Hytten, 1954
Kjeldahl	NR	0.73	NR	NR	0.76	NR	0.71	NR	Lönnerdal et al., 1976
Kjeldahl with TCA[d] precipitation	NR	1.52	NR	NR	NR	NR	NR	NR	Gross et al., 1980
Kjeldahl with TCA precipitation	1.60	NR	1.42	NR	NR	NR	NR	NR	Gross et al., 1981
Kjeldahl with TCA precipitation	1.18	1.10	1.22	0.89	0.84	0.82	NR	NR	Lemons et al., 1982
Kjeldahl with TCA precipitation	NR	1.00	NR	NR	NR	NR	NR	NR	Butte et al., 1984
Microkjeldahl	NR	1.03	NR	1.10	0.99	0.88	0.91	0.82	Kader et al., 1972
Lowry	1.51	1.50	NR	NR	NR	NR	NR	NR	Hibberd et al., 1982
Lowry with albumin standard	NR	1.44	NR	1.33	1.32	1.30	1.25	1.27	Dewey and Lönnerdal, 1983
Lowry	1.41	NR	1.10	NR	NR	0.85	NR	NR	Duncan et al., 1983
Lowry	NR	NR	NR	NR	1.09	NR	NR	1.21	Saint et al., 1986

Lipid, g/dl

Method									Reference
NR	4.0	3.0	3.3	NR	NR	NR	NR	NR	Hytten, 1954
"Agricultural method"	NR	3.6	NR	3.7	3.6	3.7	3.6	3.5	Nagra, 1989
Creamatocrit, Folch extraction	NR	4.2	NR	3.7	3.7	3.3	3.3	3.4	Prentice et al., 1983
Creamatocrit	NR	3.6	NR	NR	3.7	NR	3.2	NR	Jackson et al., 1988
Creamatocrit, Folch extraction	4.7	NR	5.3	NR	4.2	NR	NR	5.6	Neville, University of Colorado, personal communication, 1990
Modified Folch extraction	NR	4.1	NR	4.6	5.2	NR	NR	NR	Clark et al., 1982

Table C-1 continues

TABLE C-1—Continued

Nutrient, Analytic Method	Days Post Partum								Reference
	21	30	45	60	90	120	150	180	
Gravimetric	NR	3.1	NR	3.0	2.8	2.7	2.6	2.7	Brown et al., 1986
Enzymatic analysis	3.9	4.0	NR	NR	NR	NR	NR	NR	Hibberd et al., 1982
Enzymatic for triglycerides (Worthington)	NR	4.0	NR	NR	NR	NR	NR	NR	Butte and Calloway, 1981
Gravimetric	NR	2.7	NR	2.5	2.3	2.6	2.5	2.6	Lauber and Reinhardt, 1981
Gravimetric	NR	4.0	4.5	4.8	4.2	NR	NR	NR	Butte et al., 1984
Gravimetric	NR	3.6	NR	3.4	3.2	3.5	NR	NR	Butte et al., 1984
Roese-Gottlieb	NR	3.9	4.0	NR	NR	NR	NR	NR	Gross et al., 1980
Roese-Gottlieb	3.0	NR	NR	NR	NR	NR	NR	NR	Gross et al., 1981
Sulfuric acid-vanillin	3.0	3.1	3.5	NR	NR	NR	NR	NR	Lemons et al., 1982
Sulfuric acid-vanillin	NR	4.9	NR	4.6	4.6	4.6	4.4	4.3	Dewey and Lönnerdal, 1983
Sodium, mmol/liter									
Ashed, flame emission	NR	10.0	NR	NR	NR	NR	NR	NR	Atkinson et al., 1980
Dry-ash, atomic absorption	NR	6.8	6.1	5.4	6.2	NR	NR	NR	Butte et al., 1984
Special ashing, atomic absorption	NR	6.6	NR	NR	5.3	5.5	NR	NR	Picciano et al., 1981
Flame emission	NR	9.3	NR	10.9	7.6	7.2	6.8	5.5	Dewey and Lönnerdal, 1983
Flame photometry	NR	10.8	8.5	NR	NR	NR	NR	NR	Gross et al., 1980
Flame photometry	10.0	NR	NR	NR	NR	NR	NR	NR	Gross et al., 1981
Flame photometry	6.8	7.0	7.1	NR	NR	NR	NR	NR	Lemons et al., 1982
Flame photometry	7.3	NR	NR	NR	NR	NR	NR	NR	Morriss et al., 1986
Ion selective electrode	9.2	NR	7.2	NR	6.3	NR	4.8	6.0	Neville, University of Colorado, personal communication, 1990
Potassium, mmol/liter									
Atomic absorption	13.6	13.6	NR	NR	NR	NR	NR	NR	Hibberd et al., 1982
Dry-ash, atomic absorption	NR	15.0	NR	NR	NR	NR	NR	NR	Atkinson et al., 1980

Method										Reference
Special ashing, atomic absorption	NR	11.9	NR	NR	10.9	10.4	NR	NR	NR	Picciano et al., 1981
Flame photometry	NR	15.8	15.0	NR	NR	NR	NR	NR	NR	Gross et al., 1980
Flame photometry	14.0	NR	NR	NR	NR	NR	NR	NR	NR	Gross et al., 1981
Flame photometry	13.9	13.0	13.6	NR	NR	NR	NR	NR	NR	Lemons et al., 1982
Flame photometry	17.1	NR	NR	NR	NR	NR	NR	12.8	NR	Morriss et al., 1986
Flame emission photometry	NR	13.2	NR	NR	12.0	11.8	11.6	11.5	10.8	Dewey and Lönnerdal, 1983
Ion selective electode	16.2	NR	15.1	NR	NR	NR	NR	NR	13.9	Neville, University of Colorado, personal communication, 1990
Chloride, mmol/liter										
Ashing, then chloride electrode	NR	12.0	NR	NR	11.7	11.9	NR	NR	NR	Picciano et al., 1981
Colorimetric	NR	15.2	13.1	NR	NR	NR	NR	NR	NR	Gross et al., 1980
Colorimetric	15.4	NR	13.9	NR	NR	11.6	NR	14.0	NR	Neville, University of Colorado, personal communication, 1990
Electrometric titration	NR	12.0	NR	NR	NR	NR	NR	NR	NR	Atkinson et al., 1980
Electrometric titration	10.5	10.5	11.3	NR	NR	NR	NR	NR	NR	Lemons et al., 1982
Electrometric titration	11.8	NR	NR	NR	NR	NR	NR	10.5	NR	Morriss et al., 1986
Calcium, mmol/liter										
"Agricultural method"	NR	7.50	NR	NR	7.67	7.77	7.60	7.85	8.00	Nagra, 1989
Ashing, atomic absorption	NR	6.80	NR	NR	NR	NR	NR	NR	NR	Atkinson et al., 1980
Ashed, atomic absorption	6.63	6.20	NR	NR	NR	NR	NR	NR	NR	Gross et al., 1980
Dry ashing, atomic absorption	NR	NR	6.40	NR	NR	NR	5.88	NR	NR	Vaughn et al., 1979
Dry ashing, atomic absorption	NR	6.33	6.65	NR	6.43	6.48	NR	NR	NR	Butte et al., 1984
Atomic absorption	NR	7.24	NR	NR	7.31	7.14	NR	NR	NR	Picciano et al., 1981
Atomic absorption	6.48	NR	6.85	NR	NR	6.72	NR	NR	6.23	Greer et al., 1982
Atomic absorption	NR	6.50	NR	NR	6.85	6.72	6.35	6.18	6.38	Dewey and Lönnerdal, 1983

Table C-1 continues

TABLE C-1—Continued

Nutrient, Analytic Method	Days Post Partum								Reference
	21	30	45	60	90	120	150	180	
Atomic absorption	8.40	NR	NR	NR	NR	NR	7.30	NR	Morriss et al., 1986
Dilution, atomic absorption	NR	6.43	NR	6.53	6.50	6.43	6.28	6.10	Karra et al., 1988
Colorimetric	6.95	6.65	7.82	NR	NR	NR	NR	NR	Lemons et al., 1982
Colorimetric	7.66	NR	7.53	NR	7.49	NR	NR	6.30	Neville, University of Colorado, personal communication, 1990
Orthocresolphthalein	4.46	4.43	NR	NR	NR	NR	NR	NR	Hibberd et al., 1982
Magnesium, mmol/liter									
"Agricultural method"	NR	1.04	NR	1.16	1.08	1.20	0.95	1.00	Nagra, 1989
Ashing, atomic absorption	NR	1.20	NR	NR	NR	NR	NR	NR	Atkinson et al., 1980
Ashing, atomic absorption	1.20	1.04	NR	NR	NR	NR	NR	NR	Gross et al., 1980
Dry ashing, atomic absorption	NR	1.49	1.66	1.74	1.74	NR	NR	NR	Butte et al., 1984
Atomic absorption	NR	1.15	NR	1.27	1.36	NR	NR	NR	Picciano et al., 1981
Atomic absorption	1.21	NR	1.23	NR	1.29	NR	NR	1.33	Greer et al., 1982
Atomic absorption	1.44	1.44	NR	NR	NR	NR	NR	NR	Hibberd et al., 1982
Atomic absorption	1.15	1.17	1.51	NR	NR	NR	NR	NR	Lemons et al., 1982
Atomic absorption	NR	1.15	NR	1.34	1.39	1.46	1.40	1.41	Dewey and Lönnerdal, 1983
Atomic absorption	1.30	NR	NR	NR	NR	NR	1.25	NR	Morriss et al., 1986
Dilution, atomic absorption	1.68	NR	NR	1.31	NR	NR	1.27	NR	Rajalakshmi and Srikantia, 1980
Dilution, atomic absorption	NR	1.18	NR	1.33	1.42	1.43	1.45	1.45	Karra et al., 1988
Colorimetric	1.63	NR	1.65	NR	1.77	NR	NR	1.63	Neville, University of Colorado, personal communication, 1990

[a]NR = Not reported.
[b]HPLC = High performance liquid chromatography.
[c]BCA = Bicinchoninic acid.

REFERENCES

Atkinson, S.A., I.C. Radde, G.W. Chance, M.H. Bryan, and G.H. Anderson. 1980. Macro-mineral content of milk obtained during early lactation from mothers of premature infants. Early Hum. Dev. 4:5-14.

Brown, K.H., N.A. Akhtar, A.D. Robertson, and M.G. Ahmed. 1986. Lactational capacity of marginally nourished mothers: relationships between maternal nutritional status and quantity and proximate composition of milk. Pediatrics 78:909-919.

Butte, N.F., and D.H. Calloway. 1981. Evaluation of lactational performance of Navajo women. Am. J. Clin. Nutr. 34:2210-2215.

Butte, N.F., C. Garza, C.A. Johnson, E.O. Smith, and B.L. Nichols. 1984. Longitudinal changes in milk composition of mothers delivering preterm and term infants. Early Hum. Dev. 9:153-162.

Clark, R.M., A.M. Ferris, M. Fey, P.B. Brown, K.E. Hundreiser, and R.G. Jensen. 1982. Changes in the lipids of human milk from 2 to 16 weeks postpartum. J. Ped. Gastroenterol. Nutr. 1:311-315.

Dewey, K.G., and B. Lönnerdal. 1983. Milk and nutrient intake of breast-fed infants from 1 to 6 months: Relation to growth and fatness. J. Ped. Gastroenterol. Nutr. 2:497-506.

Duncan, M.E., R.R. Samson, J. McGrath, and D.B. McClelland. 1983. Humoral defence factors in the breast milk of Ethiopian women with leprosy and healthy controls. Am. J. Clin Nutr. 38:921-928.

Greer, F.R., R.C. Tsang, R.S. Levin, J.E. Searcy, R. Wu, and J.J. Steichen. 1982. Increasing serum calcium and magnesium concentrations in breast-fed infants: longitudinal studies of minerals in human milk and in sera of nursing mothers and their infants. J. Pediatr. 100:59-64.

Gross, S.J., R.J. David, L. Bauman, and R.M. Tomarelli. 1980. Nutritional composition of milk produced by mothers delivering preterm. J. Pediatr. 96:641-644.

Gross, S.J., J. Geller, and R.M. Tomarelli. 1981. Composition of breast milk from mothers of preterm infants. Pediatrics 68:490-493.

Hibberd, C.M., O.G. Brooke, N.D. Carter, M. Haug, and G. Harzer. 1982. Variations in the composition of breast milk during the first 5 weeks of lactation: implications for the feeding of preterm infants. Arch. Dis. Child. 57:658-662.

Hytten, F.E. 1954. Clinical and chemical studies in human lactation: IV. Trends in milk composition during course of lactation. Br. Med. J.:249-255.

Jackson, D.A., S.M. Imong, A. Silprasert, S. Preunglumpoo, P. Leelapat, Y. Yootabootr, Y. Amatayakul, and J.D. Baum. 1988. Estimation of 24 h breast-milk fat concentration and fat intake in rural northern Thailand. Br. J. Nutr. 59:365-371.

Kader, M.M., R. Bahgat, M.T. Aziz, F. Hefnawi, M.H. Badraoui, N. Younis, and F. Hassib. 1972. Lactation patterns in Egyptian women. II. Chemical composition of milk during the first year of lactation. J. Biosoc. Sci. 4:403-409.

Karra, M.V., A. Kirksey, O. Galal, N.S. Bassily, G.G. Harrison, and N.W. Jerome. 1988. Zinc, calcium and magnesium concentrations in milk from American and Egyptian women throughout the first 6 months of lactation. Am. J. Clin. Nutr. 47:642-648.

Lauber, E., and M. Reinhardt. 1979. Studies on the quality of breast milk during 23 months of lactation in a rural community of the Ivory Coast. Am. J. Clin. Nutr. 32:1159-1173.

Lemons, J.A., L. Moye, D. Hall, and M. Simmons. 1982. Differences in the composition of preterm and term human milk during early lactation. Pediatr. Nutr. 16:113-117.

Lönnerdal, B., E. Forsum, and L. Hambraeus. 1976. Longitudinal study of the protein, nitrogen, and lactose contents of human milk from Swedish well-nourished mothers. Am. J. Clin. Nutr. 29:1127-1133.

Morriss, F.H., Jr., E.D. Brewer, S.B. Spedale, L. Riddle, D.M. Temple, R.M. Caprioli, and M.S. West. 1986. Relationship of human milk pH during course of lactation to concentrations of citrate and fatty acids. Pediatrics 78:458-464.

Nagra, S.A. 1989. Longitudinal study in biochemical composition of human milk during the first year of lactation. J. Trop. Pediatr. 35:126-128.

Picciano, M.F., E.J. Calkins, J.R. Garrick, and R.H. Deering. 1981. Milk and mineral intakes of breastfed infants. Acta Paediatr. Scand. 70:189-194.

Prentice, A.M., S.B. Roberts, A. Prentice, A.A. Paul, M. Watkinson, A.A. Watkinson, and R.G. Whitehead. 1983. Dietary supplementation of lactating Gambian women. I. Effect on breast-milk volume and quality. Hum. Nutr.: Clin. Nutr. 37C:53-64.

Rajalakshmi, K., and S.G. Srikantia. 1980. Copper, zinc and magnesium content of breastmilk of Indian women. Am. J. Clin. Nutr. 33:664-669.

Saint, L., P. Maggiore, and P.E. Hartmann. 1986. Yield and nutrient content of milk in eight women breast-feeding twins and one woman breast-feeding triplets. Br. J. Nutr. 56:49-58.

Vaughn, L.A., C.W. Weber, and S.R. Kemberling. 1979. Longitudinal changes in the mineral content of human milk. Am. J. Clin. Nutr. 32:2301-2306.

Appendix D
Biographical Sketches of
Committee Members

Barbara Abrams, Dr.P.H., R.D., is assistant professor in the Departments of Social and Administrative Health Sciences, School of Public Health, University of California, Berkeley, and the Department of Obstetrics, Gynecology and Reproductive Sciences, School of Medicine, University of California, San Francisco. She worked as a perinatal nutritionist for more than a decade and has conducted several epidemiologic studies on maternal weight gain, nutrition, and pregnancy outcome.

Lindsay Allen, Ph.D., is professor in the Department of Nutritional Sciences at the University of Connecticut, Storrs. She has conducted research on relationships between nutrition and the outcome of human pregnancy and lactation in the United States as well as in other countries. In recent years, her special interest has been the effect of marginal malnutrition on the function of women and children in Mexico.

Kathryn Dewey, Ph.D., is associate professor in the Department of Nutrition and associate director of the program in International Nutrition at the University of California, Davis. She has conducted research related to the biological and behavioral determinants of lactation performance, the impact of early nutrition on infant growth and development, and maternal and child nutrition in industrialized and developing countries. Dr. Dewey is secretary-treasurer of the International Society for Research on Human Milk and Lactation and has served on the Expert Panel on Core Indicators of Nutritional Status in Difficult-to-Sample Populations for the Life Sciences Research Office.

Cutberto Garza, M.D., Ph.D., is director and professor of the Division of Nutritional Sciences at Cornell University. He has conducted research on milk composition, physiologic responses of full-term and preterm infants to human milk, and relationships of maternal nutritional status to milk production. Dr. Garza has served on several committees of the National Institutes of Health and on the National Academy of Sciences Committee on International Nutrition Programs.

Armond S. Goldman, M.D., is professor of pediatrics, and chief of the Division of Immunology/Allergy at The University of Texas Medical Branch in Galveston. He has conducted research on the immunology of human milk, antiinflammatory properties of human milk, effects of length of pregnancy and lactation on the immunologic system in human milk, evaluation of lactation performance, and the evaluation of human milk for banking. Dr. Goldman chaired the International Conference on the Effects of Human Milk on the Recipient Infant, which was sponsored by the National Institute of Child Health and Human Development.

Jere D. Haas, Ph.D., is professor of nutritional sciences at Cornell University. He has conducted research on the maternal, fetal, and infant responses to stresses at extreme high altitudes as well as on relationships between maternal nutritional status and fetal growth, postnatal growth, and postnatal development and morbidity in Bolivia, Peru, Guatemala, Indonesia, and the United States.

Margit Hamosh, Ph.D., is professor in the Department of Pediatrics and chief of the department's Division of Developmental Biology and Nutrition at Georgetown University Medical Center. She is also adjunct professor in the Department of Nutrition and Food Systems at the University of Maryland. She has conducted research on lung development as well as on fat digestion and absorption, lipid clearance, the composition of human milk, and the function of its components in the neonate. Dr. Hamosh has served on several committees of the National Institutes of Health.

Francis E. Johnston, Ph.D., is professor and chairman of the Department of Anthropology of the University of Pennsylvania. His research focuses on the growth, development, and body composition of children and youth, especially in relationship to nutritional status.

Janet C. King, Ph.D., is professor of nutrition and chair of the Department of Nutritional Sciences at the University of California, Berkeley. She has conducted research on nutritional needs during pregnancy and has published on the protein, energy, and zinc requirements of pregnant women. She has served on many national committees involved in establishing policies relating to prenatal care.

Ruth A. Lawrence, M.D., is professor of pediatrics and obstetrics/gynecology and the director of the Breastfeeding and Lactation Study Center at the University of Rochester School of Medicine and Dentistry. She was chair of the Surgeon General's Workshop on Breastfeeding and Lactation and has conducted research concerning motivation to breastfeed, lactation management, and maternal medications during lactation.

Charles S. Mahan, M.D., is deputy secretary for health and state health officer for Florida, director of the Robert Wood Johnson Healthy Futures Program, and professor of obstetrics and gynecology at the University of Florida College of Medicine. His special interests have been preterm birth prevention, food supplementation in pregnancy, family-centered maternity care, prevention of unnecessary cesarean deliveries, infant mortality, improved care for low-income women, and out-of-hospital birth centers.

Mary Frances Picciano, Ph.D., is professor of nutrition at The Pennsylvania State University. She has conducted research on the content, bioavailability, and metabolism of protein, iron, folacin, and selenium in human milk. Her work has also included methods of measurement and selenium content of prepared infant cereal.

Roy M. Pitkin, M.D., is professor and chair of the Department of Obstetrics and Gynecology at the University of California, Los Angeles. Before assuming this post in 1987, he was professor and head of the Department of Obstetrics and Gynecology at the University of Iowa, Ames. He previously chaired the Committee on Nutrition of the Mother and Preschool Child of the Food and Nutrition Board, National Academy of Sciences.

Sara A. Quandt, Ph.D., is associate professor of anthropology and of nutrition and food science at the University of Kentucky. She has conducted research on the interaction of breastfeeding styles, early infant growth, and maternal nutritional status. Her work has also focused on methodological issues in measuring dietary intake of infants.

Kathleen M. Rasmussen, Sc.D., R.D., is associate professor of nutrition at Cornell University and program director of a National Institutes of Health training grant in maternal and child nutrition. Her research has focused on the effects of maternal malnutrition on reproductive performance, with an emphasis on lactation.

David Rush, M.D., is professor of nutrition and community health and head of the Epidemiology Program at the USDA Human Nutrition Research Center on Aging, all at Tufts University. In the recent past, he was principal investigator of the National Evaluation of the Special Supplemental Food Program for Women, Infants, and Children (WIC).

John W. Sparks, M.D., is associate professor in the Department of Pediatrics at the University of Colorado. A neonatologist, he has served as director of Newborn Services and medical director of the Neonatal Intensive Care Unit at University Hospital, Denver. His scientific interests include the physiology, metabolism, and nutrition of the fetus and newborn.

Mervyn Susser, M.B., B.Ch., D.P.H., is Sergievsky Professor of Epidemiology and founder and director of the Sergievsky Center at Columbia University in New York. The Center is endowed for the study of the epidemiology of neurodevelopmental disorders. He has also been head of epidemiology in the Columbia University School of Public Health. His work covers several specific fields, including prenatal development and prenatal nutrition, as well as such general topics as causality and the social sciences in epidemiology.

Acronyms

AAP	American Academy of Pediatrics
ACOG	American College of Obstetricians and Gynecologists
ADA	American Dietetic Association
AFDC	Aid to Families with Dependent Children
APHA	American Public Health Association
BMI	Body mass index
BMR	Basal metabolic rate
DHHS	Department of Health and Human Services
FAO	Food and Agriculture Organization of the United Nations
FASEB	Federation of American Societies for Experimental Biology
FNB	Food and Nutrition Board
HTLV-1	Human T lymphocytotropic virus
HIV-1	Human immunodeficiency virus-1
IgA	Secretory immunoglobulin A
IOM	Institute of Medicine
IU	International unit
LH	Luteinizing hormone
NCHS	National Center for Health Statistics
NICHD	National Institute of Child Health and Human Development
RDA	Recommended Dietary Allowances
SD	Standard deviation
SEM	Standard error of the mean
USDA	United States Department of Agriculture
WHO	World Health Organization
WIC	Special Supplemental Food Program for Women, Infants and Children

Glossary

Alveolar ductal system   the infrastructure of the breast that includes both the milk-making lacteal cells and the lactiferous ducts of the mammary gland.

Amenorrhea   absence or abnormal stoppage of menses.

Anovulation   suspension or cessation of ovulation.

Anthropometric methods   methods of measurement of the size and proportions of the human body, including measurement of weight, height, circumferences, and skinfold thicknesses.

Antimetabolite   a substance that closely resembles one required for normal physiological function and that exerts its desired effect by replacing or interfering with the utilization of the essential metabolite. Antimetabolites are used therapeutically to slow or stop the growth of malignant cells.

Antineoplastic agent   a pharmacologic agent that inhibits or prevents the maturation and proliferation of malignant cells.

Areola   circular pigmented area surrounding the nipple of the breast.

Bioavailability   the proportion of a nutrient absorbed from food and available for physiologic function.

Body mass index (BMI)   an expression of body weight for height used for children and adults. In this report, metric units are used, namely, BMI = $[(kg/m^2) \times 100]$

Breast abscess   a localized collection of pus in the breast usually resulting from an inadequately treated mastitis.

Catabolism the chemical breakdown of complex substances into simpler ones.

Catalysis the speeding up of a chemical reaction by a substance, needed in only a small amount, that is not itself permanently changed in the reaction.

Ceruloplasmin a protein that carries the majority of the copper in the blood.

Colostrum the fluid secreted by the mammary gland for the first few days following parturition.

Continuance rate in this report, the percentage of women who initiated breastfeeding who were still breastfeeding when their infants reached 6 months of age.

Engorgement in this report, the distension of the breast with milk.

Enteropathogens microorganisms that cause intestinal disease.

Enzymes proteins that serve as organic catalysts.

Exclusive breastfeeding consumption of human milk as the sole source of energy.

Femoral region the thigh.

Fibronectin an adhesive glycoproprotein.

Glutathione peroxidase a selenium-containing enzyme that reduces toxic hydrogen peroxide formed within the cell.

Hemorrhagic disease of the newborn Syndrome in newborn period caused by vitamin K deficiency.

Immunoregulation control of the immune response by mechanisms such as the immunoglobulin idiotype-antiidiotype network.

Inducer a substance that causes or stimulates the start of an activity.

Lactation performance degree of success of breastfeeding, as determined by measurements such as milk volume, milk composition, duration of breastfeeding, and infant growth.

Lacteal cells cells within the mammary gland that collect and produce the nutrients that make up milk.

Lactoferrin an iron-binding protein found in secretions such as milk and in specific granules of neutrophils.

Lactogenesis the onset of copious milk secretion shortly after parturition.

Lactogenic hormones hormones that stimulate the development and growth of the mammary glands.

Lactose intolerance a condition in which the intestinal enzyme lactase, which breaks down lactose to glucose plus galactose, is lacking; this may lead to cramps and diarrhea after consumption of certain lactose-containing foods (e.g., milk).

Let-down reflex in reference to breastfeeding, the transport of milk from the alveoli of the breast to the ducts in response to sensory stimulus. Release of oxytocin and prolactin results in the contraction of myoepithelial cells and the release of milk.

Luteinizing hormone hormone essential for maturation of the ovarian follicle so that ovulation can occur.

Lymphokines a general term for soluble mediators of immune responses that are not antibodies or complement components and that are released by sensitized lymphocytes on contact with antigens.

Lysozyme an enzyme of the hydrolase class that has antibacterial properties.

Macrominerals minerals (calcium, phosphorus, and magnesium) present in relatively high concentration in the human.

Macronutrients protein, fat, and carbohydrate.

Mastitis an infectious process in the breast that produces localized tenderness, redness and heat, together with systemic reactions of fever, malaise, and sometimes nausea and vomiting.

Menaquinone vitamin K_2, the form of the vitamin synthesized by bacteria.

Milk-ejection reflex cf **let-down reflex**.

Myoepithelial cells spindle-shaped or branched contractile epithelial cells found between glandular cells and basement membrane of mammary glands and certain other glands.

Nutrient density nutrient content of food per 1,000 kcal of energy.

Oligosaccharide a compound made up of a small number of monosaccharide (simple sugar) units.

Oophorectomy excision of an ovary or ovaries.

Oral elimination challenge trial in this report, a trial period during which a suspected food allergen is eliminated from the mother's diet to determine whether her breastfed infant will become asymptomatic.

Organochlorinated compounds Insecticides such as DDT or PCB; usual term is organophosphates.

Osteoporosis reduction in the amount of bone mass, leading to fractures after minimal trauma.

Oxytocin a pituitary hormone. Among its actions is stimulation of the release of milk from the mammary glands, cf **let-down reflex**.

Parity the number of children previously born to a woman.

Partial breastfeeding consumption of human milk in combination with formula, other foods, or both.

Parturition the act or process of giving birth.

Phototherapy   the use of variously concentrated light rays for treating conditions such as hyperbilirubinemia (jaundice) of the newborn.

Phylloquinone   vitamin K_1, the form of the vitamin synthesized by plants.

Placental lactogen   a placental hormone that stimulates milk production.

Postprandial   after meals.

Progesterone   a steroid hormone obtained from the corpus luteum and placenta. Among its functions is development of the mammary glands.

Prolactin   a pituitary hormone that stimulates lactation in mammary glands.

Radiopharmaceutical   a radioactive compound that is used for medical treatment or diagnosis.

Residual milk volume   difference between the amount of milk that can be extracted by pump compared with usual infant intake.

Respiratory syncytial virus   a virus that causes epidemic acute respiratory disease that is especially serious in children (e.g., it causes bronchial pneumonia and bronchitis).

Retinol equivalent   a unit of measurement of the vitamin A value of foods. One retinol equivalent is equivalent to approximately 5 internatational units of vitamin A obtained from the typical U.S. diet in the form of retinol (from animal products) and carotenoids (from plants).

Substrate   a substance on which an enzyme acts.

Synergism   the joint action of agents so that their combined effect is greater than the algebraic sum of their individual effects.

Taurine   a sulfur-containing amino acid important to growth of brain, retina, heart, and liver; present in high concentrations in human milk.

Test weighing   in this report, a method of determining the quantity of milk consumed that involves weighing the baby before and after breastfeeding.

Thermogenesis   heat production (energy expenditure) following the ingestion of food or exposure to cold above that produced by basal metabolism.

Well nourished   for purposes of this report, this term refers to a healthy woman who is of appropriate weight for height and without notable dietary limitations.

Index

297